# Progress in Electrodermal Research

# NATO ASI Series

## Advanced Science Institutes Series

*A series presenting the results of activities sponsored by the NATO Science Committee, which aims at the dissemination of advanced scientific and technological knowledge, with a view to strengthening links between scientific communities.*

The series is published by an international board of publishers in conjunction with the NATO Scientific Affairs Division

| | | |
|---|---|---|
| **A** | **Life Sciences** | Plenum Publishing Corporation |
| **B** | **Physics** | New York and London |
| | | |
| **C** | **Mathematical and Physical Sciences** | Kluwer Academic Publishers |
| **D** | **Behavioral and Social Sciences** | Dordrecht, Boston, and London |
| **E** | **Applied Sciences** | |
| | | |
| **F** | **Computer and Systems Sciences** | Springer-Verlag |
| **G** | **Ecological Sciences** | Berlin, Heidelberg, New York, London, |
| **H** | **Cell Biology** | Paris, Tokyo, Hong Kong, and Barcelona |
| **I** | **Global Environmental Change** | |

### *Recent Volumes in this Series*

*Series A: Life Sciences*

# Progress in Electrodermal Research

Edited by

## Jean-Claude Roy

University of Lille-USTL
Villeneuve d'Ascq, France

## Wolfram Boucsein

University of Wuppertal
Wuppertal, Germany

## Don C. Fowles

University of Iowa
Iowa City, Iowa

and

## John H. Gruzelier

Charing Cross and Westminster Medical School
University of London
London, United Kingdom

Plenum Press
New York and London
Published in cooperation with NATO Scientific Affairs Division

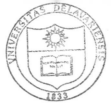

QP
372
.9
.P76
1993

Proceedings of a NATO Advanced Research Workshop on
Electrodermal Activity: From Physiology to Psychology,
held May 20–23, 1992,
in Château de Tilques, Saint-Omer. France

## NATO-PCO-DATA BASE

The electronic index to the NATO ASI Series provides full bibliographical references (with keywords and/or abstracts) to more than 30,000 contributions from international scientists published in all sections of the NATO ASI Series. Access to the NATO-PCO-DATA BASE is possible in two ways:

—via online FILE 128 (NATO-PCO-DATA BASE) hosted by ESRIN, Via Galileo Galilei, I-00044 Frascati, Italy

—via CD-ROM "NATO-PCO-DATA BASE" with user-friendly retrieval software in English, French, and German (©WTV GmbH and DATAWARE Technologies, Inc. 1989)

The CD-ROM can be ordered through any member of the Board of Publishers or through NATO-PCO, Overijse, Belgium.

Library of Congress Cataloging-in-Publication Data

Progress in electrodermal research / edited by Jean-Claude Roy ... [et al.].
        p.   cm. -- (NATO ASI series. Series A. Life sciences ; v. 249)
    "Proceedings of a NATO Advanced Research Workshop on Electrodermal Activity: From Physiology to Psychology, held May 20-23, 1992, in Château de Tilques, Saint-Omer, France"--T.p. verso.
    "Published in cooperation with NATO Scientific Affairs Division."
    Includes bibliographical references and indexes.
    ISBN 0-306-44536-0
    1. Galvanic skin response--Congresses.   I. Roy, Jean-Claude.
II. North Atlantic Treaty Organization.   Scientific Affairs Division.   III. NATO Advanced Research Workshop on Electrodermal Activity: From Physiology to Psychology, 1992 : Saint-Omer, Pas-de -Calais, France.   IV. Series.
    [DNLM: 1. Galvanic Skin Response--physiology--congresses.   WL 106 P963 1993]
QP372.9.P76   1993
612.7'91--dc20
DNLM/DLC
for Library of Congress                                                93-11397

ISBN 0-306-44536-0

©1993 Plenum Press, New York
A Division of Plenum Publishing Corporation
233 Spring Street, New York, N.Y. 10013

Printed in the United States of America

# PREFACE

Electrodermal activity refers to electrical changes across the skin in areas of the body that are psychologically responsive. The eccrine sweat glands are the primary determinant of electrodermal activity, and these are psychologically active especially on the palms of the hands and the soles of the feet. As a matter of convenience, electrodermal activity is most often recorded from the palms. Over the years, the electrodermal response has been known as the psychogalvanic reflex, the galvanic skin response, the skin resistance response, the skin conductance response, and the skin potential response. The terms psychogalvanic reflex and galvanic skin response have fallen into disuse among scientists, but are still to be found in psychology text books.

Because of its early discovery, ease of measurement, and often easily observable response to experimental manipulations, the recording of electrodermal activity is one of the most frequently used methods in psychophysiology. Indeed, in the early years following the founding of the Society for Psychophysiological Research, electrodermal research so dominated the field that people worried that the society was simply an electrodermal society. Although other psychophysiological techniques have emerged as equally strong contributors to psychophysiology, electrodermal research continues to be important throughout the world. As a result of this massive research investment, there has been great progress in understanding electrodermal phenomena, as well as major advances in recording methods since the phenomenon was discovered.

Though, at present, electrodermal research is especially concentrated in North America, Northern Europe and Germany, the discovery of the electrodermal phenomenon as a concomitant of psychological activity was made in France, where in 1888 Féré published his paper reporting a decrease in skin resistance following sensory or emotional stimulation in hysterical patients. The original concept of a commemorative scientific meeting arose out of discussions between Jean Claude Roy, Kenneth Hugdahl and Graham Turpin, during a conference at the University of Juväskylä, Finland, when it was suggested that the centenary of the discovery of electrodermal activity should be celebrated. It seemed the ideal time to reflect on the achievement of the past years and to bring researchers up to date on the current state-of-the-art. Thus, electrodermal activity returned to its homeland for one of the first scientific meetings dedicated to that particular method in its over a 100 years of history.

This conference was organized as a NATO-Advanced Research Workshop, entitled "Electrodermal Activity: from Physiology to Psychology". The scientific committee consisted of Jean-Claude Roy, Wolfram Boucsein, Don Fowles, and John Gruzelier. The title of the meeting emphasised the intention to relate together different spheres of research on electrodermal activity, and to underline the multi-disciplinary nature of research on the phenomenon. This meeting was held in the Château of Tilques, near Saint-Omer in Northern France, from May 20th to 23th 1992. The setting was comfortable and isolated, and allowed complete concentration on the theme.

We are grateful to the NATO Scientific Affairs Division for making this meeting possible by bringing together researchers from all countries, through its financial suppport. The help of the Région Nord-Pas-de-Calais, of the Fédération Universitaire Polytechnique de Lille (Département de psychologie), and the Municipalité de Villeneuve d'Ascq is gratefully acknowledged. The French CNRS (National Center for Scientific Research) granted his patronage.

We are grateful to Janick Naveteur who carried most of the burden of the practical organisation of the conference, with the logistical help of the Laboratoire de Neurosciences du Comportement at the USTL-University of Lille.

When the meeting ended, the main speakers were invited to complete their presentations in the light of the conference discussions and to write a chapter for this book, under a very tight schedule. The editors thank the authors for their diligence in respecting requests for revisions, copy, etc. in such a very short time. All the chapters were reviewed either by the editors of this book, or by others, mostly participants who agreed to do so. The editors want to thank Robert Edelberg, David Lykken, Adrian Raine and Peter Venables in that respect.

The book contains chapters by distinguished investigators  in the field of electrodermal research activity. The authors review current understanding of the use of electrodermal activity to assess cognitive processes, individual differences in human personality, and processes associated with psychopathology. It covers the material presented at the conference and provides the state-of-the-art in various fields of basic and applied research- e.g. peripheral effectors theory, methodological issues, central nervous system control of electrodermal activity, personality, psychopathology, and hemispherical asymmetry- thereby illustrating the richness of research with this measure. This volume underlines our belief that only through inter-disciplinary collaborative efforts can research into these phenomena lead to essential insights about their behavioral significance and central nervous system control.

W.Boucsein<br>
D.Fowles<br>
J.Gruzelier<br>
J.C.Roy

# CONTENTS

# ON THE CENTENNIAL OF THE DISCOVERY

# OF ELECTRODERMAL ACTIVITY

Vincent Bloch

Laboratoire de Neurobiologie de l'Apprentissage
et de la Mémoire
C.N.R.S. U.R.A. 1491 - Université de Paris-Sud
91405 Orsay Cedex
France

First, I wish to thank the organizers, and I feel honoured to have been asked to introduce this meeting. I do not deserve this honour because I was somewhat a turncoat to your field when I left electodermal research more than twenty five years ago. But I have been a member of your club for a very long time and I still feel at home in the electrodermal family.

At an acceptable error level of three per cent, we can claim that today is the anniversary of the discovery of galvanic skin response. The first paper on this topic dates back to 1889 in France and if we are a little late for this centennial it is because in 1989 France was too busy celebrating the bicentennial of the French Revolution. Now we have more time.

I have had the privilege of having heard about some main figures of this story from my boss Henri Piéron (see Piéron, 1910) who knew Romain Vigouroux personally. By the way, the story starts with Vigouroux, an electrotherapist, who was one of Charcot's co-workers at the Salpêtrière Hospital in Paris and a former student of another famous neurologist, Duchène de Boulogne, a name with a familiar ring in this part of France. For a moment, let me try to describe the atmosphere at the Salpêtrière in the latter part of the nineteenth century. Charcot was mainly involved in the treatment of hysteria and there was great hope in treatment by hypnosis. Hypnosis was the new name for what Mesmer one century earlier had called animal magnetism. Incidentally, Mesmer thought that the influence that one person can exert on another was based upon the transmission of some magnetic fluid. This view was condemned by a committee of referees at the French Academy of Sciences in 1784. Besides, these referees were Benjamin Franklin, the chemist Lavoisier, the astronomer Bailly and doctor Guillotin, the inventor of the machine which was later fatal to his last two colleagues! But in the 19th Century, the dominant materialistic trend and advances in the application of electricity both contributed to renewing interest in Mesmerism. Charcot, who used electrotherapy and metallotherapy intensively was willing to look for a physical basis for hypnotic therapy. He was actively searching for a demonstration of the influence of the hypnotizer on the electrical characteristics of the body of the hypnotised subject. So while Bernheim and the Nancy School, who had such a profound influence on Freud, argued that hypnotic action was based upon a specific psychological relationship between the physician and his patient, Charcot on the other hand believed in some form of organic fluid.

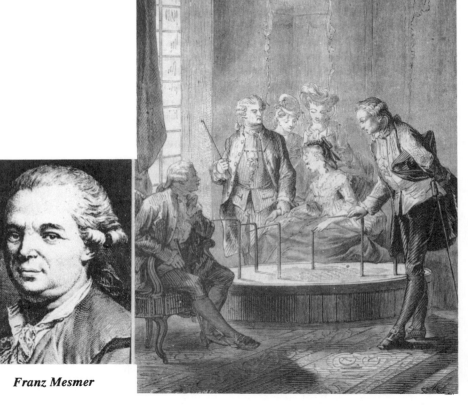

*Franz Mesmer*

*Mesmer hypnotising a lady, in an aristocratic salon, soon after his arrival in Paris in 1776. He claimed that his influence was transmitted through a magnetic fluid.*

This was the context when a certain Baron de Puyfontaine came to Charcot to present the results of his experiments. Puyfontaine had tried to exert a distant action on a highly sensitive galvanometer specially made for this purpose by Ruhmkorff, the inventor of the induction coil. He was not successful, but during the trials he observed that when he held electrodes in his hands, the galvanometer displayed deflections. Charcot asked Vigouroux to examine these results. Vigouroux was rapidly convinced that these variations in current flow observed by Puyfontaine were due to variations of contact between the skin and the electrodes. Vigouroux was in fact familiar with these problems of contact since he was engaged in research on electrical resistance of the human body for practical reasons : he believed that these resistance variations could influence the efficacy of electrotherapy and metallotherapy used in the treatment of hysteria. In addition, Vigouroux was also interested in skin resistance per se as a diagnostic tool after having observed that hysterical patients who presented a hemianaesthesia had a greater resistance value on the insensitive side of their body, compared to the normal side. He also observed a high skin resistance level in patients with hysterical hemiplegy. These observations were published in a note in 1878.

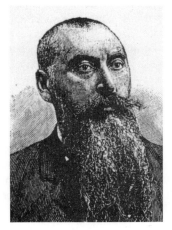
**Charles Féré**

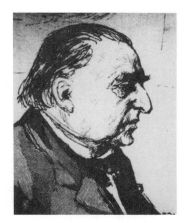
**Jean Martin Charcot**

A little later, another collaborator of Charcot, the neurologist Charles Féré made his entrance. He was the former student of Broca who was famous for his localizationist theory, but who was also interested in hypnotism. Féré became Charcot's secretary, and then the head of his experimental laboratory. Féré used the hand dynamometer as a diagnostic tool in the study of hysterical muscular contractions. He then designed an experiment in which he presented various stimuli to subjects while they gripped the dynamometer. He observed that stimulation caused an increase in pressure exerted by the subjects and that the pressure varied with intensity of the stimulus. He claimed that stimuli, regardless of modality, determined the development of what he called "psychic energy". I shall discuss this interpretation later on. Going further and inspired by Vigouroux, Féré replicated his study using the same set of stimuli, but this time he studied its effects on skin resistance of the anterior surface of the forearm rather than on muscular contractions. In hysterical patients specially chosen for being highly excitable Féré obtained a considerable increase in current flow from each discrete stimulus. In normal subjects, the responses were unfortunately much less pronounced but Féré made a very important observation concerning these subjects. Reducing stimulation, for instance by closing the eyes, diminished current flow. In this way both the elctrodermal response to stimuli and basal skin resistance levels were discovered. Féré published these observations in two notes in the Bulletin of the Société de Biologie in 1888 and this date is generally recognized as the date of discovery of GSR. But Féré considered these skin resistance data as a mere confirmation of his previous dynamometric study and additional evidence for his theory of a "psychic energy" derived from non specific sensory stimulation. This is why he can also be considered to be the ancestor of sensory activation theory which was later defended by successively Pavlov, Piéron, Bremer in his "dynamogénie sensorielle", Hebb, Lindsley and some others.

Thus, from the very beginning, electrodermal research was related to the vast problem of the intensive dimension of behavior and the general level of functioning of the brain. It is interesting to note that despite the "gratuitous" nature of EDA, gratuitous - in the sense that it is not clearly related to a main physiological function - its recording appeared as one of the best indices of an important feature of brain mechanisms (for discussion, see Bloch, 1965).

To return to the Féré experiments it is interesting to note that in these studies, Féré was helped by two prominent scientists. First, he benefited from the advice of the physicist d'Arsonval, well known among physiologists for having designed his galvanometer with a mobile frame. And incidentally, d'Arsonval interpreted Féré's resistance data as a possible effect of some cutaneous secretion while Féré himself like many workers subsequently thought that resistance varied under the influence of vasomotricity. Féré was also helped by a man who directly participated in the experiments : Alfred Binet, another student of Charcot who became famous for his further studies in suggestibility and mainly for having been the inventor of intelligence testing. Thus it is worthwhile pointing out that thirty years later a man called David Wechsler came from the University of Columbia to Paris in order to prepare a thesis at the Sorbonne with Henri Piéron and Louis Lapicque. The subject of this thesis was ..."the Psychogalvanic Reflex" (1925)! Over the course of his work Wechsler designed a superb "photogalvanograph" in a cabinet made with precious wood and I had the privilege of playing with this relic in Piéron's laboratory. Like Binet, David Wechsler became famous not for his interest in GSR but for his intelligence test. You might come to the conclusion that electrodermal research is a necessary prerequisite for entering the field of psychology of intelligence.

One year after Féré's publications, a Russian physiologist named Tarchanoff, affiliated with the French Société de Biologie, published an important note in the Comptes Rendus of this Society on - I translate from french - "Electrical discharges in human skin provoked by excitation of sensory organs and various forms of psychic activity". This 1889 paper was followed by another and one in German in the Pflügers Archiv in 1890 which is generally cited as the publication which rediscovered GSR independently of Féré. Neumann and Blanton, in a paper on the early history of EDA research (1970) claimed that Tarchanoff had followed all the Salpêtrière work but voluntarily did not quote it. Whatever the case his paper was the first to describe electrodermal responses not only to current sensory stimuli but also to suggestions for memories of these stimuli or to emotionnal stimuli and mental effort. But the name of Tarchanoff is more commonly linked to the technique of skin potential since his work was done without exosomatic current versus the studies of Féré based upon skin resistance measurements. Tarchanoff is also often cited for having been the first to propose the sweat gland hypothesis. Nevertheless much more direct evidence was put forward ten years previously by Herman. He showed in 1878 that a current occurs in cat food pads when the animal is aroused and that current is related to sweating and that this response can be obtained as well by electrical stimulation of the sciatic nerve.

It is better known that in 1904 a Swiss engineer, Müller, observed changes in skin resistance which he believed to be correlated with psychological processes. He was unaware of the earlier literature but he persuaded a psychiatrist from Zurich, Veraguth, to participate in these studies. Veraguth was probably sincerely convinced that he had discovered a new phenomenon. He proposed calling it the "psychogalvanic reflex". It happened that he was a friend of Carl Jung. Jung proposed to combine this technique with his word association method. Thus along with Jung association experiment the electrodermal response became extremely popular as a way of revealing aspects of mental life. Peterson, who came from the United States to Zurich in 1907, was extremely

4

enthousiastic about it and over popularized the technique and the instrument under the name of "psychometer" and was responsible for a period of caricatural belief in machines for reading thoughts!

Much later a new period started when EDA was studied in conjunction with other approaches of brain physiology : I would like to cite particularly the work of Chester Darrow, since by promoting polygraphy, he sparked new interest in electrodermal research by relating GSR with other indices of brain functioning, specially electroencephalography. At this point we enter the beginning of the modern era where you are currently the authors.

# REFERENCES

Bloch, V., 1965, Le Contrôle Central de l'Activité Electrodermale, Masson, Paris.

Darrow, C.W., 1950, A new frontier : neurophysiological effects of emotion on the brain, in: "Feelings and Emotions", M.L. Reymert, ed., McGraw Hill Book Company, New York.

Féré, C., 1888, Modifications de la résistance électrique sous l'influence des excitations sensorielles et des émotions, C. R. Soc. Biol., 5:217.

Hermann, L., and Luchsinger, B., 1878, Über die secretionsstrome der Haut bei der Katze, Pflügers Arch. ges. Physiol., 17:310.

Müller, E.K., 1904, Das elektrische Leitvermögen des menschlichen Körpers als Masstab für seine Nervosität, Schweiz. Blat. Electrotechn. 9:321.

Neumann, E., and Blanton, R., 1970, The early history of electrodermal research. Psychophysiol., 6:453.

Peterson F., 1907, The galvanometer as a measurer of emotion, Brit. med. J., 2:804.

Piéron, H., 1910, Les variations physio-galvaniques comme phénomène d'expression des émotions, Rev. Psychiat., 14:486.

Tarchanoff, J., 1889, Décharges électriques dans la peau de l'homme sous l'influence de l'excitation des organes des sens et de différentes formes d'activité psychique, C. R. Soc. Biol., 41:447.

Tarchanoff, J., 1890, Über die galvanischen Erscheinungen an der Haut des Menschen bei Reizung des Sinnesorgane und bei verschiedenen Formen des psychischen Tätigkeit. Pflügers Arch. ges. Physio., 46:46.

Veraguth, O., 1909, Das Psychogalvanische Reflexphenomen, Karger, Berlin.

Vigouroux, R., 1868, De l'action du magnétisme et de l'électricité statique sur l'hémianesthésie hystérique, C. R. Soc. Biol., 5:64.

Vigouroux, R.., 1879, Sur le rôle de la résistance électrique des tissus dans l'électro-diagnostic, C. R. Soc. Biol., 31:336.

Wechsler, D., 1925, The measurement of emotional reactions, Arch. Psychol., 12:5.

# ELECTRODERMAL MECHANISMS: A CRITIQUE OF THE

# TWO-EFFECTOR HYPOTHESIS AND A PROPOSED REPLACEMENT

Robert Edelberg

Department of Psychiatry
UMDNJ-Robert Wood Johnson Medical School
Piscataway, NJ 08854-5635
USA

Although response amplitude and response rate have served as the primary electrodermal measures in behavioral research, several lines of evidence have given hope that in addition to these quantitative indicators, electrodermal activity might provide qualitative indices as well. When one examines the behavioral correlates of the electrodermal reflex, it becomes evident that EDA may be associated with very different adaptations, e.g. tactual exploration, grasping, thermoregulation, or ambulation (Darrow, 1927; Edelberg, 1973a; Fowles, 1986; Boucsein, 1988), as well as the abstracted representation of such actions, for example information intake. The reviews elsewhere in this volume by Roy et al and by Sequeira-Martinho and Roy, covering the neurophysiological systems underlying these adaptations, reveal the existence in the CNS of at least two relatively independent descending pathways that control electrodermal activity (EDA), one of reticular origin under cortical and sensory influences (Bloch, 1965), the other a direct corticospinal system, suggesting that different cutaneous adjustments may follow activation of these respective areas. If true, a two-effector system may be an effective means of accomplishing such adjustments.

This chapter will review briefly the origins of the two-effector hypothesis, discuss the evidence supporting it and challenging it, will propose a substitute single-effector model, and will test some of its predictions.

## EVOLUTION OF THE MEMBRANE MODEL

An early indication that the electrodermal response (EDR) was more than a unitary process came from the work of Richter, who in 1929 reported that while the palmar response originated in sweat glands and was elicited by emotional activity, responses from the dorsal surface of the hand originated in an epidermal membrane and were associated with motor activity. Darrow and Freeman (1934) properly challenged Richter's assertion and demonstrated that both palmar and non-palmar activity originated in sweat glands. They viewed these areas as representing different adaptations: the glands in non-palmar areas mediating thermoregulatory adjustments associated with motor activity, those in palmar areas maintaining the adhesiveness and pliability essential for tactual acuity and grasping in situations associated with anticipation, alertness, apprehension.

Both Darrow and Richter had focussed on the exosomatic measure of skin reactivity, namely resistance change. During the same period Forbes and Bolles (1936) examined the characteristics of the endosomatic measure. They found that the negative potential component tended not to habituate while the positive component showed clear habituation over repeated shock or startle trials. They concluded that these two components were mediated by different systems. The two effector hypothesis was indeed germinating.

Their conclusion was in part confirmed by Wilcott (1958) who demonstrated that the two potential components were differentially affected by exsanguination, the positive alone being eliminated. He further claimed (1959), on the basis of experiments involving puncture of the epidermis and measurements with subepidermal electrodes, that the potential response of the skin originates in an epidermal structure, not in the sweat glands. Takagi and Nakayama (1959) examined simultaneous potential and resistance changes from a single site and concluded that the negative skin potential response (SPR) originates in the sweat gland, the positive in the corium (dermis). The additional findings that the positive component can be differentially altered by a variety of procedures, including elevated temperature (Nakayama and Takagi, 1958; Yokota et al, 1959), high currents (Wilcott, 1964), and exposure to various cations (Edelberg et al, 1960), led to the view that it was an independent phenomenon and that it might arise at a different site.

The membrane model was now beginning to emerge as the second effector in the two-component model. The earlier finding by Gildemeister (1915), that skin resistance response (SRR) amplitude diminished when a high frequency alternating current was used as a voltage source, reinforced the membrane idea, although as will be discussed later, this interpretation was probably spurious. Rein's demonstration (1929) of a cation-selective membrane within the skin, probably at the boundary between the stratum corneum and the germinating layer, gave further support to this notion.

The membrane hypothesis did not remain unchallenged. Darrow and his coworkers (1957) noted that positive SPRs occur only when sweat can be observed emerging from the pores. They believed that the sweat gland gave rise to a positive potential response, but that only when the sweat column connected this source with the surface could it be observed. The negative component was seen as resulting from linked activity on the outside of the sweat gland. As will be shown, although Darrow had his polarities reversed, there was some validity to his idea. Wilcott (1959), although one of the five coauthors on Darrow's paper, later took exception to this interpretation and argued that the positive-going potential arises in an epidermal membrane somewhere between the germinating layer and the vascular bed of the dermis. A more conservative interpretation by Trehub et al (1962) viewed the positive component as a passive epidermal process triggered by the surge in surface negativity initiated by sweat gland activity (Trehub et al, 1962).

Strong support for the participation of an active membrane, was provided by the findings of Edelberg, Burch and Greiner (1960) who showed that various multivalent ions like aluminum produced a marked polarity-dependent potentiation of electrodermal response amplitude, while very low concentrations of detergents as well as highly acid or alkaline media caused a marked reduction in response amplitude. These observations were consistent with known effects on membrane structure. The marked effects

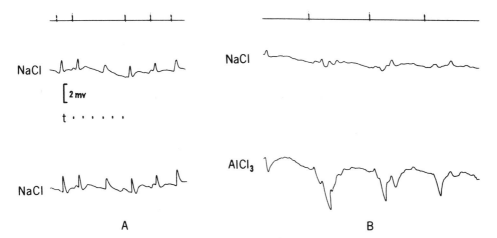

**Figure 1.** Potentiation of positive SPR from the palm by 1 M AlCl₃. Panel A: Control (upper) and experimental sites in 0.1 M NaCl. Panel B: Control site (upper) changed to fresh 0.1 M NaCl. Experimental site changed to 1 M AlCl₃. From "Electrical activity of the skin" by R. Edelberg. In N.S. Greenfield and R.A. Sternbach (eds), *Handbook of Psychophysiology,* Chap 9. New York: 1972. Reproduced by permission of Holt, Rinehart and Winston.

demonstrated on the resistance response were equally as conspicuous for the positive potential response (Fig. 1).

   While these findings pointed to the involvement of a membrane there was at that time no sound basis for chosing between the secretory coil of the sweat gland and some epidermal layer as its locus. Subsequently Shaver, Brusilow and Cooke (1965), using microelectrodes placed in the sweat duct of the cat footpad, showed that potential responses could be observed when the electrode tip was located in the epidermal duct but not in the dermal duct. With this evidence, the case for viewing the secretory membrane of the sweat gland as the site of the resistance and potential changes in the EDR was seriously weakened.

   The additional findings that EDR amplitude was frequently independent of sweat activity (Edelberg, 1964; Wilcott, 1964) lent further support for the two-effector model, which was gaining dominance. Nakayama and Takagi (1958), on the basis of various procedures that showed dissociation of their effects on EDA components concluded that a two-component system was needed to account for their data. Martin and Venables (1966), after assessing the available evidence concluded that the assumption of a two-component process is warranted, but that both components probably reside in the sweat gland. Wilcott (1966; 1967) also defended the two-effector hypothesis but focussed on the potential response, viewing the positive wave as evidence of depolarization associated with sweating, the negative with increased polarization of the epidermis. Based in part on the strong linkage between EDA and tactile sensitivity (Edelberg, 1961), he suggested that the epidermal process involved sensitization of tactile or pain receptors.

   Another phenomenon that pointed toward membrane activity was the so-called "reabsorption reflex" (Edelberg, 1966). When a special sensor is used to monitor the hydration of the outer layer of the corneum, a sudden reduction in hydration can often be observed soon after onset of an EDR (Fig. 2). This was attributed to an active

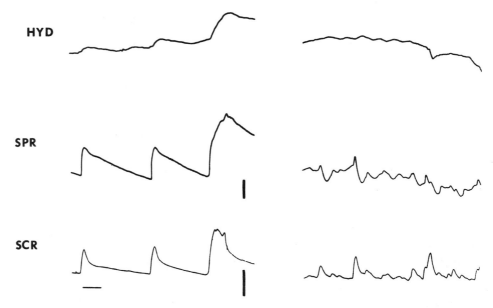

**Figure 2.** Relation of surface hydration to potential and conductance responses. Right panel recorded 30 minutes after left panel shows change of hydration to "reabsorption", appearance of positive SPRs, and acceleration of SCR recovery.

reabsorption of water at a deeper level, possibly the germinating layer. Its close association with positive SPR activity at a nearby site, suggested that both the positive SPR and the reabsorption process originated in the same active membrane (Edelberg, 1973b).

There was yet another indication of the two-effector character of EDA. On the basis of the palmar/dorsal differences found by Richter and by Darrow and the array of evidence suggesting that EDA depends on activity of both sweat glands and a membrane, presumably epidermal, Edelberg and Wright (1964) proposed a unifying model. They hypothesized that both sweat gland and epidermal activity occurred at the same electrodermal site, but that because of the difference in sweat gland densities, the palmar finger site reflected more of the sweat gland component, the dorsal more of the epidermal. Their results supported the stimulus response specificity of these two areas, but not in the direction hypothesized. In keeping with the predictions of the model, the ratio of sweat response amplitude to SRR amplitude, both from palmar sites, also demonstrated response specificity though to a weaker extent than did the palmar/dorsal measure. Some degree of response specificity of the palmar and dorsal areas was subsequently demonstrated by Katkin et al (1967), Mordkoff et al (1967), Mordkoff (1968), and Sorgatz (1978) in a variety of paradigms.

Some investigators have considered the possible role of myoepithelial contraction as a mechanism for some degree of response specificity, a supposition that was especially attractive because of the early evidence that these fibers were adrenergic. This would suggest dual innervation of the sweat gland, but Venables and Christie (1973) argued that since atropine abolishes all activity, any dual control must be completely cholinergic. Sato (1977) evaluated his own impressive studies and those of others and concluded that the myoepithelial fibers are cholinergic, and further that they probably serve as support structures rather than for the expulsion of sweat. The picture is further complicated by a study by Jenkinson et al (1978) who showed that in the human, neurotransmitters released by sympathetic fibers innervating nearby blood vessels very likely stimulate adrenergic receptors in the secretory coil. Also provocative is the finding by Stevens and Landis (1988) that the cholinergic' or adrenergic character of sympathetic nerves to a sweat gland is determined during development by the type of target cells that they innervate. This observation may have relevance to the controversy on the innervation of myoepithelial cells.

## ALTERNATIVES TO THE MEMBRANE MODEL

During the period of growing evidence for a membrane component, there were other studies that put into question the membrane hypothesis. One was the series of elegant experiments by Adams and his coworkers (Adams, 1966; Adams and Vaughan, 1965; Stombaugh and Adams, 1971) that showed that the independence of the electrodermal response and sweat output demonstrated by Edelberg (1964) and by Wilcott (1964) could be explained by the hydration and electrolyte content of the corneum and by the **"hydraulic capacitance" of the skin**. In Adams' model the sweat duct contents empty in large part by lateral diffusion into the corneum which in turn is drained by continuous reabsorption into the dermis. Because the takeup capacity of the reservoir in the corneum varies, the output of sweat at the surface appears to be independent of SCR amplitude. Unfortunately, some of his most crucial experiments were performed on the cat footpad, which does not produce a positive SPR, (Shaver et al, 1965; Edelberg, 1973a; Yamazaki et al, 1975) and whose sweat glands have no sodium reabsorption mechanism, so there is some question about the extent to which his conclusions can be generalized.

Another mechanism, one that explained the positive potential response without the requirement for an active membrane was the **mosaic (voltage-divider) model** (Edelberg, 1968). This model took into consideration the fact that the epidermis consists of two sources of voltage, the sweat gland, whose duct has a high negative potential with respect to the inside of the body, and the corneum whose potential is also negative with respect to the inside of the body but less so than the sweat duct. For the purposes of this discussion, it is not important to know where these potentials would arise, but it should be recognized that this relationship has been experimentally demonstrated (Edelberg, 1968). An internal current (Fig.3) flows between these two voltage sources through the resistance of the sweat duct and that of the corneum, the two being relatively insulated by the duct wall.

This circuit constitutes an internal voltage divider which operates such that the potential observed at the surface is determined not only by the strength of the voltage sources, but by the relative magnitudes of the two resistance legs. If the resistance of the sweat gland decreases, the surface potential goes more negative; if that of the corneum decreases the surface potential goes more positive. Thus as the sweat duct fills, there is a negative voltage swing at the surface, but as sweat diffuses into the corneum, negativity decreases and there may even be a positive swing in potential, i.e. a positive SPR. These occur even if there is no change in either voltage source. In keeping with the predictions of this model, it was demonstrated that increasing the resistance of the corneum, by applying an external dehydrating agent such as polyethylene glycol, would increase surface negativity.

Fowles et al (Fowles and Johnson, 1973; Fowles and Rosenberry, 1973; Fowles and Schneider, 1974; Fowles and Schneider, 1978) subsequently directed their attention to this model, testing its implications with a series of media having graded hydrating effects on the skin. They hypothesized that if the corneum were well hydrated, no positive SPR would occur, because it is not possible to further hydrate an already fully hydrated site.

Of special significance, they showed that positive SPRs at a highly hydrated site are dramatically depressed. In general they found their results to be in good agreement with the predictions of the voltage-divider model. They also focussed on the role of poral closure in explaining their results, since several authors have reported that the corneum swells when exposed to dilute solutions (Robbins and Fernee, 1983; Potts, 1986), and others have shown that such swelling is often adequate to close the sweat pores and to prevent emission of sweat (Peiss and Randall, 1957; Brebner and Kerslake, 1964; Sarkany et al 1965; Rushmer et al 1966). This effect had been previously disputed by Fowles and Venables (1970). Fowles also properly called attention to the fact that the original voltage-divider model would work just as well if one of the two voltage sources were zero, i.e. even if there were only one voltage source. Moreover he argued (Fowles, 1974) that for it to be complete, the model should include another voltage source and resistance in the duct wall.

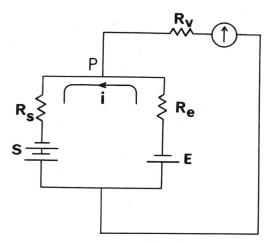

**Figure 3.** Voltage-divider circuit in the skin. $R_S$, resistance of sweat duct; $R_e$, resistance of extaductal epidermis; S, standing potential in sweat duct; E, standing potential in epidermis; $R_V$, input resistance of voltage amplifier. From R. Edelberg, Biopotentials from the skin surface: the hydration effect, Annals of the New York Academy of Sciences, 1968, **148**, 252-262. Reproduced by permission of the New York Academy of Sciences.

Many observations are explained by the voltage-divider model and in general it stands up to rigorous testing. There is, however, one common observation that it has difficulty explaining, namely the very sudden interruption in the negative SPR followed by a jet-like positive wave (Figs. 2, 6, 7). The speed of the diffusion process from the duct into the corneum is apparently too slow to explain this sudden shift. Schulz et al (1965) have observed that saline trapped in the duct takes approximately 10 minutes to empty into the corneum. In view of the difficulty of explaining these fast positive SPRs by the one recognized non-membrane mechanism, Fowles (1986) still had reservations about discarding the two-effector hypothesis.

Another model, one useful for interpreting the impedance results of Gildemeister (1915) without postulating the participation of an active membrane is the **parallel resistance-capacitance circuit** proposed by several investigators including Montagu and Coles (1966). In this model an ohmic resistance, comprising that of the sweat ducts and corneum, is in parallel with a capacitance. Boucsein (1988) has adopted this model as a practical approach to dealing with EDA without having to resolve the "membrane" issue. The model can also explain the results by Lykken et al (1966) in which they concluded, using impedance measurements, that only a small fraction of the EDR can be explained by ohmic changes. In this and many similar demonstrations, the relatively high capacitance of the corneum causes it to act as a low reactance shunt when high frequency energizing currents are used. Under such conditions, the surface reflection of changes in the impedance of the sweat gland (i.e. the major source of the ohmic component) is greatly attenuated. Lykken (1971) recognized this when he interpreted his later work on the impedance characteristics of the skin.

The various passive mechanisms capable of explaining the characteristics of the electrodermal response were consistent with experimental observations and were generally not challenged. The membrane hypothesis was neither precluded nor supported by these additional models. Left unexplained, however, were several observations that, despite these passive models, seemed to require participation of an active membrane. These included:

- the fast positive SPR
- the reabsorption reflex
- polarity-dependent potentiation of the EDR by various ions
- attenuation of the SCR by detergents and high or low pH
- acceleration of SCR recovery rate when positive SPRs occur

## PROBLEMS FOR THE MEMBRANE MODEL

On the other hand there were some serious problems with the membrane model, having to do with the location of the hypothesized membrane, the mechanism of the reabsorption response, and the consistency of the behavioral adaptations postulated in the interpretation of membrane activity.

Ion effects are readily explained in terms of an excitable, selective membrane. But where is the membrane and who has demonstrated its excitability? How do the surface electrolytes reach this area? A clue to its identity should be provided by considering those sites that may be accessible to the ions that produce the marked effects described above. As has been discussed elsewhere (Edelberg, 1973a), entry of ions through the sweat ducts is not a likely option. True, some studies with $AlCl_3$ had shown that $Al^{+++}$ can enter the duct (Papa and Kligman, 1967; Quatrale et al, 1985) but they involved 24 hour exposures with long periods in which there was no flushing of the sweat glands, whereas the ion effects described above could be detected readily within 5 minutes after exposure. Further, the effects on EDA could be reversed within 5 minutes after substituting water or dilute saline for the experimental solution. This argued against any deep penetration of the duct, a conclusion consistent with that of Flesch et al (1951) who viewed the sweat duct as an improbable route of entry.

The corneum also seems an unlikely pathway, as summarized elsewhere (Tregear, 1962; Rushmer et al, 1966; Edelberg, 1971), because numerous investigators had demonstrated the low permeability of the corneum to ions. Accordingly we are left with the inevitable conclusion that either the target "membrane" is very superficial or some other mechanism is at play. It should also be pointed out that this author demonstrated with microhygrometric measurement (Edelberg, 1979) that skin exposed to water for 10 minutes undergoes only superficial hydration of the corneum, i.e. down to a depth of about 25 microns. The thickness of the palmar corneum is typically about 0.5 mm.

Still another observation that presented problems was the reabsorption "reflex". This sudden, superficial reduction in hydration was supposedly caused by active reabsorption of water across a membrane at a much deeper level. In view of the slow rate at which changes in hydration at this deeper level could be transmitted through the corneum to the surface layer, it seems inconceivable that these responses, which have a time course similar to some of the fast components of the SCR or SPR, could be registered so soon after onset of the EDR, e.g. 1 second (Edelberg, 1966).

A problem also arises in attempting to reconcile the behavioral correlates of the positive SPR, which is considered to originate in the membrane component, with the results of the palmar/dorsal study in which the membrane component was supposedly represented predominantly in dorsal activity. The membrane model views membrane activity as functioning in the tuning up of the skin surface and tactile apparatus for optimum discrimination (Edelberg, 1961; Wilcott, 1967). Since the forearm is a particularly active source of positive SPRs and, unlike the palm, can hardly be said to participate in fine tactile performance, this relation appears to be paradoxical.

## VARIATION IN RECOVERY AS EVIDENCE FOR MEMBRANE INVOLVEMENT

These various considerations seemed to leave the two-effector hypothesis very much in limbo. Such was the state of affairs when attention was directed to the recovery limb of the skin conductance response (SCR). Darrow (1932) had noted the variation in rate of recovery as a function of level of excitation. Other authors (Freeman and Katzoff, 1942; Mednick and Schulsinger, 1965; 1968) had examined the behavioral correlates of recovery rate and had interpreted it in terms of the homeostatic capacity of the CNS . This author (Edelberg, 1970) had observed that recovery rate accelerates when there is increased activity of positive SPRs or reabsorption reflexes (Fig. 2). Since the theoretical framework underlying the membrane hypothesis assumed that the positive SPR was generated by an epidermal membrane, this observation suggested that responses dominated by the membrane component had faster recovery than those in which sweat activity played a greater role. Of particular importance was the demonstration that the application of high currents slowed SCR recovery rate markedly (Edelberg, 1973b) as would be predicted if recovery depended on the action of an active membrane that was inactivated by this procedure (Fig. 4). Boucsein and Hoffmann (1979), using resistance and conductance measures to study recovery rate, observed differences in rates between the two and also interpreted their results in terms of membrane behavior.

In the course of these investigations it was found that the recovery measure could differentiate goal-oriented activity from non-task situations in which arousal was just as high (Edelberg, 1970) and that the measure could also distinguish defensive from goal-oriented behavior (Edelberg, 1972a). A series of papers from other laboratories appeared, in each case with confirmation of the robust quality of the measure as a differentiator (e.g. Bull and Nethercott, 1972; Lockhart, 1972; Waid, 1974). The measure rapidly gained use in distinguishing response patterns, especially defensive vs orienting (e.g. Furedy, 1972; Öhman et al, 1978; Dimberg, 1990), and also in sorting groups, in particular those with high vs low antisocial behavior (e.g. Siddle et al, 1976; Hare ,1978), or schizophrenics and normals (e.g. Ax and Bamford, 1970; Gruzelier and Venables, 1972, 1974; Maricq and

Edelberg, 1975; Patterson, 1976; Zahn et al, 1976).  While the recovery measure was finding application as a useful behavioral tool, its continued success was also viewed as evidence in support of the membrane hypothesis.  This support was viewed as especially convincing since, unlike the palmar/dorsal differences which possibly represented differences in regional innervation, the discriminating index was derived from a single site. Furthermore it fit well with the predictions of the two-component model.

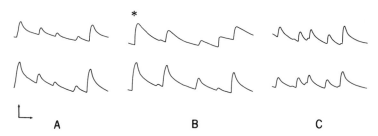

**Figure 4.** Slowing of recovery rate by high current. Upper and lower traces are simultaneously recorded from the palm. Panel A, control; panel B, upper trace recorded shortly after exposure to 22.5 V for 2 minutes; panel C, upper site has been exposed to 22.5 V for 4 minutes and allowed to recover for 3 minutes.

In 1974, **Bundy** reported a study that put in question the interpretation of recovery limb data.  He showed that the studies purporting to demonstrate the stimulus-specificity of recovery rate were flawed in that the stimulus schedule could possibly have biased the results.  He further demonstrated that recovery rate could be predicted by an assessment of immediately preceding electrodermal activity in terms of recency and amplitude (Bundy's X); the greater and more recent the activity, the faster the recovery rate (Bundy and Fitzgerald, 1975).  His findings were subsequently confirmed (Edelberg and Muller, 1981).  Moreover these authors showed that by manipulating the Bundy X by stimulus and task scheduling it was possible to alter recovery rate predictably.  Although X accounted for only 20% of the variance in recovery rate, its reliability as a predictor convinced this author that recovery rate was not an indication of the selective activation of two electrodermal effectors.

Despite this, on an operational basis, various laboratories continued to use the measure as a device for differentiating groups or response patterns.  Some authors provided data that indicated that when controls were introduced to account for Bundy's X, differences in recovery rate persisted.  Venables and Fletcher (1981) pointed out, that a substantial portion of the total variance was not removed by the Bundy procedure and that the measure had considerable value as a subject variable.  Janes (1982; Janes et al, 1985) published studies which showed that recovery rate was retarded as stimulus significance increased, even though prior EDA was held constant.  Levander et al (1980) examined their data on the relationship of recovery rate to various indices of socialization in a criminal population and concluded that antecedent activity could not account for their results.  Nevertheless, Bundy's findings placed the two-component hypothesis in serious doubt.  Complete abandonment of that model was not warranted, however, in the light of the failure of any proposed alternative to account for all major observations.

# THE FOWLES MODEL: TWO COMPONENTS WITH ONE INNERVATION

Fowles, in a careful evaluation of the status of the mechanism of the electrodermal response (Fowles, 1986) concluded that an effector system that included the sweat gland operating in conjunction with the voltage-divider model could explain most of the existing findings. He pointed out that if the alleged membrane and sweat components of the EDR were independent, they would require separate innervation, something that has never been satisfactorily demonstrated. He proposed five phases of activity in the sudomotor unit during an electrodermal response: the secretion of sweat, the reabsorption of sodium in the dermal duct, the rise of sweat in the epidermal duct, the movement of sweat across the duct wall into the corneum, and if sweat secretion is strong enough, the stretching of the duct at the epidermal level. This stretching could serve as a trigger to activate the ductal membrane. If the stretch were to reach trigger threshold, the sudden increase in permeability across the duct wall would cause an increase in conductance beyond that produced by the rise of sweat in the ducts. Moreover because repolarization of the duct wall is presumably rapid, producing a sudden fall in conductivity, it would account for faster recovery. One attractive aspect of his model was that it accounted for the membrane characteristics of the electrodermal effector without requiring a separate innervation.

In the event the pores were closed by hydration of the corneum, stretching would be greater because of the higher levels of hydrostatic pressure attained. However, these effects would be less observable at the surface because of the shutting down of the conductance pathway through the pores. While for the most part discounting the likelihood of a separately controlled membrane, he acknowleged that two still unexplained observations dictated against final ruling out of this possibility. One of these was the marked potentiating effect of certain ions like $Ca^{++}$ or $Al^{+++}$ on the amplitude of the SCR or the positive SPR. The other was the fast positive SPR.

# THE PORAL VALVE MODEL

In examining an array of passive mechanisms that could explain existing findings, this author also found most of them, including his own (Edelberg, 1973a), either inadequate or lacking experimental demonstration. Such was also the case for Fowles' proposed model in that ductal permeability changes associated with stretching or sodium triggering were hypothetical. There is, however, a model which does seem to fit the needs of a passive replacement. In brief, it is essentially the same as the Fowles model up to the point at which stimulation of the duct wall is considered, but in contrast **it makes no assumption about a change in the duct wall**. It focusses instead on the predictable effects of the **high intraductal pressures** that have been demonstrated to develope in the filled sweat gland either because the pores are closed (hydrated condition), or because an appreciable resistance is encountered in exiting the duct.

## Nature of Sweat Duct Filling

Before discussing the sequence of events that comprise the EDR, it is helpful to consider certain aspects of the sweat gland unit underlying these events. They relate to the manner in which the sweat duct fills and empties. Any hydrostatic column that exists in the duct is actually of negligible effect because it extends less than 1 mm. Furthermore the palms in most cases face downward. Once secretion has stopped, there is no reason to view the duct as containing a column of fluid that continues from the secretory area up to some distance from the pore. Rather the contained sweat, during the resting period, should as a result of tissue pressure and capillarity distribute itself throughout the length of the duct up to the level of the pore. It should be pointed out that Jeje and Koon (1989) have taken an opposite view, namely that the sweat column ends in a meniscus at some level below the pore.

The second notion also concerns the state of an unfilled sweat duct. One must ask the question as to what replaces the sweat as it drains out of the duct into the corneum after secretion ceases. If the pores are open it is possible that electrode medium or air is drawn into the duct (Maricq, 1972; Braham et al, 1979). With pores closed, however, since the duct contents can not be replaced, **partial collapse of the duct** wall must occur. Kuno (1956, p.16) in fact shows the sweat duct as evolving from an open lumen in the germinating layer to a flattened one in the corneum. Sato (1977) has described expansion and collapse in the sweat duct as secretion occurred and abated, but it should be emphasized that his observation were on the straight duct in the dermis.

Finally it is helpful to consider the question of what drives sweat out of the duct into the corneum. The vapor pressure difference between the sweat duct and the corneum is a relatively ineffective driving force as evidenced by Schulz' observations that sweat ducts in the corneum took about 10 minutes to empty. This also indicates that **the permeability of the duct wall is limited**. A more potent driving force is the **hydraulic pressure difference** that may develope across the wall. The eccrine sweat gland can develope very high intraductal (hydraulic) pressures, e.g. 250 mm Hg (Schwartz, 1960) to 500 mm Hg (Schulz, 1969). Such pressures produce relatively high filtration rates even across a duct wall that is relatively impermeable, since rate of filtration is directly proportional to pressure differential, much the same as filtration in the kidney glomerulus increases with increasing arterial pressure. This great augmentation of the rate of movement of sweat into the corneum (possibly by 6 to 10 times) should be kept in mind when one considers the generation of a positive SPR.

If the superficial layer of the corneum is initially well hydrated, the sweat pore and probably the most distal portion of the sweat duct will be collapsed by the pressure exerted by the surrounding corneum. I have not been able to find data on the tissue pressure exerted by hydrated corneum. However the forces due to swelling pressure have been measured in various gels as they imbibe water and for the most part attain pressures of the order of 20 mm Hg (Guyton, 1971). The swelling pressure of the corneum may be considerably greater, but is probably far less than the pressure of 225 mm Hg to 500 mm Hg that may develope within the duct.

## Sequence of Events in the Electrodermal Response

For a hydrated site, with ducts initially empty, the early sequence of events is essentially that proposed in earlier models. It is likely that some or most of the pores are closed. At the start of the response, if there is a change in membrane potential or conductance in the secretory coil, it is not observed at the surface (Shaver, Brusilow and Cooke, 1965). As sweat fills the duct, laterally as well as axially, it provides a more conductive path through the relatively resistant corneum, causing an increase in conductance and, due to the internal voltage-divider, an increased negative potential at the surface (Fig. 5, B). The negative potential probably arises in the duct wall at the level of the germinating layer and may well originate as a result of the sodium reabsorption mechanism (Fowles and Venables, 1970; Sato, 1977; Fowles, 1986).

If the ducts are filled to the limits of their limp capacity and secretion continues, intraductal pressure will start to build up, causing **hydraulic-driven movement of sweat into the corneum**. Due to the voltage-divider effect, this should ordinarily cause a positive swing in surface potential. However because of the hydrated state of the outer layer of corneum, any movement of water into that region would have only a weak effect in changing the state of the voltage-divider. Moreover, due to the tissue pressure exerted by the swollen corneum, this region of the duct may be collapsed along with the pores. At a somewhat deeper layer, however, dryer conditions often prevail (Suchi, 1958; Edelberg, 1979). During this phase increasing hydration of the deeper levels of the corneum could contribute to the positive potential response. Despite the movement of sweat into the corneum, the sweat ducts will remain full as long as secretion continues; it is not the duct component but the increasing hydration of the deeper levels of the corneum that then contributes to rising conductance (Stombaugh and Adams, 1971).

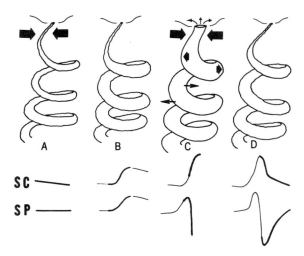

**Figure 5.** Diagram of the sequence in a sweat response at a hydrated site, starting with unfilled ducts and collapsed poral segment in panel A. Panel B, secretion has partially filled ducts; panel C, secretion has filled ducts to limit of capacity and has generated sufficient intraductal pressure to open poral "valve"; panel D, escape of sweat has reduced intraductal pressure to collapse point. Associated skin conductance and potential responses (SC and SP) are shown at the bottom.

**Dilation**

If secretion is strong enough, it may generate an intraductal pressure that is greater than the tissue pressure of the corneum. In that case the collapsed portion of the distal duct will reopen, as will the pore, and will become filled with sweat. As the terminal portion of the duct opens, the conductance increase will be augmented (Fig. 5, C). Sweat will be forced out through the sweat pore but will continue to move laterally into the corneum as well. As before, at some depth below the surface, the hydraulic "pump" will continue to increase the hydration of the corneum, and will augment the rapidly developing positive SPR.

## Collapse

Secretion may or may not stop at this point. As sweat leaves the duct, unless secretory rate can keep up with the loss of volume, intraductal pressure will fall. When it falls below external tissue pressure, the pore and terminal duct will again collapse, causing a rapid fall in conductance (Fig. 5, D). The acceleration of recovery that attends the positive SPR is in part a reflection of this rapid fall. Because of the increase in the resistance of the sweat duct leg of the voltage-divider induced by the collapse, surface potential swings still more positively, thus potentiating the positive SPR. The sudden increase in surface resistance occasioned by the collapse likely explains the "reabsorption" response as well.

At this point one must take into consideration another phenomenon, one discussed by Burton (1962) for small blood vessels. When a vessel surrounded by tissue is collapsed by tissue pressure, it takes more internal pressure to open that vessel than to close it. This follows from the geometrical relation of the vessel to the surrounding tissue. This principle would apply to the sweat duct as well, so that once open, the pore would not close as soon as the pressure diminished; rather it would remain open until intraductal pressure fell below a lesser value. This would delay collapse and prolong emptying time.

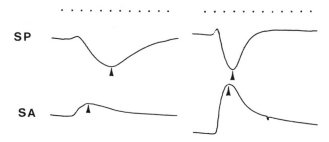

**Figure 6.** Simultaneous skin potential and skin admittance (135 Hz) recorded from a single palmar sites on each of two subjects. Arrowheads show start of recovery of positive SPRs and of admittance. Tracings demonstrate slow (left) and fast positive SPRs. Differences may reflect levels of intraductal pressure attained. Time ticks are at 1 sec intervals.

Still to be accounted for is the **recovery of the positive limb of the SPR** and the continuing recovery of the SCR. As sweat from the corneum is reabsorbed into the dermis, or diffuses away from the periductal area, the resistance of the corneum rises (Adams, 1966). Its relatively high initial rate probably reflects diffusion away from the periductal area. For some reason, possibly the binding of water further from the duct where the keratin is drier, and the attraction of ions by the charged side-chains of the keratin, the conductance of the corneum appears to become less as the same total amount of sweat is more evenly distributed. Due to the voltage-divider effect, surface potential becomes more negative, i.e. the positive SPR recovers. Of interest is the fact that a fairly rapid skin conductance recovery continues during this period (Fig. 6, right panel). Here admittance at 135 Hz has been used instead of conductance to enable simultaneous registration of exosomatic and endosomatic EDRs from a single site, i.e. under precisely the same conditions. If this effect depends on diffusion from the periductal region, one might expect the recovery pattern described in the "interrupted decay" hypothesis (Edelberg and Muller, 1981). Since recovery of the positive skin potential wave is an indication that the resistance of the corneum is increasing, the recovery of the SCR during this phase implies that increasing resistance of the corneum is contributing substantially to this recovery. Implicit in this is that **hydration of the corneum can contribute considerably to the SCR**.

This sequence of events seems inconsistent with the results reported by Fowles and his coworkers in which SPR activity was commonly abolished at a hydrated site in most subjects. Some of my own studies, however, did show conspicuous positive SPR activity at hydrated sites. Moreover the Fowles and Schneider (1974) study which used female subjects showed appreciable positive SPR activity in the early phase of testing.

## Open Pore Condition

If a dehydrating medium is used, the pores may be open. In such a case, starting with the unfilled condition, events will be the same up to the point at which the ducts become full. At this point continuing secretion may merely empty the duct contents through the pore with little additional effect on EDA. However, **if secretion rate exceeds the emptying capacity of the pores, intraductal pressure will rise**. The sequence of events will then depart from the pores-closed condition in several ways. First, because the superficial region of the corneum is dehydrated, the expression of sweat into the outer corneum will be more effective in producing positive SPRs. Secondly, because there is no episode of poral dilation and closure, "reabsorption responses" will not be observed and recovery will be slower than at a hydrated site. Retardation of recovery has in fact been demonstrated when polyethylene glycol is applied for a long enough period to dehydrate the site (Edelberg, 1977). This effect is opposite to the acceleration of recovery observed when a dehydrating agent of intermediate strength, e.g. 1 M $AlCl_3$, is used. The difference is presumably due to the dilation/collapse cycle that occurs in the latter case.

## Summary of Poral Valve Sequence

The sequence of events when a hydrating medium is used to record EDA may be summarized as follows:

Starting with relatively empty ducts, whose pores are closed, the partial filling of the ducts at each response causes an increase in conductance and negative surface potential. These are the initial steps of the staircase in the early section of figure 7. Subsequent responses ultimately achieve the "full ducts" condition. Further secretion builds up intraductal pressure which drives sweat into the deeper corneum at an accelerated rate, causing a further increase in conductance and a sharp positive SPR. Intraductal pressure may become high enough to exceed the tissue pressure of the corneum, causing the poral region, including the collapsed terminal portion of the duct, to dilate, thereby increasing conductance further. As sweat escapes, the fall in pressure enables the tissue pressure of the corneum to collapse the duct once again. The consequent increase in the resistance of the superficial duct, coupled with the closure of the pore, causes an added positive shift in surface potential, a sharp decrease in skin conductance, seen as accelerated recovery, and a sudden increase in the horizontal resistance near the surface which may appear as a "reabsorption" response. Diffusion of sweat from the periductal area causes slower but still relatively rapid recovery of the SCR and the positive SPR. Tonic reabsorption into the dermis or outward diffusion into the electrode medium, slowly dehydrates the corneum, causing slow emptying of the sweat ducts and slow drift in baseline potential and conductance. If the pores are open, dilation and collapse will not occur, and very fast recovery and "reaborption" will consequently not be in evidence. However, strong secretion may overwhelm the emptying capacity of the pores, causing the development of high intraductal pressure, and therefore of rapid positive SPRs and some acceleration of recovery.

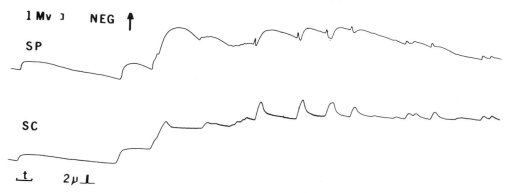

**Figure 7.** Transition from condition of relatively empty ducts to full ducts. SPRs show evolution from negative responses to biphasic. SCRs show buildup of skin conductance level and acceleration of recovery as poral dilation/collapse is reached. From "Electrical activity of the skin" by R. Edelberg. In N.S. Greenfield and R.A. Sternbach (eds), *Handbook of Psychophysiology*, Chap 9. New York: 1972. Reproduced by permission of Holt, Rinehart and Winston.

## OBSERVATIONS EXPLAINED BY THE PORAL VALVE MODEL

The above sequence is consistent with various features of an EDR. It must also be tested against other findings.

### Ion Effects

If the above model is correct, how does one explain the ionic effects in which large, highly hydrated, ions cause dramatic polarity-dependent potentiation of SCR amplitude? These effects are seen to be mediated by the dehydrating effect of the lyophilic series on the corneum. In the original study on "membrane" properties (Edelberg et al, 1960), it was pointed out that the effects of these ions were in the same order as the Hofmeister lyotropic series, i.e. in the order of their affinity for water. Evidence for interpreting at least one ion effect as originating in its effect on hydration is seen in the work of Fowles and Johnson (1973) who kept the vapor pressure of various concentrations of KCl constant by the addition of sucrose and found that the marked effect of concentration on the potentiation of SPR by KCl disappeared.

If these ions were exerting their effect by virtue of their dehydration of the corneum surrounding the sweat pore, the most hydrophilic ions would be most effective. Potentiation of the SCR would occur because in the dehydrated state the corneum has a smaller shunting effect on any changes in duct resistance (Edelberg, 1983). Dehydration of the corneum would also account for the potentiation of the positive SPR by the voltage-divider effect. Any dehydrating influence exerted by the ion population of a hydrating medium (e.g. 1 M $AlCl_3$) would lower the threshold for pore opening, causing a greater frequency of poral opening episodes, and therefore of collapsing episodes. The consequent increase in positive SPR amplitude at intermediate levels of hydration contrasts with the situation at a completely dehydrated site. There the pores would be open and unless secretion were intense, high intraductal presures would not develope. A similar explanation may account for the U-shaped curve alluded to by Fowles and Schneider (1974) in relation to hydration effects on SCR amplitude.

At a cathodal site the cations would be pulled away from the corneum by electrostatic action, reducing the degree of dehydration, thus accounting for the polarity dependence. To explain the attenuation of SCR produced by detergents or by high or low pH, one may consider their well-recognized effects in increasing the hydration of the corneum (Yates, 1971; Putterman et al, 1977; Rhein et al, 1986).

**Reabsorption "Reflex":**

From the sequence of events in the hydrated condition, one may understand how a so-called "reabsorption reflex" may occur. The sensor used to study the water-reabsorption phenomenon consists of two closely-spaced parallel wires. The current between them, unlike the case with widely-spaced electrodermal electrodes, passes laterally and traverses a shallow depth (Fig. 8). As intraductal pressure dilates the collapsed poral segments, filling them with sweat, such a sensor will record a small increase in conductance, since the parallel wires include a number of sweat ducts between them. As these ducts again collapse, the sensor will encounter the rapid increase in resistance that has been erroneously described by this author as the "reabsorption reflex". The collapse effect will generally be greater than the dilation effect because the final volume after a period of sweat loss throught the open pores will be diminished.

It is noteworthy that such "reabsorption responses" have been found only after hydration of the site and have been associated with positive SPRs and rapid SCR recovery, conditions which this model predicts when the poral region collapses.

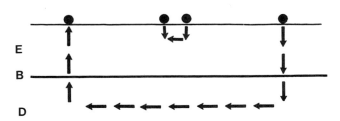

**Figure 8.** Principle of surface hydration sensor. Pathway between closely spaced wires at center is confined to superficial layer of epidermis (E). High lateral resistance between widely spaced pair prevents lateral movement until current crosses barrier (B) and reaches low resistance of dermis (D).

In the original paper on reabsorption (Edelberg, 1966), other types of sensors were used to demonstrate that this "reabsorption reflex" was not an artifact of electrical circuitry. One of these, the stagnant chamber, recorded prominent, sudden reductions in vapor pressure at the same time as a nearby site showed SCRs of especially high amplitude. If these observations are valid, one would have difficulty in reconciling them with the poral valve model. However when rate of sweat flow increases, there is less time for reabsorption of sodium in the dermal duct and the salt level in the excreted sweat becomes more concentrated (Schwartz and Thaysen, 1956). Calculation of the change in vapor pressure associated with a concentration change from 0.03 M NaCl to 0.08 M NaCl, one that might occur during rapid secretion, shows it to produce a change in vapor pressure about 8 times as great as that which would be needed to account for the "reabsorption responses" observed.

**Other Observations**:

The poral valve model explains the generation of uniphasic positive SPRs. If the ducts are full when the response starts, and the attained intraductal pressure is insufficient to open the pores, the initial phase will be isometric, i.e. hydraulic driving of sweat into the corneum will occur without substantial ductal volume change, hence without the negative component. The model also accounts for the manner in which Fowles and Schneider (1974) were able to manipulate the SCR recovery rate of their subjects, since it predicts the **acceleration of recovery** when EDRs are elicited at a hydrated site under conditions of full ducts.

It appears that this model deals adequately with various observations with which it must be reconciled. It is also consistent with a large number of other reports in the literature. For example, it makes clear why there is a synchrony between the occurrence of the positive SPR and the visual appearance of sweat on the surface (Darrow et al 1957) and why there is a positive correlation between recovery rate and the magnitude of perspiration (Darrow, 1932). It also explains why the application of high current to the skin causes slower recovery (Fig. 4), since the associated reduction in secretory activity would reduce the maximum level of intraductal pressure attained, thereby reducing the frequency of episodes of dilation and collapse.

In another example, as habituation occurs in a series of EDRs, initial filling of the ducts for each response will diminish progressively, as the amplitude of the preceding response decreases. Since high intraductal pressure would then be less likely to develope, this would cause the sequence of events to progress from one with positive SPR components and fast SCR recovery to one with uniphasic negative SPRs and slower recovery. An apparent habituation of the positive but not of the negative SPR would result (e.g. Forbes and Bolles, 1936). As another example, if one reduces sweat activity by arterial occlusion or exsanguination (Edelberg, 1964), responses would not likely reach the stage of high intraductal pressure and there would be an apparent selective inactivation of the positive SPR (Wilcott, 1958). It would also explain those reports in which a given result occurred only with large amplitude responses (e.g. Hygge and Hugdahl, 1985), i.e. those in which high intraductal pressures developed only when intense secretion occurred.

## CONCLUSIONS

The operation of this passive mechanism can clearly be modified by the pattern of neural activity that activates the sweat gland. Thus, if the discharge pattern consists of relatively frequent bursts of low level activity, the consequences on EDA characteristics will be considerably different than those of less frequent, large magnitude bursts. Given a site prepared with a hydrating medium, these two patterns will determine the likelihood that high intraductal pressures are developed and that poral opening occurs. If the responses to different classes of stimuli are mediated by different CNS structures whose characteristic neural discharge pattern are different, one might expect to note signs of response specificity even in this one-effector system. Lang et al (1964) have in fact reported that the form of the EDR in the cat varies as a function of location and intensity of stimuli to the amygdala and brainstem structures. Differences in efferent pattern may perhaps account for the finding that the ratio of sweat to conductance change from palmar sites varies as a function of stimulus (Edelberg and Wright, 1964).

On the other hand if the neural response pattern of one subject is characteristically different from that of another, differences in their EDA pattern, such as frequency of positive SPR activity or rate of recovery may emerge. Thus, although the effect of antecedent activity on recovery rate can be explained by this model in terms of the likelihood of the ducts being full, the added influence of neural discharge pattern may be the determining factor in properly designed experiments. Such appears to be the case in the demonstrations of recovery rate differences in which antecedent activity has been controlled.

This model predicts that even with open pores, the nature of the efferent neural volley can influence the ensuing events in the skin. Small bursts in rapid succession would tend to send most of the sweat to the surface. Large concentrated bursts could momentarily exceed the emptying capacity of the pore, build up intraductal pressure, and divert a larger portion into the corneum. This would hold even in the absence of electrode medium. It is tempting to consider the possibility that the CNS uses these differential effects in an adaptive fashion.

With this passive model it is no longer necessary to make any assumptions about the participation of an active membrane in the electrodermal response. Nor, if one adopts the voltage-divider model to explain changes in potential observed at the surface, is there any need to hypothesize changes in the transductal potential. The consistency of a large array of observations with the predictions of this passive model, coupled with the serious deficiencies of the two-effector hypothesis, appears to warrant abandonment of the older model, at least until such time as flaws may be discovered in these various arguments.

# REFERENCES

Adams, T., 1966, Characteristics of eccrine sweat gland activity in the footpad of the cat, *J. Appl. Physiol.* **21,** 1004-1012.

Adams, T. and Vaughan, J.A., 1965, Human eccrine sweat gland activity and palmar electrical skin resistance, *J. Appl. Physiol.* **20,** 980-983.

Ax, A.F. and Bamford, J.L., 1970, The GSR recovery limb in chronic schizophrenia, *Psychophysiol.* **7,** 145-147.

Bloch, V., 1965, Le contrôle central de l'activité électrodermale: étude neurophysiologique et psycho-physiologique d'un indice sympathique de l'activation réticulaire, *J. Physiol. (Paris)* **57,** Suppl. 13, 1-132.

Boucsein, W., 1988, "Electrodermale Aktivität: Grundlagen, Methoden und Anwendungen," Springer-Verlag, Berlin.

Boucsein, W. and Hoffmann, G., 1979, A direct comparison of the skin conductance and skin resistance methods, *Psychophysiol.* **16,** 66-70.

Braham, J., 1979, Skin wrinkling on immersion of hands: a test of sympathetic function, *Arch. Neurol.* **36,** 113-114.

Brebner, D.F. and Kerslake, D.McK., 1964, The time course of the decline in sweating produced by wetting the skin, *J. Physiol. (London)* **175,** 295-302.

Bull, R.H.C. and Nethercott, R.E., 1972, Physiological recovery and personality, *Br. J. Soc. Clin. Psychol.* **11,** 297.

Bundy, R.S., 1974, The effect of previous responses on the skin conductance recovery limb, *Psychophysiol.* **11,** 221-222, (abstr).

Bundy, R.S. and Fitzgerald, H.E., 1975, Stimulus specificity of electrodermal recovery time: an examination and reinterpretation of the evidence, *Psychophysiol.* **12,** 406-411.

Burton, A.C., 1962, Physical principles of circulatory phenomena: the physical equilibria of heart and blood vessel, Chap. 6 *in*: "Handbook of Physiology," Section 2, "Circulation," Amer. Physiol. Soc., Wash. D.C.

Darrow, C.W., 1927, Sensory, secretory and electrical changes in the skin following bodily excitation. *J. Exp. Psychol.* **10**, 197-226.

Darrow, C.W., 1932, The relation of the galvanic skin reflex recovery curve to reactivity, resistance level, and perspiration, *J. Gen. Psychol.* **7**, 261-273.

Darrow, C.W., 1937, Neural mechanisms controlling the palmar galvanic skin reflex and sweating: a consideration of available literature, *Arch. Neurol. Psychiat.* **37**, 641-663.

Darrow, C.W. and Freeman, G.L., 1934, Palmar skin-resistance changes contrasted with non-palmar changes, and rate of insensible weight loss, *J. Exp. Psychol.* **17**, 739-748.

Darrow, C.W., Wilcott, R.C., Siegel, A., Wilson, J., Watanabe, K., and Vieth, R., 1957, The mechanism of diphasic skin potential response, *Electroenceph. Clin. Neurophysiol.* **9**, 169, (abstr).

Dimberg, U., 1990, Facial electromyographic reactions and automonic activity to auditory stimuli, *Biol. Psychol.* **31**, 137-147.

Edelberg, R., 1961, The relationship between the galvanic skin response, vasoconstriction, and tactile sensitivity, *J. Exp. Psychol.* **62**, 187-195.

Edelberg, R., 1963, Electrophysiologic characteristics and interpretation of skin potentials, *Sch. Aerospace Med. Tech. Doc. Rpt. 63-95*.

Edelberg, R., 1964, Independence of galvanic skin response amplitude and sweat production, *J. Invest. Derm.* **42**, 443 448.

Edelberg, R., 1966, Reponse of cutaneous water barrier to ideational stimulation: a GSR component, *J. Comp. Physiol. Psychol.* **61**, 28-33.

Edelberg, R., 1968, Biopotentials from the skin surface: the hydration effect, *Ann. N. Y. Acad. Sci.* **148**, 252-262.

Edelberg, R., 1970, The information content of the recovery limb of the electrodermal response, *Psychophysiol.* **6**, 527-539.

Edelberg, R., 1971, Electrical properties of skin, Chap. 15 *in:* "Biophysical Properties of the Skin," H.R. Elden, ed., Wiley, New York.

Edelberg, R., 1972a, Electrodermal recovery rate, goal-orientation, and aversion, *Psychophysiol.* **9**, 512-520.

Edelberg, R., 1972b, The electrodermal system, Chap. 9 *in:* "Handbook of Psychophysiology," N.S. Greenfield and R.A. Sternbach, eds., Holt, Rinehart and Winston, New York.

Edelberg, R., 1973a, Mechanisms of electrodermal adaptations for locomotion, manipulation, or defense, *in:* Progress in Physiological Psychology," Vol 5, E.Stellar and J.M. Sprague, eds., Academic Press, New York, pp. 155-209.

Edelberg, R., 1973b, The role of an epidermal component in control of electrodermal recovery rate. Paper presented at the 13th Annual Meeting of the Society for Psychophysiological Research, Galveston. *Psychophysiol.* **11**, 221 (abstr).

Edelberg, R., 1977, The status of the electrodermal recovery measure: a caveat. Paper presented at the 17th Annual Meeting of the Society for Psychophysiological Research, Philadelphia. *Psychophysiol.* **15**, 283-284 (abstr).

Edelberg, R., 1979, More on the mechanism of electrodermal recovery. Paper presented at the 19th Annual Meeting of the Society for Psychophysiological Research, Cincinanati. *Psychophysiol.* **17**, 305-306 (abstr).

Edelberg, R., 1983, The effects of initial levels of sweat duct filling and skin hydration on electrodermal response amplitude, *Psychophysiol.* **20**, 550-557.

Edelberg, R., Greiner, T., and Burch, N.R., 1960, Some membrane properties of the effector in the galvanic skin response, *J. Appl. Physiol.* **15**, 691-696.

Edelberg, R. and Muller, M., 1981, Prior activity as a determinant of electrodermal recovery rate, *Psychophysiol.* **18**, 17-25.

Edelberg, R. and Wright, D.J., 1964, Two galvanic skin response effector organs and their stimulus specificity, *Psychophysiol.* **1**, 39-47.

Flesch, P., Goldstone, S.B., and Urbach, F., 1951, Palmar pore patterns: their significance in the absorption of dyes, *Arch. Derm. Syphilol.* **63**, 228-231.

Forbes, T.W. and Bolles, M.M., 1936, Correlation of the response potentials of the skin with "exciting" and non"exciting" stimuli, *J. Psychol.* **2**, 273-285.

Fowles, D.C., 1974, Mechanisms of electrodermal activity, Chap. 9 *in*: "Bioelectric Recording Techniques," R.F. Thompson and M. Patterson, eds., New York, Academic Press.

Fowles, D.C., 1986, The eccrine system and electrodermal activity, Chap 4 *in:* "Psychophysiology: Systems, Processes, and Applications," M.G.H. Coles, E. Donchin, and S.W. Porges, eds., Guilford Press, New York.

Fowles, D.C. and Johnson, G., 1973, The influence of variations in electrolyte concentration on skin potential level and response amplitude, *Biol. Psychol.*, **1**, 151-160.

Fowles, D.C. and Rosenberry, R., 1973, Effects of epidermal hydration on skin potential responses and levels, *Psychophysiol.* **10**, 601-611.

Fowles, D.C. and Schneider, R.E., 1974, Effects of epidermal hydration on skin conductance responses and levels, *Biol. Psychol.* **2**, 67-77.

Fowles, D.C. and Schneider, R.E., 1978, Electrolyte medium effects on measurements of palmar skin potential, *Psychophysiol.* **15**, 474-482.

Fowles, D.C. and Venables, P.H., 1970, The effects of epidermal hydration and sodium reabsorption on palmar skin potential, *Psychol. Bull.* **73**, 363-378.

Freeman, G.L. and Katzoff, E.T., 1942, Methodological evaluation of the galvanic skin reflex with special reference to the formula for R. Q. (recovery quotient), *J. Exp. Psychol.* **31**, 239-248.

Furedy, J.J., 1972, Electrodermal recovery time as a supra sensitive autonomic index of anticipated intensity of threatened shock, *Psychophysiol.* **9**, 281-282.

Gildemeister, M., 1915, Der sogenannte psychogalvanische Reflex und seine physikalischchemische Deutung. *Pflüg. Arch. ges. Physiol.*, **162**, 489-506.

Gruzelier, J.H. and Venables, P.H., 1972, Skin conductance orienting activity in a heterogeneous sample of schizophrenics: possible evidence of limbic dysfunction, *J. Nerv. Ment. Dis.* **155**, 277-287.

Guyton, A.C., Granger, H.J., and Taylor, A.E., 1971, Interstitial fluid pressure, *Physiol. Rev.* **51**, 527-563.

Hare, R.D., 1978, Electrodermal and cardiovascular correlates of psychopathy, *in:* "Psychopathic Behavior: Approaches to Research," R.D. Hare and D. Schalling, eds., Wiley, London.

Hygge, S. and Hugdahl, K., 1985, Skin conductance recordings and the NaCl concentration of the electrolyte, *Psychophysiol.* **22**, 365-367.

Janes, C.L., 1982, Electrodermal recovery and stimulus significance, *Psychophysiol.* **19**, 129-135.

Janes, C.L., Strock, B.D., Weeks, D.G., and Worland, J., 1985, The effect of stimulus significance on skin conductance recovery, *Psychophysiol.* **22**, 138-146.

Jeje, A. and Koon, D., 1989, An analysis on the rates and regulation of insensible water loss through the eccrine sweat glands, *J. Theor. Biol.* **141**, 303-324.

Jenkinson, D.M., Montgomery, I., and Elder, H.Y., 1978, Studies on the nature of the peripheral sudomotor control mechanism, *J. Anat.* **125**, 625-639.

Katkin, E.S., Weintraub, G.S. and Yasser, A.M., 1967, Stimulus specificity of epidermal and sweat gland contributions to GSR, *J. Comp. Physiol. Psychol.* **64**, 186-190.

Kuno, Y., 1956, "Human Perspiration," Charles C. Thomas, Springfield, p. 16.

Lang, H., Tuovinen, T. and Valleala, P., 1964, Amygdaloid afterdischarge and galvanic skin response, *Electroenceph. Clin. Neurophysiol.* **16**, 366-374.

Levander, S.E., Schalling, D.S., Lidberg, L., Bartfai, A., and Lidberg, Y., 1980, Skin conductance recovery time and personality in a group of criminals, *Psychophysiol.* **17**, 105-111.

Lockhart, R.A., 1972, Interrelations between amplitude, latency, rise time, and the Edelberg recovery measure of the galvanic skin response, *Psychophysiol.* **9**, 437-442.

Lykken, D.T., 1971, Square-wave analysis of skin impedance, Psychophysiol. 7, 262-275.

Lykken, D.T., Miller, R.D., and Strahan, R.F., 1966, GSR and polarization capacity of the skin, *Psychonom. Sci.* **4**, 355 356.

Maricq, H.R., 1972, The effect of stripping on sweat ducts observed by intravital microscopy, *J. Invest. Derm.* **59,** 375-379.

Maricq, H.R. and Edelberg, R., Electrodermal recovery rate in a schizophrenic population, 1975, *Psychophysiol.* **12,** 630-633.

Martin, I. and Venables, P.H., 1966, Mechanisms of palmar skin resistance and skin potential, *Psychol. Bull.* **65,** 347-357.

McCleary, R.A., 1950, The nature of the galvanic skin response, *Psychol. Bull.* **42,** 97-117.

Mednick, S.A. and Schulsinger, F., 1965, A longitudinal study of children with a high risk for schizophrenia: a preliminary report, *in:* "Methods and Goals in Human Behavior Genentics," S. Vandenberg, ed., Academic Press, New York.

Mednick, S.A. and Schulsinger, F., 1968, Some premorbid characteristics related to breakdown in children with schizophrenic mothers, *in:* "Transmission of Schizophrenia," D. Rosenthal and S.S. Kety, eds., Pergamon Press, London.

Montagu, J.D., 1958, The psychogalvanic reflex: a comparison of A.C. skin resistance and skin potential changes, *J. Neurol. Neurosurg. Psychiat.* 21, 119-128.

Montagu, J.D. and Coles, E.M., 1966, Mechanism and measurement of the galvanic skin response, *Psychol. Bull.* **65,** 261-279.

Mordkoff, A.M., 1968, Palmar-dorsal skin conductance differences during classical conditioning, *Psychophysiol.* **5,** 61-66.

Mordkoff, A.M., Edelberg, R., and Ustick, M., 1967, The differential conditionability of two components of the skin conductance response, *Psychophysiol.* **4,** 40-47.

Nakayama, T. and Takagi, K., 1958, Two components involved in galvanic skin response, *Jap. J. Physiol.* **8,** 21-30.

Öhman, A. Nordby, H., and D'Elia, G., 1989, Orienting in schizophrenia: habituation to auditory stimuli of constant and varying intensity in patients of high and low skin conductance responsivity, *Psychophysiol.* **26,** 48-61.

Papa, C.M. and Kligman, A.M., 1967, Mechanisms of eccrine anidrosis. II The antiperspirant effect of aluminum salts, *J. Invest. Derm.* 49, 139-145.

Patterson, T., 1976, Skin conductance recovery and pupillometrics in chronic schizophrenia, *Psychophysiol.* **13,** 189-195.

Peiss, C.N. and Randall, W.C., 1957, The effect of vapor impermeable gloves on evaporation and sweat suppression in the hand, *J. Invest. Derm.* **28,** 443-448.

Potts, R.O., 1986, Stratum corneum hydration: experimental techniques and interpretation of results, *J. Soc. Cosmet. Chem.* **37,** 9-33.

Putterman, G.J., Wolejsza, N.F., Wolfram, M.A., and Laden, K., 1977, The effect of detergents on swelling of stratum corneum, *J. Soc. Cosmet. Chem.* **28,** 521-532.

Quatrale, R.P., Thomas, E.L., and Birnbaum, J.E., 1985, The site of antiperspirant action by aluminum salts in the eccrine sweat glands of the axilla, *J. Soc. Cosmet. Chem.* **36,** 435 440.

Rein, H., 1929, Der Electrophysiologie der Haut, in:"Handbuch der Haut und Geschlechtskrankheiten, 1/2," J. Jadassohn, ed., Springer, Berlin. Cited by S. Rothman, 1954, "Physiology and Biochemistry of the Skin," Univ. Chic. Press, Chicago.

Rhein, L.D., Robbins, C.R., Fernee, K. and Cantore, R., 1986, Surfactant structure effects on swelling of isolated human stratum corneum, J. Soc. Cosmet. Chem. 37, 125-139.

Richter, C.P., 1929, Physiological factors involved in the electrical resistance of the skin, *Amer. J. Physiol.* **88,** 596-615.

Richter, C.P., 1930, Galvanic skin reflex from animals with complete transection of the spinal cord, *Amer. J. Physiol.* **93,** 468-472.

Robbins, C.R. and Fernee, K.M., 1983, Some observations on the swelling of human epidermal membrane, *J. Soc. Cosmet. Chem.* **34,** 21-34.

Rushmer, R.F., Buettner, K.J.K., Short, J.M. and Odland, G.F., 1966, The skin, *Science* 154, *343-348.*

Sarkany, I., Shuster, S. and Stammers, M.C., 1965, Occlusion of the sweat pore by hydration, *Brit. J. Derm.* **77,** 101-104.

Sato, K., 1977, The physiology, pharmacology, and biochemistry of the eccrine sweat gland, *Rev. Physiol. Biochem. Pharm.* **79**, 51-131.

Schulz, I., Ullrich, K.F., Frömter, e., Holzgreve, H., Frick, A., and Hegel, U., 1965, Mikropunktion und electrische Potentialmessung an Schweisdrü sen des Menschen, *Pflüg. Arch. ges. Physiol.* **284**, 360-372.

Schulz I.J., 1969, Micropuncture studies of the sweat formation in cystic fibrosis patients, *J. Clin. Invest.* **48**, 1470-1477.

Schwartz, I.L., 1960, Extrarenal regulation with special reference to the sweat glands, *in:* "Mineral Metabolism," Vol. 1, C.L. Colmar and F. Bronner, eds., Academic Press, New York. Cited in Fowles, D.C. and Venables, P.H., 1970, The effects of epidermal hydration and sodium reabsorption on palmar skin potential, *Psychol. Bull.* **73**, 363-378.

Schwartz, I.L. and Thaysen, J.H., 1956, Excretion of sodium and potassium in human sweat, *J. Clin. Invest.* **35**, 114-120.

Shaver, B.A., Brusilow, S.W. and Cooke, R.E., 1965, Electropyhysiology of the sweat gland: intraductal potential changes during secretion, *Bull. Johns Hopkins Hosp.* **116**, 100-109.

Siddle D.A.T., Mednick, S.A., Nicol, A.R. and Foggitt, R.H., 1976, Skin conductance recovery in antisocial adolescents, *Brit. J. Soc. Clin. Psychol.* **15**, 425-428.

Sorgatz, H., 1978, Components of skin impedance level, *Biol. Psychol.* *6, 121-125.*

Stevens, L.M. and Landis, S.C., 1988, Developmental interactions between sweat glands and the sympathetic neurons which innervate them: effects of delayed innervation on neurotransmitter plasticity and gland maturation, *Devel. Biol.* **130**, 703-720.

Stombaugh, D.P. and Adams, T., 1971, Skin electrical phenomena, sweat gland activity, and epidermal hydration of the cat footpad, *Amer. J. Physiol.* **221**, 1014-1018.

Suchi, T., 1955, Experiments on electrical resistance of the human epidermis, *Jap. J. Physiol.* **5**, 75-80.

Takagi, K. and Nakayama, T., 1959, Peripheral effector mechanism of galvanic skin reflex, *Jap. J. Physiol.* **9**, 1-7.

Tregear, R.T., 1962, The structures which limit the penetrability of the skin, *J. Soc. Cosmet. Chem.* **13**, 145-151.

Trehub, A, Tucker, I., and Cazavelan, J., 1962, Epidermal beta waves and changes in basal potentials of the skin, *Amer. J. Psychol.* **75**, 140-143.

Venables, P.H. and Christie, M.J., 1973, Mechanisms, instrumentation, recording techniques, and quantification of responses, Chap. 1, *in:* "*Electrodermal Activity in Psychological Research,*" W.F. Prokasy and D.C. Raskin, eds., Academic Press, New York.

Venables, P.H. and Fletcher, R.P., 1981, The status of skin conductance recovery time: an examination of the Bundy effect, *Psychophysiol.* **18**, 10-16.

Waid, W.W., 1974, Degree of goal-orientation, level of cognitive activity and electrodermal recovery rate, *Percept. Mot. Sk.* **38**, 103-109.

Wang, G.H., 1964, "The Neural Control of Sweating," Univ. Wisc. Press, Madison.

Wilcott, R.C. 1958, Effects of local blood removal on skin resistance and potential, *J. Comp. Physiol. Psychol.* **51**, 295-300.

Wilcott, R.C., 1959, On the role of the epidermis in the production of skin resistance and potential, *J. Comp. Physiol. Psychol.* **52**, 642-649.

Wilcott, R.C., 1964, The partial independence of skin potential and skin resistance from sweating, *Psychophysiol.* **1**, 55-66.

Wilcott, R.C., 1966, Adaptive value of arousal sweating and the epidermal mechanism related to skin potential and skin resistance, *Psychophysiol.* **2**, 249-262.

Wilcott, R.C., 1967, Arousal sweating and electrodermal phenomena, *Psychol. Bull.* **67**, 58-72.

Yamazaki, K., Tajimi, T., Okuda, K., and Niimi, Y., 1975, Skin potential activity in rats, cats and primates (including man): a phylogenetic point of view, *J. Comp. Physiol. Psychol.* **89**, 364-370.

Yates, J.R., 1971, Mechanism of water uptake by skin, Chap. 14 *in:* "*Biophysical properties of the skin,*" H.R. Elden, ed., Wiley, New York.

Yokota, T, Takahashi, T., Kondo, M. and Fujimori, B., 1959, Studies on the diphasic wave form of the galvanic skin reflex, *Electroenceph. Clin. Neurophysiol.* **11,** 687-696.

Zahn, T.P., Carpenter, W.T., and McGlashen, T.H., 1976, Autonomic variables related to short term outcome in acute schizohrenic patients, *Psychophysiol.* **13,** 166 (abstr).

# METHODOLOGICAL ISSUES IN ELECTRODERMAL MEASUREMENT

Wolfram Boucsein

Physiological Psychology
University of Wuppertal
5600 Wuppertal 1
Germany

Electrodermal recording has been extensively used for more than a century, but serious attempts to standardize recording and evaluation have not been performed since the early seventies. The Society for Psychophysiological Research has published a consensus of an expert committee (Fowles, Christie, Edelberg, Grings, Lykken, & Venables, 1981). Despite this, conflicting methodology still persists in electrodermal research and application. Perhaps this is in part the result of the committee's concentration on electrodes, jelly, placement, and preparation of sites. On the other hand, some central issues which had been raised by Edelberg (1967) and by Lykken and Venables (1971), have not attracted much attention of the commission. The aim of this paper is to bring up these issues again, in order to discuss recommendations given earlier with respect to more recent empirical work.

## 1. ENDOSOMATIC VERSUS EXOSOMATIC RECORDING

Electrodermal recording using an external current is by far the more prevalent. Endosomatic recording has been extensively used only in research performed by our British colleagues. However, either method has its advantages and disadvantages, as outlined by Edelberg (1967). Exosomatic recording has the following main advantages:

(1) Exosomatic measures are always unidirectional and therefore easier to analyze. This is not the case for biphasic or triphasic potential reactions which are inseparably composed of negative and positive waves.

(2) Exosomatic recording is less affected by electrode artifacts such as bias potentials or drift.

(3) When constant current is used in exosomatic recording, considerably less amplifier gain is required as compared to endosomatic recording (which is not the case in the majority of studies).

(4) Abrasion of a site to provide an inactive reference electrode is unnecessary. Abrasion may cause pain and the danger of infection.

(5) The sensitivity of conductance level to hydration effects is probably less than that of potential level.

(6) Much more is known about the psychological correlates of exosomatic measurements, since the majority of studies have used this method.

Endosomatic recording has the following main advantages:

(1) Endosomatic recording is regarded as being more "physiological", since the skin is not influenced by application of an external current. This is especially an advantage in long-term runs.

(2) Electrode polarization is prevented as no external current is applied.

(3) Skin potential can be measured by using ordinary bioamplifiers. Though DC amplification should be preferred to gain exact values for positive and negative SPR components, amplifiers with long time constants will be sufficient in most cases. Special circuitry such as an EDA coupler is not required.

(4) Endosomatic recordings are not affected by variations in contact area, as long as skin areas with different potentials are not connected together.

If there are not only disadvantages but also advantages to using skin potential recording, why has it essentially fallen out of use? The SPR committee, being not primarily concerned with basic EDA research but rather with the typical user who wants to apply EDA as a tool to study psychphysiological behavior, treated this entire issue in a 15-line paragraph. They recommended conductance over potential recording, unless there is a specific interest in comparing one's results with the literature on skin potential. Their central argument seemed to be the difficulty in interpreting biphasic skin potential reactions.

However, Forbes and Bolles (1936), as well as Edelberg (1967) suggested that the positive and negative potential waves may have independent behavioral significance. Furthermore, testing physiological models of the skin requires potential recording as well. From the present author's point of view, endosomatic recording should be revitalized, not for general application but in basic research, as an aid to gaining a better theoretical understanding of electrodermal phenomena.

## 2. CONSTANT CURRENT VERSUS CONSTANT VOLTAGE RECORDINGS

Another issue that had been regarded as already decided in 1981 is, whether to use constant current or constant voltage in exosomatic recording. However, the discussion on this topic suffered from not clearly separating recording methods and measurement units.

As a simple matter of fact, the use of constant current will result in resistance values, while recording with constant voltage gives conductance values. Reporting the latter ones is in accordance with the SPR commission's recommendations. However, as long as the corresponding tonic values are recorded as well, resistance scores can be easily transformed into conductance units.

The advantages and disadvantages of either recording method have been discussed by Edelberg (1967). Constant current recording has the following main advantages:

(1) They need less amplification than constant voltage techniques, by about a factor of 10. This is especially advantageous in field polygraphy where electrical noise is more probable.

(2) The density of the current flowing through the electrodes is limited which reduces the danger of electrode polarization.

(3) An unknown series resistance (e.g. a dry corneum) has a less serious effect in a constant current as compared to a constant voltage system.

Constant voltage recording has the following main advantages:

(1) High voltages over single sweat glands resulting from current concentration on a few ducts are avoided, thus reducing the danger of sweat gland damage.

(2) In a certain sense, the system is self-correcting with respect to the peripheral influence of the electrodermal level upon the reaction amplitude.

(3) The reference resistance, over which the amplifier measures the voltage, is low and constant, which leads to a good, constant relationship of the system and input impedances of the amplifier.

(4) Results are immediately expressed in conductance units and do not have to be transformed if one prefers reporting conductance values.

Recommendations in favor of constant voltage are somewhat contrary to common practice in electronic engineering. Here the constant current sources are generally preferred, since they are more easily stabilized and display much smaller tolerances than constant voltage sources.

In their proposal for standardization, Lykken and Venables (1971) took up some of the points raised by Edelberg. In particular, they concentrated on the first advantage of constant voltage recording as shown above. It was argued that by using a constant voltage system, both voltage and current densities can be kept within tolerable limits, thus avoiding non-linearities in the current-voltage relationship. None of the above arguments have been taken up by the SPR committee. Instead, in a footnote, their report simply referred to the recommendation given by Lykken and Venables for the use of conductance instead of resistance units, which seemed to imply the method of recording. Unfortunately, Lykken and Venables also did not directly distinguish between method and unit, since most of their arguments for skin conductance units referred to the advantages of the constant voltage method.

However, despite the committee's recommendations, constant current techniques did not disappear from the scene. As a matter of fact, they are preferred in field studies because of their greater robustness. Even in scientific laboratories, constant current technique persisted because of the expense involved in renewing equipment.

When psychophysiologists in Germany inaugurated annual meetings in the early seventies, one of the topics was to standardize EDA methodology. A review of literature revealed that direct empirical comparisons of constant current and constant voltage methodology were rare and not convincing. Therefore, it was decided to perform such a study in the present author's laboratory (Boucsein & Hoffmann, 1979). In this study, records were taken simultaneously from pairs of sites on each hand, one constant current, one constant voltage during a series of 30 white noise stimuli covering a wide range of intensities (i.e. 60 to 110 dB). No differences were found between EDA parameters obtained with the two methods, except for recovery times being shorter when measuring with constant voltage. This was interpreted by us in terms of the membrane component in Edelberg's model being differentially influenced by the two methods. However, Sagberg (1980) showed that this was a mathematical rather than a methodological effect. Since reliabilities and correlations with stimulus intensities rated by the subjects were also equivalent, no recommendation could be given for either recording technique.

To clarify the psychological significance of recording methods and units of measurement, the data from this study were reanalyzed by Boucsein, Baltissen, and Euler (1984). Electrodermal reactions (EDRs) obtained with constant current were transformed into conductance reactions and vice versa. Courses of conductance reactions and resistance reactions obtained with either recording method were in good accordance, as shown by the interactions and trend analyses (cf. Boucsein et al, 1984, Tab. 1). EDA parameters of orienting and habituation turned out to be widely independent from the recording method applied. The observed differences in courses of amplitudes over trials turned out to be clearly dependent on the unit (i.e. skin resistance versus conductance) and not on the recording method (i.e. constant current versus constant voltage). It was therefore concluded that the unit of measurement is more important for the phenomenon under investigation than the particular recording method.

From the present author's point of view, there is no need in general to switch from constant current to constant voltage recording. Both recording methods have certain advantages and disadvantages, and it is therefore recommended simply using the technique available. However, at least in EDA research, the constant voltage method is to be preferred in behalf of standardization. In field applications, the advantages of constant current may justify its continued use. If the expression of results in terms of conductance is preferred, a transformation can easily be performed provided data on electrodermal level have been retained (Boucsein, 1992).

## 3. UNIT OF MEASUREMENT

Despite the availability of more refined models, considerations on the adequate unit of measurement were based on rather simple electrical models, for example the Montagu- Coles model, using parallel resistors connected in series with another resistor, and disregarding the capacitance in parallel (cf. Boucsein et al., 1984, Fig. 4a). If a voltage is applied to resistors connected in parallel, the total resistance cannot be calculated simply by adding the individual resistors, as can be shown by applying Ohm's Law. However, if conductance values (i.e. their reciprocals) are considered instead, adding the values of the single conductors will result in the total conductance. As a consequence, the total change in conductance during an EDR will be proportional to the sum of conductance changes of the elements, which is not true for the total change in resistance.

The results from a study by Thomas and Korr (1957) have often been cited as evidence for the linear relationship between skin conductance and the number of active sweat glands. However, their experiment was performed with dry electrodes and heated skin, so that the upper layers of the corneum were dried out, and no contact existed between incompletely filled sweat gland ducts and the electrode. In contrast, normally the skin surface and thereby the electrode will also have electrical contact with incompletely filled sweat gland ducts through the moistened corneum. Here, the all-or-none principle of connected parallel resistors can no longer be applied. Instead, the part of resistance that can be traced back to sweat gland activity depends on the degree of duct filling. In this case the relationship between the decrease of the resistance and the height of the duct filling would be linear. Thus, resistance and not conductance would be the adequate unit of measurement.

Furthermore, the secretory processes of the sweat glands may be too slow to account for the relatively fast changing EDR signal. Edelberg (1971) presumed that EDRs having a slow recovery rate may be attributed to duct filling, while EDRs with shorter recovery times should be attributed to changes in permeability of the sweat gland membranes. Hence, the above discussion on resistances resulting from duct filling may not be of central importance for modelling the EDR. Instead, considering other structural properties of the skin such as parallel-connected membranes which behave similarly to capacitors, a simple addition of the single capacitances would be valid again, and thus conductance is an adequate measure for the EDR. Hence, contrary demands seem to exist for the measurement unit of choice for the slow and fast recovering EDA components.

It has to be concluded that the modelling of electrodermal phenomena as attained today does not provide a theoretical answer to the question of adequate units of measurement. If the argument that conductance is more "physiological" is disregarded, since it in fact relates to the method and not to the unit of measurement, the question of the adequate measurement unit should be treated empirically. Distributional characteristics and level dependencies may serve as criteria here, and the psychological meaning of the parameters obtained should also be taken into account.

As a general result from the 1984 reanalysis of the Boucsein and Hoffmann (1979) study, values obtained from either constant current or constant voltage recordings that were transformed into the other unit were equivalent to those obtained with the method providing the appropriate values directly. However, a critical difference has been found between results expressed in conductance and resistance units: With high stimulus intensities (i.e. the stimulation level exceeding 90 dB), sensitization was only found when results were expressed in conductance units. In contrast, skin resistance reactions showed habituation even with stimulus intensities of 100 dB and above where normally sensitization should have been expected.

Thus, from an empirical point of view, the use of conductance instead of resistance units appears to be justified. However, this has to be stated cautiously since the appropriate database is still small. Another topic which has also been used to gain arguments for conductance units will be treated in the next section.


## 4. LEVEL DEPENDENCY

Psychophysiological level dependencies are usually discussed with reference to the so-called Law of Initial Values (LIV), as formulated by Wilder (1931). However, EDA does not satisfy the conditions underlying the function of this law. This has been empirically shown by Hord, Johnson, and Lubin (1964), who considered EDA as belonging to the "slow equilibrium variables", where - because of the missing parasympathetic counter-regulation - Wilder's Law would not operate.

Nevertheless, a large number of studies investigating its validity have been performed by using EDA recording. Maybe this is due to a misunderstanding. Normally, resting values have to be obtained by specific sampling methods in order to get baseline recordings for testing the LIV. This does not seem to be a necesarry procedure when testing EDA for LIV effects, since electrodermal baseline values are easily determined as the level recorded immediately prior to each single reaction.

However, simply combining tonic with phasic EDA measures cannot fit Wilder's idea of underlying homeostatic processes, since different physiological mechanisms may be responsible for electrodermal reaction and level. Instead, investigations of a possible baseline dependency from the standpoint of the LIV have to make use of the same class of parameters for baseline and reaction scores. Therefore, the proposal made by Levey (1980) to clearly distinguish between at least two tonic levels - the baseline prior to any stimulation versus the EDL during interstimulus intervals - should be followed.

Results of studies on electrodermal level dependency are extraordinarily inconsistent. Firstly, it seems that different level dependencies may result from situational characteristics. Furthermore, differing level dependencies appear for within-subjects versus between-subjects correlations, as found by Martin and Rust (1976). In an habituation experiment with 21 loud tones, the between-subjects correlation of the mean response scores with the mean preceding level was .62, while the pooled within-subjects correlation yielded only .08.

The Boucsein et al. (1984) study yielded throughout positive average between-subjects correlations for the conductance reaction and the respective level, which however decreased with rising intensity of the applied stimuli (from .61 at 60 dB to .32 at 110 dB white noise). The corresponding within-subject correlations, calculated over all 30 stimuli including all levels of intensity, averaged only .06 and covered a large range. Note that in both studies the between-subjects correlations were in apparent contradiction to what would have been predicted by the LIV. This result is in line with Block and Bridger (1962) who found that the form of the interindividually determined regression of the skin resistance reaction amplitude on the preceding level was not predictable from the regression among the single subjects over the trials.

Frequently, corrections of the EDR using the EDL were conducted with the aim of eliminating tonic-phasic dependencies. However, when such corrections are used without a careful investigation of individual data structures, important properties of EDA parameters may get lost, and erroneous interpretations of the electrodermal system's properties might result. According to Grings (1974), two cases should be distinguished from each other when matching the EDR to the EDL:

(1) Both scores can be regarded as correlating indicators of the phenomenon under investigation, both of them explain specific variance components. In this case no baseline correction should be made; instead, the information from both scores should be combined. An example here are canonical correlations between "electrodermal behavior" on one hand, and personality dimensions on the other.

(2) The investigation focuses on EDRs, whereby the influence of differing EDLs is regarded as erroneous and thus should be eliminated. An example is the use of the EDR as an indicator for an orienting or for a conditioned reaction. In this case corrections taking regard of varying EDLs may be applied. However, it should be carefully ensured that the differing EDLs do not appear themselves as a consequence of the experimental manipulation (Edelberg, 1972).

It is both theoretically and practically important that the level dependency of the EDR is not invariant during a transformation of resistance into conductance data and vice versa. This has been pointed out by Johnson and Lubin (1972), and has also been found by Boucsein et al. (1984). Here, the correlations between resistance reaction and resistance level increased with stimulus intensity, while the correlations between conductance reaction and conductance level behaved inversely. Moreover the within-subject tonic-phasic correlations for resistance, as determined across the different stimulus intensities, were significantly higher than those for conductance. Rather high standard deviations of the correlations pointed to large interindividual variations in the level dependencies found.

This differential level dependency of resistance and conductance units has been used to find the "true" electrodermal behavior behind the different trends of responses over trials as shown in the raw data. Using the empirically determined level dependency for both measures, different correction factors were obtained for each. When the amplitudes were corrected by the respective factors, the difference in the trends disappeared (cf. Boucsein et al., 1984, Fig. 3).

One possible explanation of this differential level dependency with the use of either conductance or resistance can be given using a simplified Montagu-Coles model (Fig. 1).

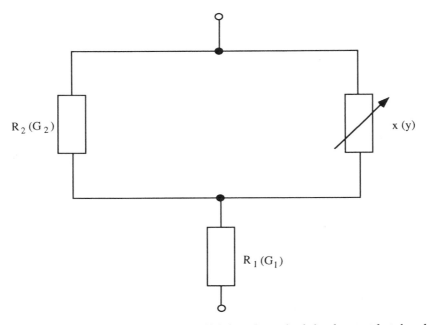

**Figure 1.** A simplified Montagu-Coles model in which the resistors simulating the sweat ducts have been replaced by a variable resistor x. The respective conductance values are given in parentheses.

In this model, proposed by Montagu and Coles (1966), $R_1$ and $R_2$ (the resistances of the dermis and of the corneum) are regarded as mostly responsible for the EDL, and a variable resistance x (which can be traced back to sweat gland activity) as being responsible for the response component. The total resistance R of the system can be calculated by using the rule for adding two resistors in parallel on $R_2$ and x, and adding $R_1$, according to the more simple rule for resistors in series as given by Equation (1a):

Equation (1a)

$$R = R_1 + \frac{R_2 x}{R_2 + x}$$

Similarly, the total conductance amounts to:

Equation (1b)

$$C = \frac{C_1(C_2 + y)}{C_1 + C_2 + y}$$

Now it is possible to compute the variation dR of the total resistance R due to small variations dx by differentiation:

Equation (2a)

$$dR = \frac{R_2^2}{(R_2 + x)^2} dx$$

On the other hand, differentiation of the total conductance C by y yields:

Equation (2b)

$$dC = \frac{C_1^2}{(C_1 + C_2 + y)^2} dy$$

As can be inferred from the equivalent Equations (2a) and (2b), the resistance reaction and the conductance reaction are not only dependent upon the "true" resistance and conductance variations dx and dy. They are multiplied by factors that include resistance levels in different branches of the model. This results in different nonlinear dependencies of resistance and conductance reactions on their respective levels. Such differential level dependencies may lead to even contrary results when conductance or resistance units are used.

How cautiously such level dependencies should be treated can be shown with the following two examples. Lykken and Venables (1971) used fictitious data to show that uncorrelated tonic and phasic conductance scores may display an almost perfect positive correlation after being transformed into resistance units. This is shown in the left-hand panel of Table 1.

In the right-hand panel of Table 1, uncorrelated resistance level and resistance reaction scores were produced in the same manner and were transformed into conductance units, which then displayed almost the same positive correlation due to the reciprocal

38

relationship between conductance and resistance. Thus, it cannot be inferred from that particular example that conductance units are to be preferred because of a non-existent tonic-phasic dependency.

Another example is taken from Bull and Gale (1974). Their aim was to avoid habituation effects while recording the EDR in response to only one single stimulus on 10 different days; this only worked with 7 out of their 15 subjects. Use of the constant current method (but without the necessary adaptation time for the electrode skin system) displayed a clear inverse relationship between the resistance reaction and the immediately preceding resistance level. This was interpreted by the authors as an undesirable effect of the Wilder's LIV when using resistance scores. This was not the case when using conductance, since the observed tonic-phasic connection got lost after a transformation into conductance scores, and even a trend to the contrary appeared.

Table 1. Fictitious examples of generating correlative dependencies between formerly independent EDRs and EDLs after transformation from SC into SR and vice versa. Example A: from Lykken and Venable (1971, page 669). Example B: Contrary example generated for SR.

| Trial | Example A: | | | | Example B: | | | |
|---|---|---|---|---|---|---|---|---|
| | SCL | SCR | SRL | SCR | SRL | SRR | SCL | SCR |
| | $\mu S$ | $\mu S$ | $k\Omega$ | $k\Omega$ | $k\Omega$ | $k\Omega$ | $\mu S$ | $\mu S$ |
| 1 | 10 | 1 | 100 | 9.09 | 100 | 10 | 10 | .11 |
| 2 | 11 | 1 | 91 | 7.57 | 90 | 10 | 11 | .13 |
| 3 | 12 | 1 | 83 | 6.41 | 80 | 10 | 13 | .18 |
| 4 | 13 | 1 | 77 | 5.49 | 70 | 10 | 14 | .24 |
| 5 | 14 | 1 | 71 | 4.76 | 60 | 10 | 17 | .33 |
| 6 | 15 | 1 | 67 | 4.17 | 50 | 10 | 20 | .50 |
| 7 | 16 | 1 | 62 | 3.68 | 40 | 10 | 25 | .83 |
| Correlation EDA/EDL | .000 | | .998 | | .000 | | .985 | |

However, this result can be easily inferred from the transformation used and cannot, especially in view of the narrow database provided, be used as a general argument for conductance as the more adequate unit of measurement.

In summary, an empirical explanation of the relationship between tonic and phasic EDA has not yet been reached, and the application of baseline correlations of the EDR using the EDL is problematical. Furthermore, the connection of questions concerning level dependency to those concerning an adequate unit of measurement for exosomatic EDA is not justified on the basis of the existing data.

# 5. CONCLUDING REMARKS

The methodological discussion on EDA recording and evaluation still remains unresolved (see Boucsein, 1992, for a summary). Neither the physiological models available until now, nor the overall low empirical evidence supporting the different points of view, will really help us to finally decide the issues raised. A proposal on how to circumvent most of the problems discussed here is given by Schaefer (this volume).

## REFERENCES

Block, J. D., & Bridger, W. H. (1962). The law of initial value in psychophysiology: A reformulation in terms of experimental and theoretical considerations. *Annals of the New York Academy of Sciences, 98,* 1229-1241.

Boucsein, W. (1992). *Electrodermal activity.* New York: Plenum Press.

Boucsein, W., Baltissen, R., & Euler, M. (1984). Dependence of skin conductance reactions and skin resistance reactions upon previous level. *Psychophysiology, 21,* 212-218.

Boucsein, W., & Hoffmann, G. (1979). A direct comparison of the skin conductance and skin resistance methods. *Psychophysiology, 16,* 66-70.

Boucsein, W., Schaefer, F., & Neijenhuisen, H. (1989). Continuous recording of impedance and phase angle during electrodermal reactions and the locus of impedance change. *Psychophysiology, 26,* 369-376.

Bull, R., & Gale, M. A. (1974). Does the law of initial value apply to the galvanic skin response? *Biological Psychology, 1,* 213-227.

Cole, K. S., & Cole, R. H. (1941). Dispersion and absorption in dielectrics. *Journal of Chemical Physics, 9,* 341-351.

Edelberg, R. (1967). Electrical properties of the skin. In C. C. Brown (Ed.), *Methods in psychophysiology* (pp. 1-53). Baltimore: Williams & Wilkins.

Edelberg, R. (1971). Electrical properties of skin. In H. R. Elden (Ed.), *A treatise of the skin, Vol. 1: Biophysical properties of the skin* (pp. 519-551). New York: Wiley.

Edelberg, R. (1972). Electrical activity of the skin. In N. S. Greenfield, & R. A. Sternbach (Eds.), *Handbook of Psychophysiology* (pp. 367-418). New York: Holt.

Forbes, T. W., & Bolles, M. M. (1936). Correlation of the response potentials of the skin with "exiting" and non-"exiting" stimuli. *The Journal of Psychology, 2,* 273-285.

Fowles, D. C., Christie, M. J., Edelberg, R., Grings, W. W., Lykken, D. T., & Venables, P. H. (1981). Publication recommendations for electrodermal measurements. *Psychophysiology, 18,* 232-239.

Grings, W. W. (1974). Recording of electrodermal phenomena. In R. F. Thompson, & M. M. Patterson (Eds.), *Methods in Physiological Psychology. Vol. 1: Bioelectric recording techniques. Part C: Receptor and effector processes* (pp. 273-296). New York: Academic Press.

Hord, D. J., Johnson, L. C., & Lubin, A. (1964). Differential effect of the law of initial value (LIV) on autonomic variables. *Psychophysiology, 1,* 79-87.

Johnson, L. C., & Lubin, A. (1972). On planning psychophysiological experiments: Design, measurement, and analysis. In N. S. Greenfield, & R. A. Sternbach (Eds.), *Handbook of Psychophysiology* (pp. 125-158). New York: Holt.

Levey, A. B. (1980). Measurement units in psychophysiology. In I. Martin, & P. H. Venables (Eds.), *Techniques in psychophysiology* (pp. 597-628). New York: Wiley.

Lykken, D. T., & Venables, P. H. (1971). Direct measurement of skin conductance: A proposal for standardization. *Psychophysiology, 8,* 656-672.

Lowry, R. (1977). Active circuits for direct linear measurement of skin resistance and conductance. *Psychophysiology, 14,* 329-331.

Martin, I., & Rust, J. (1976). Habituation and the structure of the electrodermal system. *Psychophysiology, 13*, 554-562.

Montagu, J. D., & Coles, E. M. (1966). Mechanism and measurement of the galvanic skin response: An addendum. *Psychological Bulletin, 60*, 74-76.

Sagberg, F. (1980). Dependence of EDR recovery times and other electrodermal measures on scale of measurement: A methodological clarification. *Psychophysiology, 17*, 506-509.

Thomas, P. E., & Korr, I. M. (1957). Relationship between sweat gland activity and electrical resistance of the skin. *Journal of Applied Physiology, 10*, 505-510.

Wilder, J. (1931). Das "Ausgangswert-Gesetz" - ein unbeachtetes biologisches Gesetz; seine Bedeutung für Forschung und Praxis. *Klinische Wochenschrift, 41*, 1889-1893.

# A NEW APPROACH TO CIRCUMVENTING THE CONDUCTANCE-RESISTANCE CHOICE: RECORDING OF PHASE ANGLE BETWEEN ALTERNATING-CURRENT AND -VOLTAGE

Florian Schaefer

Physiological Psychology
Unversity of Wuppertal
5600 Wuppertal 1
Germany

Electrodermal Responses (EDRs) recorded by the exosomatic technique are usually described as either Skin Conductance Responses (SCRs in µmho units) or as Skin Resistance Responses (SRRs in kΩ units). These two measures, though transformable into each other, are not equivalent when parameters are extracted from the raw data. Response magnitude is affected by changes of tonic level in a different manner when conductance is used instead of resistance. Therefore it is difficult to compare results obtained the two methods, and the question of the more appropriate measure is discussed in the literature. However, up to now there is no satisfactory solution of that problem. In order to make results obtained from different recording techniques comparable it is necessary to express results always in the same unit. Lykken and Venables (1971) have recommended that this should be conductance. Thus, when data are obtained in resistance units by using the constant current technique, all values have to be transformed into their reciprocal before any addition or subtraction is performed. Furthermore, the subtraction of the tonic level from superimposed phasic responses by offset compensation or an alternating-current amplifier with a time constant cannot be done before transformation. Therefore, if phasic responses are recorded separately with high resolution, information on level has to be recorded additionally to enable later transformation from resistance to conductance.

To circumvent these problems, we started to test a new measure for EDR description which is derived from our research on alternating current (AC) technique in electrodermal recording.

It is important to keep in mind that it is not an electrical unit like conductance or resistance we are interested in, but the physiological changes of sweat gland activity. However, since this activity is accompanied by changes of the electrical properties of the skin, it is accessible to non-invasive measurement, and an electrical unit by which these changes can be indicated sufficiently and which is easy to handle in registration and statistical computation is required. In order to decide which electrical measure is the appropriate one, we should first consider how many possibilities there are.

In the light of systems theory, an exhaustive analysis of the electrical properties of the skin can only be obtained by AC-measurement techniques using a sine-wave function as a probe signal (Fig. 1). Similar to DC-measurement, level of either voltage or current can be kept constant. When using an operational amplifier according to Lowry (1977), the constant voltage technique is applied when the skin is used as the impedance $Z_1$ between the probe voltage at the amplifier's inverting input while a fixed value resistor is used as the feedack impedance $Z_2$. The constant current technique is applied when the skin is used as $Z_2$ in the feedback loop between amplifier output and inverting input while $Z_1$ at the

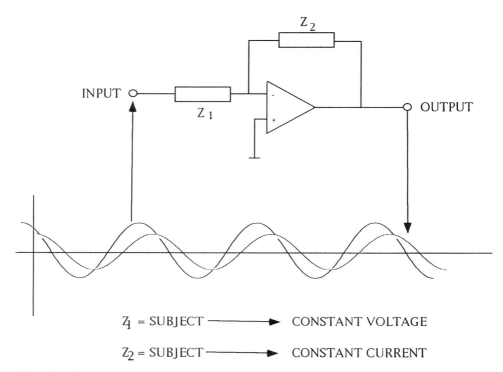

**Figure 1.** AC-recording technique by using an operational amplifier and a sine-wave probe signal. During an EDR the output signal changes its amplitude and phase angle.

amplifier's input is kept constant. The output signal of the amplifier is described by the amplitude, which is proportional to the absolute skin impedance for constant current technique, or to the admittance for the constant voltage technique. In addition there is a phase shift between input and output signal. This is due to the capacitance of the skin residing in the stratum corneum which induces a phase shift relative to the applied AC voltage.

This means that the output of AC-recording of EDA has to be described as a complex value: Admittance with the real component conductance and the imaginary component susceptance, or impedance with the components resistance and reactance (Fig.2).

To obtain an exhaustive description of an electrical transducer, the frequency of the probe sine wave has to be varied over a wide range. Because the transmission of capacitances depends on frequency, vector length and phase angle are changed, and the top of the vector moves on a circular arc (Cole & Cole, 1941). Using such a locus of frequency obtained with an AC-phase-voltmeter the electrical properties of any electrical network can be characterized.

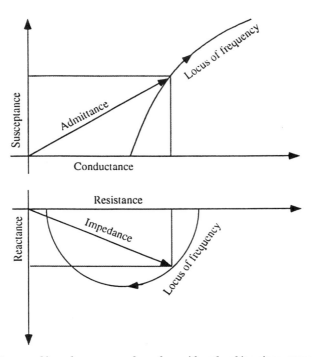

**Figure 2.** Admittance and impedance as complex values with real and imaginary component. When the probe signal frequency is changed the vector moves along the locus of frequency.

When using DC-measurement, recordings are restricted to the real components conductance and resistance. This is only a partial description of the phenomenon in question since the electrical properties caused by the polarisation capacitance are not included.

From a psychophysiological point of view, the important question is whether there is any gain of information by working with complex EDA parameters. This depends on the existence of capacitive fluctuation within the skin in addition to the well known ohmic changes during an EDR.

This question was investigated by Boucsein, Schaefer, & Neijenhuisen (1989). EDRs were recorded using a high resolution phase voltmeter with the constant current technique at a frequency of 100 Hz. Recordings were transformed data point by data point to conductance and susceptance in order to get separate response curves for the real and the imaginary component, respectively. The results showed that complex EDRs are mainly determined by a fluctuation of conductance. Additionally, small changes in susceptance could be found, when the scale of the imaginary component was enlarged sufficiently. These fluctuations are of great interest for understanding the physiological mechanisms of EDR and are further investigated. Since these changes are very small they can be neglected from the quantitative aspect. The well known EDR is indeed mainly due to ohmic changes. Thus, due to the arithmetical dependencies of the other measures, the typical EDR curves can be found in each of the remaining parameters (cf. Boucsein et al., 1989, Fig. 4). The cross correlation between the different measures exceeds .96, which means that each curve indicates the same phenomenon from a different point of view.

Apparently, there is no need for a two-dimensional description of EDR in terms of complex parameters since the information in the different curves is equivalent. EDRs can be sufficiently described by a single parameter. However, this does not necessarily have to be conductance or resistance.

This vector diagram in Figure 3 shows all possible EDR parameters together with their mathematical relations. Vector $Y_1$ is the admittance level and vector $Z_1$ is the corresponding impedance level at the beginning of an EDR. $Y_2$ and $Z_2$ are the values at the response maximum. The response amplitudes can be described by one of the following parameters:

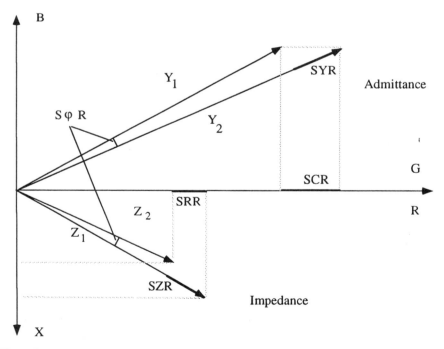

**Figure 3.** Different electrical parameters describing the same EDR and its geometrical relation in the complex plane.

**Skin Conductance Response (SCR)** can only be recorded directly using the DC constant voltage technique. **Skin Resistance Response (SRR)** can only be recorded directly using the DC constant current technique.

When using AC-techniques the following parameters can be obtained directly: **Skin Admittance Response (SYR)** with AC constant voltage technique and **Skin Impedance Response (SZR)** with the AC constant current technique. These AC-measures have been used in some studies in order to avoid electrode polarisation.

**Skin Phase Angle Response (SΦR)** is the only measure which can be directly recorded with AC constant voltage as well as with the constant current technique (Tab. 1). As shown in Figure 3 the phase angle is changed only in its sign when the recording technique is switched, since impedance is the complex conjugate vector of admittance. Thus, results from constant voltage and constant current recordings are directly comparable without any transformation because the same unit is already used at the measurement level. Thus, level information is not needed to compare response amplitude between different recording techniques. This means when using the Φ–measure as a standard unit in all studies on EDA the problem of unit transformation would not occur any more.

**Table 1.** Recording techniques with the use of DC or AC and their results.

| Parameter | Unit | technique |
|---|---|---|
| DC-recording | | |
| Skin Conductance Response SCR | µSiemens | constant voltage |
| Skin Resistance Response SRR | kOhm | constant current |
| | | |
| AC-recording | | |
| Skin Admittance Response SYR | µSiemens | constant voltage |
| Skin Impedance Response SZR | kOhm | constant current |
| | | |
| Skin Phase Angle Response SΦR | degree | constant voltage or constant current |

In addition, there are some other advantages of the SΦR measure: The phase angle can only vary between 0 and 90 degrees, whereas the scale of the other units is open in one direction. Because of this, Φ has properties similar to an absolute scale. This may be the reason for the findings in our laboratory that level drifts during an experimental session are relatively smaller for phase angle than for conductance.

Thus, turning away from the psychophysiological tradition of electrodermal recording, the application of phase angle Φ as the standard unit for EDA measurement, would have many advantages.

The technical realisation of an appropriate phase-detection device has been facilitated by modern integrated circuits. In our lab we use a SΦR-coupler built by a Phase-Locked-Loop (PLL) circuit as used for FM demodulation in broadcast systems. As compared to the use of SCR or SRR couplers, problems of gain adjustment and temperature drifts are reduced, since only the temporal delay between input and output signal is to be quantified. Amplification of the output signal has to be kept sufficient but need not be calibrated exactly.

In addition, the $\Phi$–measure could provide a new possibility for coping with interindividual level differences. As mentioned above the phase angle depends on the frequency of the probe signal. Unlike conductance or resistance, phase angle does not reflect the electrical properties of the skin as a fixed value but as a function of frequency. This means that although skin capacitance is interindividually different, a probe signal frequency exists where the phase angle is the same. This enables a trade-off between skin capacitance and measuring frequency. Thus, instead of measuring all the subjects with one arbitrarily fixed frequency we could adjust the frequency for each subject according to the individual skin type. Using this method, one could move on the locus of frequency to a point where tonic phase angle has a fixed value for all subjects. This equalisation of initial values is not reached by subtraction of an off-set but by a trade-off between skin capacitance and measuring frequency. To keep measuring frequency low and to avoid the adjustment of too different values between the subjects, small initial phase angles should be chosen, a procedure that moves the vector to that part of the locus near the abscissa.

All these aspects should be taken into consideration when discussing a standardisation of electrodermal recording and evaluation.

**REFERENCES** see Boucsein (this volume)

# ELECTRODERMAL ACTIVITY AND PSYCHOPATHOLOGY:

# THE DEVELOPMENT OF THE PALMAR SWEAT INDEX (PSI)

# AS AN APPLIED MEASURE FOR USE IN CLINICAL SETTINGS

Graham Turpin[1] and Keith Clements[2]

[1]University of Sheffield
Department of Psychology
POB 603 Western Bank
Sheffield S10 2UR, U.K.

[2]University of Plymouth
Department of Psychology, Drakes Circus
Plymouth PL4 8AA, U.K.

## INTRODUCTION

Measures of electrodermal activity (EDA) have frequently been adopted within studies of psychopathology. Indeed, the origins of EDA measurement are intimately associated with studies of hysteria at the Saltpêtrière and the pioneering work of Vigouroux and Féré (see Bloch, this volume). The purpose of this chapter is to review briefly their validity and utility, and to examine the development of the Palmar Sweat Index (PSI) as a possible substitute index reflecting EDA which might be better suited to more applied or clinical settings. Previous research involving the PSI is reviewed and various methodological issues identified. Results from a series of current studies designed to examine reliability, concurrent and construct validity, and clinical utility of the PSI are presented.

It should be stressed that this chapter has been written from the perspective of clinical assessment, and seeks to address the question as to the benefits and practicality of EDA measurement within clinical settings. It should, therefore, be read as a supplement to the many authoritative chapters within this book which address basic questions of clinical research. The criteria adopted in order to judge the utility of EDA measurement are derived from models of behavioural assessment (see Turpin, 1991 a, b) and concern basic psychometric properties of reliability and validity, together with issues of the conceptual validity and clinical utility of an applied clinical measure.

*Progress in Electrodermal Research*, Edited by
J.-C. Roy *et al*. Plenum Press, New York, 1993

## RATIONALES UNDERLYING CLINICAL APPLICATIONS OF THE PSI

Given the widespread adoption of electrodermal measures, the question must be posed as why develop an alternative measure such as the PSI. Essentially, there are three answers. First, it will be argued that both measures potentially share common variance and hence might be used interchangeably. Second, it will be claimed that although electrodermal measures have proved useful in advancing fundamental research within the area of psychopathology, their clinical utility has been limited. Thirdly, it will be suggested that the PSI might have certain practical advantages in relation to EDA measures, which might enhance their clinical utility within certain applied clinical settings.

### Relationship Between Electrodermal Measures and the PSI

Although EDA measures are the most widely adopted, it must be recognised that psychophysiologists have also employed a variety of non-electrocutaneous indices of sudorific activity. A common rationale, therefore, can be identified underlying the use of EDA and other sudorific measures which relates to their use as indirect indices of the interaction between the autonomic nervous system (sudorific activity) and certain emotional-cognitive psychological processes. Accordingly, it can be assumed that there is some common variance associated with these processes, across the various different measures of sudorific activity. Hence the arguments in support of the PSI as a measure are not concerned with any unique measurement properties of the PSI but relate to the possibility that the PSI and EDA share common variance as regards indexing certain psychophysiological processes. Moreover, there will be certain specific properties associated with each measure which will be unrelated. The degree to which one measure reflects the other is reflected by their concurrent validity, the extent to which they mutually reflect psychological processes will determine their construct validity. The concurrent and construct validity of both these measures has to be assessed empirically. These studies are reviewed in the second half of this chapter.

### Clinical Utility of Electrodermal Measures

Two essential criteria, conceptual validity and clinical utility, have to be satisfied when evaluating the contribution of a measure to behavioural assessment (cf. Turpin, 1991 a, b). The former addresses contributions to psychological understanding gained by a measure whereas the latter describes the ability of a measure to predict treatment outcome and clinical improvement.

The present volume contains many excellent examples of the use of EDA as a clinical research measure in areas of psychopathology as diverse as schizophrenia, anxiety, criminality and psychopathy, bipolar affective disorder and many more. To a large degree, this research has focused on fundamental questions concerning the aetiologies and mechanisms underlying specific disorders. Accordingly, the conceptual validity of EDA is high. The application of EDA measurement to the assessment and treatment of individuals within the clinical setting, however, has not been established. Indeed, Venables (this volume) asserts that the major value to be gained from EDA is its ability to reflect underlying psychological processes and central neurophysiological substrates as opposed to supplementing routine clinical or behavioural diagnostic markers. Undoubtedly, this position reflects the contribution which EDA has made to the literature, and will continue to do so in the future. Nevertheless, it may also be fruitful to explore the utility of EDA measurement within more clinically-based situations in order both to examine its potential as a clinical measure, and also to derive additional data from the clinical situation which might inform more fundamental research questions and theory development.

Unfortunately, the clinical utility of the PSI has seldom been demonstrated. Despite early attempts to adopt measures of emotional sweating as makers of therapeutic change (e.g. Mowrer, 1953), the use of EDA as a clinical assessment tool has been neglected (see Turpin, 1989). Although chapters in the current book have identified EDA correlates for schizophrenia, depression, anxiety and many other disorders, their direct use in clinical situations is most uncommon. Occasionally, electrodermal measures have been adopted within treatment outcome studies of anxiety in order to assess the effectiveness of relaxation based interventions (e.g. Paul, 1966), but these examples are most unusual.

There would appear to be a contradiction between the established conceptual validity of these measures and their limited clinical utility. We have previously discussed this paradox (Turpin and Clements, 1992) specifically in relation to schizophrenia, and have concluded that two issues need to be addressed. The first concerns the development of adequate theoretical models which address the role of EDA measurement within clinical research. We would argue that recent advances in psychophysiological theories provide rationales upon which such applications can be based. The second set of issues concern the practical implementation of clinical psychophysiological measures. Factors identified here which might present obstacles to the clinical application of EDA measurement concern the relative sophistication and technical requirements of EDA measurement, its laboratory basis, the general unavailability of psychophysiological expertise and training to clinicians, and the problem of generalizability from the laboratory to clinic situations (Turpin, 1989, 1990; Turpin and Clements, 1992).

**The Practical Utility of the PSI**

The question can be posed, therefore, whether the practical obstacles detailed above are sufficient to prevent the application of EDA measures to clinical assessment and to restrict its use solely to clinical research? Given the potential of EDA in gaining some greater understanding of the processes underlying the development of psychopathology, such a limited approach would appear unfortunate. For example, recent developments in vulnerability research into schizophrenia suggest a role for EDA in the prediction and early intervention for relapse within schizophrenia (e.g. Clements and Turpin 1992, Dawson 1990; Nuechterlein, 1987; Tarrier and Turpin, 1992; Turpin and Clements, 1992). The aim, therefore, becomes a methodological one as to how practical difficulties concerning access to EDA measurement may be reduced. Essentially, there are three approaches that need to be considered. Firstly, the development of ambulatory measures (e.g. Turpin, 1985) so as to allow unrestricted monitoring of EDA. Second, the use of less restricted laboratory situations such as pioneered by Tarrier and colleagues in assessing EDA within video-studios or home settings (see Tarrier and Turpin, 1992). A third approach is the development of measures of sweating which can be used efficiently outside the confines of the EDA laboratory. This would require simple but reliable indices of sweating which could be readily obtained in clinic and field settings without the need for expensive or specialized equipment, and by experimenters with limited training or experience of psychophysiological measurement. Such an approach will be the focus of the remainder of this chapter.

**THE PALMAR SWEAT INDEX**

As discussed previously, a wide range of techniques other than EDA have been employed to assess general sweating. These included total body weight change due to evaporative loss (Darrow and Freeman, 1934), collection of sweat in previously weighed pads (Weiner, 1945), assessment of vapour content of gas passed over the skin (Edelberg, 1964; Wilcott, 1962) and the assessment of sweat conductivity using the "sweat bottle" (Strahan et al., 1974). In addition, specific techniques have been devised to estimate the number of active sweat glands and have included direct observation (Jurgensen, 1924; Netsky, 1948), the use of chemical indicators such as ferrous chloride or starch/iodine (eg Wada and Takagaki, 1948; Silverman and Powell, 1944a; Mowrer, 1953), and the use of plastic impressions of the skin, preserving the holes corresponding to water droplets (Sutarman and Thomson, 1952; Harris, Polk and Willis, 1972).

Although colorimetric techniques based on chemical indicators have been previously adopted in psychopathology research (Mowrer, 1953; Silverman and Powell, 1944) their use has been widely superseded by the plastic impression method due to both ease of measurement and greater accuracy (Harris et al., 1972). Indeed, these methods, generally termed the Palmar Sweat Index (PSI) will be the sole focus of this review. Developed by Sutarman and Thomson (1952), this measure is quick and easy to use, highly portable and may be less intrusive than traditional measures of EDA. The PSI consists of a count of the number of active sweat glands in an area 4 mm x 4 mm centred on the central whorl of a fingertip. The print is obtained using a plastic solution, which produces an impression of the fingertip. Since the solution is immiscible in water, the droplets of sweat which occur at the opening of active sweat glands produce holes in the film. The film is removed from the finger using a clear adhesive tape, such as "Sellotape", and the print is examined at low magnification (x 40, (or less)) under a microscope. The technique also allows closed or "inactive" glands to be counted since the graphite which is included within the plastic solution to increase the visual contrast of the prints, tends to pool in the pores of the inactive glands giving rise to distinctive dark areas. Open or "active" glands appear as bright, round holes within the print.

Since its development some forty years ago, the PSI has been adopted by both physiologists and psychologists. This work will be briefly reviewed in an attempt to summarize the existing status of the measure with respect to its reliability and validity. A series of current studies by the present authors will be reviewed which were designed to examine further the potential application of the PSI to psychopathology research. Finally, the clinical utility of the PSI will be critically summarized and some recommendations made for future research and practice.

## Previous Research

The PSI has been adopted in a wide range of studies concerned with hormonal influences on sweating through to applications within social and educational psychology. The purpose of this review is to examine findings which might influence the decision to adopt the PSI as an applied measure for psychopathological research. Accordingly, we will focus on assessing the reliability and validity of the measure.

**Reliability and Stability.** Several studies report inter-rater reliability coefficients for the scoring of individual prints (Johnson and Dabbs, 1967; Kleinknecht and Bernstein, 1979; Koehler et al., 1990; Landers, Bauer and Feltz, 1978; Martens and Landers, 1970; Melamed and Siegel, 1975; Weisenberg et al., 1976). All agree that inter-rater reliability is very high.

Johnson and Dabbs report inter-rater reliabilities ranging from .87 to .98, however, all raters scored the same area and these correlations were between change scores. When one rater scored the same prints several days apart the correlation was .99. Similarly, Melamed and Siegel found that when two raters scored the same area the correlation between their ratings was .93. By scoring the same area variation across the fingertip is excluded from the reliability estimate. Thus, these two studies probably overestimate the reliability of the PSI.

Other studies make no mention of any attempt to ensure that raters were scoring the same area. This would be assumed to give a more realistic estimate of the reliability of the PSI. Weisenberg et al. report a range of reliabilities for single counts from .93 to .99. Koehler et al. (1990) report a mean inter-rater reliability of .87 and range from .70 to .96 using a 2 mm x 2 mm scoring area. The use of a smaller area would be expected to reduce the reliability of the technique. The other studies all report single correlations between .95 and .99. Thus, the literature implies that sweat prints can be reliably scored.

With regard to stability or test - retest reliability, few findings are available. In an unpublished article, M Johnston (pers. comm., 1984) reported retest reliabilities over a thirty minute period ranging from .55 to .83. These were calculated from previously published data from MacKinnon and Harrison (1961). Kleinknecht and Bernstein (1979) report reliabilities of .6 to .7 for colorimetric methods used across several days but report no stability data for the PSI. Although not a direct measure of stability, reliabilities calculated across different fingers or hands at the same time of measurement do exist. Again, these coefficients tend to average at around .7 (Voegele et al., 1988, Koehler et al., 1990).

**Subject Variables.** Several studies report decreasing PSI counts with increasing age (Bailes, 1983; Catania et al., 1980; MacKinnon, 1954), whereas the opposite relationship is said to exist within the first few years of life (Ferreira and Winter, 1965). It is likely that these effects can be accounted for by developmental changes in finger size, sweat gland density and reduced hydration of the corneum with ageing (Catania et al., 1980).

Sex differences have also been reported for the PSI, women generally have higher levels than men (e.g. Weisenberg et al., 1976; Kleinknecht and Bernstein, 1979). Moreover, MacKinnon and colleagues (e.g. MacKinnon and Harrison, 1961) report that the PSI is lower during the luteal phase of the menstrual cycle and during the first and third trimesters of pregnancy. Furthermore, intramuscular injections of progesterone lead to suppression of sweating.

Findings regarding ethnic or cultural differences in the PSI have been inconsistent. Negative results were obtained by Weisenberg et al. (1976) and Johnson and Landon (1965). However, other studies using both electrodermal and colorimetric techniques have found sweating to be lower in black or dark skinned subjects than in white subjects (Bailes, 1983; Juniper and Dykman, 1967; Malmo, 1965).

In summary the PSI generally appears to reflect subject differences consistent with those reported in the electrodermal literature. It is likely that these effects may reflect a combination of maturational and gender differences in sweat gland density, hormonal changes, social interaction and experimenter effects (Venables and Christie, 1973).

**Concurrent and Construct Validity.** In order to assess the suitability of the PSI as a more applicable index of EDA, it is essential to examine its concurrent and construct validity. Several studies have reported on the relationship between PSI and electrodermal measures obtained within the same situation. Early studies report only modest correlations (below .4) between PSI and EDA (Bailes, 1983; Johnson and Landon, 1965; Venables and Martin, 1967). More recent studies (Koehler et al., 1990; Voegele et al., 1988; Voegele and Steptoe, 1986) report larger correlations (between .4 and .6) between the PSI and a variety of EDA measures. A recent study by Koehler and Troester (1991) has reported within subject correlations between the PSI and SCL and NS-SCRs ranging between .37 - .62, and .67 - .74 respectively. Between subject correlations ranged between .13 - .35 for

NS-SCRs but were non-significant for SCL. In summary, research to date has produced inconsistent but modest relationships between the PSI and EDA.

The construct validity of the PSI has been assessed with regard to several diverse psychological constructs. Limitations of space prevent a comprehensive review of this area. Accordingly, only the major proposed relationships between PSI activity and psychological constructs will be mentioned. Generally, the PSI has been employed as a measure of physiological stress/strain to a variety of psychological or physical stressors. Early research by MacKinnon and her colleagues (Harrison et al., 1962; Harrison and MacKinnon, 1963; Harrison, 1964; MacKinnon, 1964) observed a depression in the PSI to a variety of stressors including surgical operations, straight leg raising, threat of injections etc. which they termed the "anhidrotic response to stress". It was also further suggested that this response was mediated by circulating catecholamines.

The proposal that sweating might decrease in response to stressful situations is contrary to many findings involving electrodermal measures, and therefore, deserves careful attention. Generally, the effects of surgery have been replicated (Johnson et al., 1970; Lindeman and Stetzer, 1973; Voegele and Steptoe, 1986). These later studies also indicate that the reduction in the PSI is associated with a drop in skin conductance level and changes in various self-report scales of mood and distress. However, more recent studies which have investigated non-surgical stressors such as physical exercise (Johnston and Johnston, pers. comm.1984), examinations (Johnson and Dabbs, 1967), aircraft flights (Dabbs et al., 1969), cognitive tasks (Dabbs et al., 1968; Koehler and Troester, 1991; Voegele et al., 1988), distressing films (Koehler et al., 1990) have all tended to demonstrate increases in PSI activity to psychological challenge. Moreover, studies which have examined the psychological anticipatory response to surgery (e.g. Melamed and Siegel, 1975) or dental treatment (e.g. Brandon and Kleinknecht, 1982, Early and Kleinknecht, 1978; Kleinknecht and Bernstein, 1979; Weisenberg et al., 1976) have generally found increased sweating prior to surgical/dental procedures which is related to self-reported fear or distress. These data might suggest, therefore, that either prior to or during stressful procedures the PSI is elevated, whereas the 'anhidrotic response' might be a specific post-operative response primarily related to the physical trauma of the surgery.

Other areas of study which have employed the PSI have included manipulations of threat of electric shock (e.g. Dabbs et al., 1969) and social facilitation and audience effects (e.g. Martens, 1969; Cohen, 1979; Carver and Scheirer, 1981).

In summary, the PSI has been employed within a variety of studies which have generally tended to manipulate conditions purporting to be related to various forms of "psychological stress or arousal". Although the findings are generally indicative of the PSI being positively associated with psychological activation, many studies are limited by the lack of independent measures, such as self-report or performance measures, other than the PSI with which the validity of the experimental manipulation can be assessed. Moreover, the experimental protocols differ with respect to the frequency and timing of the PSI during and following experimental tasks. Some investigators obtain the PSI during experimental manipulations, whereas other researchers have clearly treated the PSI as a slowly changing tonic measure and have relied only on *post-task* assessments of change relative to baseline. These methodological shortcomings limit the validity of many of the above findings.

**Current Studies**

The PSI has currently been reappraised as an applied measure within clinical psychology (Clements, 1992). A series of studies were designed to assess the reliability, concurrent and construct validity, together with the clinical utility of the measure. A brief and preliminary overview of these findings will be summarized below.

**Reliability.** This was examined in a number of ways. Firstly, a random selection of 120 prints were chosen from a laboratory study which examined the effects of a cognitive reasoning task under different conditions of monetary incentive and disincentive upon the PSI (Clements and Turpin, 1988). These were scored by two independent raters, half the prints with the scoring area marked and the remaining sample with an unspecified scoring area. The PSI was scored both as an absolute measure of the total number of active sweat glands ($PSI_A$) and as the ratio of active to inactive sweat glands ($PSI_R$). The following inter-rater reliabilities were obtained for identified sites: .90 ($PSI_A$) and .92 ($PSI_R$) and non-identified sites: .82 ($PSI_A$) and .87 ($PSI_R$). In addition, inter-rater correlations were calculated separately for PSIs obtained under resting (.80 ($PSI_A$) and .87 ($PSI_R$)) and mid-task (.90 ($PSI_A$) and .90 ($PSI_R$)) conditions. Although there was a tendency for inter-rater reliabilities derived from the ratio measure, from identified sites, and under activation conditions to be higher, there were no statistically significant differences between these correlations.

Secondly, PSI scores were compared between manual scoring methods and an automated scoring system relying on the "Quantimet" image analysis system. Although the "Quantimet" system allows more precise measures of sweat gland distribution across the print area to be obtained, together with shape and diameter indices of individual active glands, the overall resolution of the system compared to a second independent manual scorer was lower. Inter-rater reliabilities obtained with the "Quantimet" system when compared to manual scoring, ranged from .68 to .82 across a range of studies. Moreover, calculation of effect sizes (omega squared; Dodd and Schultz, 1973) from a public speaking study indicated the superiority of manual scoring ($PSI_A$: .095; $PSI_R$: .147) over an automated system ($PSI_A$: .051). However, it should be stressed that greater difficulties were encountered with the image analysis system in obtaining prints of sufficient quality to allow automated scoring. Hence, the proportion of missing data was considerably higher for the "Quantimet" system and hence poses a significant disadvantage compared with the less stringent requirements of manual scoring.

Thirdly, interhand correlations were obtained for the PSI on both a between (.66) and within subject (.56) basis indicating significant correlations between hands. However, the size of these correlations were lower than for other EDA variables (between $\underline{S}$s: .71 (NS-SCR) and .66 (SCL); within $\underline{S}$: .77 (NS-SCR) and .81 (SCL)).

Finally, stability of measurement was assessed in a number of ways. In a longitudinal study of examination-related changes in PSI within an undergraduate sample, the consistency of PSI measures across time were investigated using Kendall's coefficient of concordance. This provides an index of the extent to which subjects maintained their ranking of overall PSI activity across five measurement sessions spanning approximately ten weeks. For both resting PSIs (w = .51, p < .001) and post-cognitive task PSIs (w = .55, p < .001) highly significant measures of concordance were obtained. In a subsequent laboratory based study, correlations between initial test and post-test recovery periods were found to be .68 for the PSI, compared to .65 for NS-SCRs and .95 for SCL

**Concurrent Validity.** If the PSI is to be considered as an alternative measure to EDA for use in field settings, it should demonstrate reasonable correlations with EDA measures, and respond similarly to experimental manipulations. This was examined in two studies. The first involving the effects of monetary incentives on performance on a cognitive reasoning task (N = 72) and the second study (N = 40) concerning habituation to auditory stimuli, together with performance of a cognitive task (Digit Symbol Substitution). Both between $\underline{S}$s and within $\underline{S}$ correlations were calculated between the PSI and various EDA parameters across a variety of resting, recovery and task conditions. In the first study, a total of 21 between $\underline{S}$s correlations were calculated. The mean coefficients were as follows: $PSI_A/SCL = .509$; $PSI_A/NS\text{-}SCRs = .528$ and $SCL/NS\text{-}SCRs = .55$. A total of 72 individual within $\underline{S}$ correlations were obtained and the following mean coefficients observed: $PSI_A/SCL = .43$; $PSI_A/NS\text{-}SCRs = .54$ and $SCL/NS\text{-}SCRs = .45$. In the second study, mean coefficients for between $\underline{S}$s (N = 10) and within $\underline{S}$ (N = 39) were respectively for $PSI_A/SCL = .41$ and $.44$; $PSI_A/NS\text{-}SCRs = .61$ and $.51$ and $SCL/NS\text{-}SCRs = .54$ and $.43$. From these patterns of correlations, it emerges that coefficients are consistently higher between PSI/NS-SCRs than PSI/SCL. Moreover, the range of values between PSI and EDA variables, is comparable to the range of coefficients observed between the two EDA measures of SCL and NS-SCRs. Within the second study, the relationship between PSI and EDA measures of habituation was also investigated. This revealed the following significant correlations (p < .001) between resting values and the total number of SCRs observed within an habituation sequence: $PSI_A = .58$; $SCL = .48$ and $NS\text{-}SCRs = .49$. Again, the values of the coefficients between the PSI and other EDA measures were comparable. Low resting values of the PSI, SCL and NS-SCRs were associated with non-response or fast habituation, high values with non-habituators.

Finally, the time course of the PSI response was ascertained by obtaining a continuous count of sweat glands using a microscopic video-recording technique. This revealed that the change in activity of directly observed sweat glands was comparable to phasic changes in the SCR. Repeated measures MANOVA for video counts of active sweat glands and SCR amplitudes from 2 sec before to 7 sec after the auditory stimulus revealed significant effects (Video $\underline{F}$ (1,17) = 9.4, p = .007; SCR $\underline{F}$ (1,19) = 6.46, p = .02) due to time of measurement. The appearance of a change in conductance preceded the observation of sweat at the top of the duct by about half a second. These results suggest that the PSI should perhaps be considered more as a phasic than a tonic measure.

## SUMMARY

Both previous research and current studies (Clements, 1992) would suggest that the PSI behaves in a similar fashion to traditional measures of EDA. Inter-correlations between those measures are essentially similar and assuming that they are related to a common construct relating to psychological activation associated with palmar sweating, there would appear to be no grounds for distinguishing between the PSI and measures of SCL or NS-SCRs. Moreover, their sensitivity to experimental manipulations would also appear comparable. Nevertheless, the PSI cannot be considered a truly substitute measure for EDA since it represents a discontinous and more obtrusive measure.

As regards clinical applications, its psychometric properties would suggest that it might be employed within clinical situations where EDA measure have been previously adopted within clinical research laboratories. Indeed, several collaborative studies (Clements, 1992: Clements, Romer, Turpin and Hahlweg, in press) have already employed this measure and have revealed results generally consistent with those previously obtained with electrodermal methods. However, to date, no clinical studies assessing EDA and PSI in parallel have been performed. Until these data are obtained, caution should be exercised as regards the clinical application of the PSI. Nevertheless, its ease of measurement and application would argue for further research into its potential application as an applied clinical measure for use in field settings.

## REFERENCES

Bailes, K., 1983, "Factors underlying ethnic, sex and developmental differences in skin conductance and heart rate responsivity to auditory stimuli," unpublished PhD. thesis, University of York.

Brandon, R.K., and Kleinknecht, R.A., 1982, Fear assessment in a dental analogue setting, *J. Beh. Assess.* 4:317-325.

Carver, C.S., and Scheier, M.F., 1981, The self-attention-induced feedback loop and social facilitation, *J. Exp. Soc. Psychol.* 17:545-568.

Catania, J.J., Thompson, L.W., Michaelewski, H.A., and Bowman, T.E., 1980, Comparisions of sweat gland counts, electrodermal activity and habituation behaviour in young and old groups of subjects, *Psychophysiology* 17:146-152.

Clements, K., 1991, The validity of the PSI as an alternative to Electrodermal activity (EDA), *J. Psychophysiol.* 5:201-202.

Clements, K., 1992, The Development of the Palmar Sweat Index as an Applied Measure in Clinical Pyshology, unpublished PhD thesis, Polytechnic South West.Clements, K., and Turpin, G., 1988, The validity of the Palmar Sweat Index: Effects of feedback-induced anxiety and task difficulty of measures of palmar sweating, *J. Psychophysiol* 2:76.

Clements, K., and Turpin, G., 1992, Vulnerability models and schizophrenia: The assessment and prediction of relapse, *in*: "Innovations in the Psychological Management of Schizophrenia," M. Birchwood and N. Tarrier, eds., Wiley, Chichester.

Clements, K., Romer, M., Turpin, G., and Hahlweg, K., in press, Symptomatic correlates of palmar sweat gland activity in schizophrenic individuals, *Psychophysiology* 27.

Cohen, J.L., 1979, Social Facilitation: Increased evaluation apprehension through permancency of record, *Motivation and Emotion* 3:19-33.

Dabbs, J.M., Johnson, J.E., and Leventhal, H., 1968, Palmar sweating: A quick and simple measure, *J. Exp. Psychol.* 28:347-350.

Dabbs, J.M., Leventhal, H., and Hornbeck, F.W., 1969, Palmar sweating and control of danger, *Psychosom. Sci.* 16:329-330.

Darrow, C.W., and Freeman, G L., 1934, Palmar skin-resistance changes contrasted with non-palmar changes, and rate of insensible weight loss, *J. Exp. Psychol.* 17:739-748.

Dawson, M.E., 1990, Psychophysiology at the interface of clinical science, cognitive science and neuroscience, *Psychophysiology* 27:243-255.

Dodd, D.F., and Schultz, R.H., Jr., 1973, Computational procedures for estimating magnitude of effect for some analysis of variance designs, *Psychol. Bull.* 79:391-395.

Early, C.E., and Kleinknecht, R.A., 1978, The palmar sweat index as a function of repression-sensitization and fear of dentistry, *J. Consul. Clin. Psychol.* 46:184-185.Edelberg, R., 1964, Independence of galvanic skin response amplitude and sweat production, *J. Invest. Dermatol.*, 42:443-448.

Ferreira, A.J., and Winter, W.D., 1965, Age and sex differences in the palmar sweat print, *Psychosom. Med.* 27:207-211.Harris, D.R., Polk, B.F., and Willis, I., 1972, Evaluating sweat gland activity with imprint techniques, *J. Invest. Dermatol.* 58:78-84.Harrison, J., 1964, The behaviour of the palmar sweat glands in stress, *J. Psychosom. Res.* 8:187-191.

Harrison, J., and MacKinnon, P.C.B., 1963, Central effect of epinephrine and norepinephrine on the palmar sweat index, *Amer. J. Physiol.* 204:785-788.

Harrison, J., MacKinnon, P.C.B., and Monk-Jones, M.E., 1962, Behaviour of the palmar sweat glands before and after operation, *Clin. Sci.* 23:371-377.

Johnson, J.E., and Dabbs, J.M., Jr., 1967, Enumeration of active sweat glands: A simple physiological indicator of psychological changes, *Nurs. Res.* 16:273-276.

Johnson, J.E., and Landon, M.M., 1965, Eccrine sweat gland activity and racial differences in resting skin conductance, *Psychophysiology* 1:322-329.

Johnson, J.E., Dabbs, J.M, Jr., and Leventhal, H., 1970, Psychosocial factors in the welfare of surgical patients, *Nurs. Res.* 19:18-29.

Juniper, K., and Dykman, R.A., 1967, Skin resistance, sweat gland counts, salivary flow and gastric secretion: Age, race and sex differences and intercorrelations, *Psychophysiology* 4:216-222.

Jurgensen, E., 1924, Mikrobeobachtungen der schwisssekretion der haut des menschen unter Kontrastfarbung, *Duetsches Archiv fur Klinishe Medizin*, 144:193.

Kleinknecht, R.A., and Bernstein, D.A., 1979, Short-term treatment of dental avoidance, *J. Beh. Ther. Exp. Psychiat.* 10:311-315.

Koehler, T., and Troester, U., 1991, Changes in the palmar sweat index during mental arithmetic, *Biol. Psychol.* 31:143-154.

Koehler, T., Weber, D., and Voegele, C., 1990, The behaviour of the PSI (Palmar Sweat Index) during two stressful laboratory situations, *Psychophysiology* 4:281-287.

Landers, D.M., Bauer, R.S., and Feltz, D.L., 1978, Social facilitation during the initial stage of motor leaning: A rexamination of Martnes' audience study, *J. Mot. Beh.* 10:325-337.

Lindeman, C.A., and Stetzer, S.L., 1973, Effect of preoperative visits by operating room nurses, *Nurs. Res.* 22:4-16.

MacKinnon, P.C.B., 1954, Variations with age in the number of active palmar digital sweat glands, *J. Neurosur. Psychiat.* 17:124-126.

MacKinnon, P.C.B., 1964, Hormonal control of the reaction of the Palmar Sweat Index to emotional stress, *J. Psyschosom. Res.* 8:193-195.

MacKinnon, P.C.B., and Harrison, J., 1961, The influence of hormones associated with pituitary-adrenal and sexual-cycle activity on palmar sweating, *J. Endocrino.* 23:217-225.

Malmo, R.B., 1965, Finger-sweat prints in the differentiation of low and high incentive, *Psychophysiology* 1:231-240.

Martens, R., 1969, Palmar sweating and the presence of an audience, *J. Exp. & Soc. Psychol.* 5:371-374.

Martens, R., and Landers, D.M., 1970, Motor performance under stress: A test of the inverted-U hypothesis, *J. Pers. Soc. Psychol.* 16:29-37.

Melamed, B.G., and Siegel, L., 1975, Reduction of anxiety in children facing hospitalization and surgery by use of filmed modelling, *J. Con. Clin. Psychol.* 43:511-521.

Mowrer, O.H., 1953, "Psychotherapy: Theory and Research", Ronald, New York.

Netsky, M.G., 1948, Studies on sweat secretion in man, *Arch. Neurol. Psychiat.* 60:279-287.

Nuechterlein, K.H., 1987, Vulnerability models for schizophrenia: State of the art *in* "Search for the Causes of Schizophrenia", H. Hafner, W.F. Gattaz, and W. Janzarik, eds., Springer, Berlin, Heidleberg.

Paul, G.L., 1966, "Insight Versus Desnsitization in Psychotherapy", Stanford University Press, Stanford.

Silverman, J.J., and Powell, V.E., 1944a, Studies on palmar sweating: I A Technique for the study of palmar sweating, *Amer. J. Med. Sci.* 208:297-299.

Silverman, J.J., and Powell, V.E., 1944b, Studies on palmar sweating: II The significance of palmar sweating, *Amer. J. Med. Sci.* 208:299-305.

Strahan, R.F., Todd, J.B., and Inglis, G.B., 1974, A palmar sweat measure particularly suited for naturalistic research, *Psychophysiology* 11:715-720.

Sutarman, and Thomson, M.L., 1952, A new technique for enumerating active sweat glands in man, *J. Physiol.* 117:51-52.

Tarrier, N., and Turpin, G., 1992, Psychosocial factors, arousal and schizophrenic relapse: A review of the psychophysiological data, *Brit. J. Psychiat.* 161:3-11.

Turpin, G., 1985, Ambulatory psychophysiological monitoring: Techniques and applications, *in*: "Clinical and Experimental Neuropsychophysiology," D. Papakostopolous, S. Butler and I. Martin, eds., Croom Helm, London.

Turpin, G., 1989, An overview of clinical psychophysiological techniques: Tools or theories?, *in*: "Handbook of Clinical Psychphysiology," G. Turpin, ed., Wiley, Chichester.

Turpin, G., 1990, Ambulatory clinical psychopathology: an inroduction to techniques and methodological issues, *J. Psychophysiol.* 4:299-304.

Turpin, G., 1991a, Psychophysiology and behavioural assessment: Is there scope for theoretical frameworks, *in*: "Handbook of Behaviour Therapy and Psychological Science: An Integrative Approach," P. Martin, ed., Pergammon Press, New York.

Turpin, G., 1991b, The psychophysiological assessment of anxiety disorders: Three-Systems measurement and beyond, *Psychological Assessment: A Journal of Consulting and Clinical Psychology* 3:366-375.

Turpin, G., and Clements, K., 1992, Psychophysiological contributions to clinical assessment and treatment, *in*: "Schizophrenia: An Overview and Practical Handbook," D. Kavanagh, ed., Chapman and Hall, London.

Turpin, G., Tarrier, N., and Sturgeon, D., 1988, Social psychophysiology and the study of biopsychosocial models of schizophrenia, *in*: "Social Psychophysiology: Theory and Clinical Applications," H.L. Wagner, ed., John Wiley, Chichester.

Venables, P,. and Martin, I., 1967, The relationship of palmar sweat gland activity to level of skin potential and conductance, *Psychophysiology*, 3:302-311.

Venables, P.H., and Christie, M.J., 1973, Mechanisms, instrumentation, recording techniques and quantification of responses, *in*: "Electodermal Activity in Psychological Research," W.F. Prokasy, and D.C. Raskin, eds., Academic Press, New York.

Voegele, C., and Steptoe, A., 1986, Physiological and subjective stress responses in surgical patients, *J. Psychosom. Res.* 30:205-215.

Voegele, C., Burchett, C., Koehler, T., 1988, "Palmar sweat gland activity (PSI) under laboratory stress conditions. An examination of some methodological problems," paper presented at the 16th Annual Meeting of the Psychophysiology Society, (U.K.), London.

Wada, M., and Takagaki, T., 1948, New method for detecting sweat secretion, *Tohuku J. Exp. Med.* 49:284.

Weiner, J.S., 1945, The regional distribution of sweating, *J. Physiol.* 104:32-40.Weisenberg, M., Kreindler, M.L., Schachat, R., and Werboff, J., 1976, Interpreting palmar sweat prints: A not-so-simple measure, *J. Psychosom. Res.* 20:1-6.

Wilcott, R.C., 1962, Palmar sweating versus palmar skin resistance and skin potential, *J. Comparat. Physiol. Psychol.* 55:327-331.

# ELECTRODERMAL ACTIVITY AS A TOOL FOR DIFFERENTIATING PSYCHOLOGICAL PROCESSES IN HUMAN EXPERIMENTAL PREPARATIONS: FOCUS ON THE PSYCHE OF PSYCHOPHYSIOLOGY

John J. Furedy

Department of Psychology
University of Toronto
Toronto, Ontario, M5S 1A1
Canada

The last quarter century has brought tremendous technical advances in psychophysiology. In the area of physiological recording, developments in electronics have enabled us to pick up many more physiological functions. So, to take cardiac performance as an example, we have moved from measuring heart rate as the sole index to being able to assess such additional aspects as cardiac output, pulse transit time, and pulse ejection period. In addition, we have also been able to assess dependent-variable changes in more refined ways. Computerization developments have allowed us to measure cardiac-cycle effects in the electrocardiogram instead of being to look only at the inter-beat interval as the only chronotropic measure.

These technical aspects of psychophysiology are important, but sometimes concentration on technical matters can result in a certain loss of focus on the central issues of an area of enquiry. These central issues, in my view, have to do with psychological processes. And to the extent that attention to technical matters has produced a neglect of these processes, i.e., the psyche of psychophysiology, there has to be, as suggested in my title, a refocussing of some of our attention.

The context of my argument is a definition of psychophysiology that views the field as the use of physiological measures to study psychological processes. Reasons for this view have been detailed elsewhere (Furedy, 1983, 1984); criticisms of my position are available (e.g., Stern, 1984), and Obrist (1976, 1981) has advanced a more physiologically-oriented view of psychophysiology. Applying my view of "focussing on the psyche" of psychophysiology to EDA implies that EDA is essentially a tool for differentiating among psychological processes. Moreover, the utility of the tool is lies in the fact that changes in EDA are not available to consciousness. Hence EDA-based measures will be less confounded than those based either on questionnaires (i.e., introspection) or on behavioral observation.[1] These sources of potential confounding stem from the demand characteristics of the human experimental preparation, especially when the subjects involved are students of psychology themselves.

# THE ROLE OF PHYSIOLOGICAL ISSUES IN EMPLOYING EDA AS A PSYCHOPHYSIOLOGICAL TOOL

In arguing for a psychological focus, I do not mean to imply that physiological considerations are irrelevant. In particular, knowledge of elementary physiological distinctions like that between the two branches of the autonomic nervous system (ANS) is useful for psychophysiological differentiation, even though, for sophisticated physiological purposes, such distinctions may be over simplified. The physiological sympathetic (SNS) vs. parasympathetic (PNS) distinction may be relevant, for example, in drawing the psychological distinction between stimuli that result in increases in stress, and those that result (merely) in increases in attention. This psychological distinction, of course, is of relevance to such physiologically-related phenomena as susceptibility to sudden cardiac death, for which an index that discriminates stress from attention is useful. Because (at least peripherally) EDA is known to reflect predominantly SNS activity, an increase in electrodermal level (ECL) might be reasonably used as an index of stress. In contrast, heart-rate (HR) changes, which can reflect only PNS activity (especially when these changes are relatively small, i.e., less than about 10% of base level), would reflect only an increase in attention (in the case of HR deceleration) or preparation for a stressful task without the involvement of stress itself (in the case of HR acceleration coupled with no change in ECL).

Even the relatively simplistic SNS/PNS distinction, moreover, may need to be supplemented by other similarly simple physiological distinctions in the elucidation of psychological mechanisms involved in the results of psychophysiological experiments. Consider, for example, an electrodermal differentiation-of-deception paradigm (DDP) in which, as reported recently (Furedy, Davis, & Gurevich, 1988; Furedy, Posner, & Vincent, 1991; Vincent & Furedy, 1992), deceptively answered questions produce larger skin-conductance responses (SCRs) than (equivalent) honestly answered questions. In the earliest version of the paradigm, Heslegrave (1982), it was reported also that, in addition to the enhancement of SCRs, there was also an enhancement of HR decelerations. These HR results appear to contradict the SCR results, because this phasic form of EDA is also generally considered to be an index of SNS activity.

However, although the peripheral mechanisms (e.g., the final pathway to the eccrine glands) of EDA are sympathetic (for details, see Heslegrave, 1981, pp. 210-211), there is evidence of some central parasympathetic control, based on animal preparations examining such loci as the anterior hypothalamus (Bloch & Bonvallet, 1960). This means that at least some aspects of EDA may be viewed as centrally or functionally parasympathetic.[2] Moreover, the SCRs in question are not only small magnitude, but (probably more importantly) they are short-duration, phasic changes compared to the longer-duration, tonic changes in ECL. Accordingly, the enhanced SCRs to deceptive items in the DDP may reflect PNS withdrawal, which may, in turn, indicate a "hiding" response involved in deception rather than any SNS excitation, i.e., the "fight-or-flight" response.

Still, there are physiological issues which, though of considerable interest in physiological terms, do not have to be resolved before psychophysiological advances can be made. Such an essentially physiological issue is the question of the exact nature of the peripheral mechanisms involved in EDA. In the view of certain physiologically- oriented psychophysiologists (e.g., Obrist, 1976, 1981), a physiological index cannot be used to answer psychological questions until the physiological basis of the index is completely understood. We (e.g., Furedy, 1987; Furedy, Heslegrave, & Scher, 1992; but see Contrada, 1992) have argued against this position, when the specific issue concerned the assessment of the psychophysiological utility of the cardiac-performance index, T-wave amplitude

(TWA). It is no accident that, in our argument concerning TWA we chose, as the most powerful counter-example to the physiological-mechanisms focus, the "GSR". This phasic, small-magnitude change in EDA, which is elicited by almost any level of stimulation, has been informative to experimental psychologists for well over half a century, and continues to be a useful, if at times puzzling, dependent variable. Yet the physiological mechanisms that are involved are far from fully understood. And that full physiological understanding is clearly not necessary (although it may provide additional illumination) for the utility of the GSR as a psychophysiological measure.

Moreover, it is also important to recognize that, when certain physiological findings are established, they should not be used to impose methodological rules that are inappropriate for purposes of the experiment. In this connection, it has become obvious that considerable physiological consensus has emerged from the work of Edelberg and his associates (e.g., Edelberg, 1967) that, whatever may be the ultimate mechanisms that underlie EDA, these are likely to be described in conductance rather than resistance terms. However, a more recent committee-report paper in Psychophysiology (Fowles, Christie, Edelberg, Grings, Lykken, & Venables, 1981) has extended this consensus to formulating a general methodological measurement rule, according to which non-potential EDA changes should be expressed only in conductance and not in resistance units. The vast majority of the (non-potential) EDA literature concerns the phasic changes that occur from about 1-5 seconds following stimulus onset, i.e., the GSR, rather than longer-term, relatively-tonic changes in levels. Accordingly, the major impact of the Fowles et al. (1981) rule has been that these GSR papers have expressed their measures in terms of units of SCR rather than the lower-tech (because it requires less amplification than SCR) SRR (skin-resistance response).

When applied to between-subject comparisons, this rule has a sound empirical basis that rests on non-physiological evidence gathered in the forties (e.g., Haggard, 1945). That evidence indicated that whereas the correlation between SRR and skin-resistance level (SRL) in between-subject comparisons was considerable, the same correlation between SCR (obtained in those days mostly by mathematical transformation rather than by electronic instrumentation) and skin-conductance level (SCL) was close to zero. Accordingly, if one's interest was in comparing phasic GSR magnitude between experimental conditions, the conductance transformation was useful for controlling individual-difference-based, between-subject factors as represented by differences in tonic levels of resistance (and, of course, its reciprocal, conductance). However, as noted by experimenters of the early fifties (e.g., Bitterman, Reed, & Krauskopf, 1952), in within-subject comparisons of GSR magnitude, where there were no differences in tonic levels, the conductance transformation was unnecessary[3]. Yet current experience (including my own) with editors and referees of Psychophysiology indicates that, even when all relevant comparisons are within subjects, there is great reluctance to accept resistance-based specification of GSR data. In this context the "rule" against SRR units of measurement seems to function more like a ritual than as an evidence-based assertion, and contravenes the principle that dependent-variable specification should be governed only by the requirements of the comparisons made in the particular psychophysiological experiment that has been performed.


## THREE CURRENT ZEITGEIST-INDUCED UNSOUND OVER-GENERALIZATIONS ABOUT THE SCR

In using EDA to differentiate between and study psychological processes I favor a data- or evidence sensitive approach. This is not to argue for some form of dustbowl empiricism, according to which theorising is eschewed. The investigation of psychological phenomena is a complex enterprise, and in this quest it is essential to have a set of guiding hypotheses. However, these hypotheses need to be treated as empirical generalizations to be tested, rather than universal principles that are accepted without question. When they are treated as universal principles, the investigators' sensitivity to evidence becomes less than even that of the intelligent proverbial man in the street. The three current over-generalizations that I shall briefly treat in this question are all instances of the Zeitgeist gone wild, where, instead of investigating the conditions under which a certain hypothesis holds true, we have come to simply accept the hypothesis as universally true without any regard for unequivocal evidence to the contrary.

## The Signal-elicited SCR as the Universal Protector

When an organism receives a signal (e.g., a 5-second tone) about a noxious event (e.g., shock) which, however, is unmodifiable, it is attractive to suppose that the SCR elicited by the tone which precedes the shock (i.e., the anticipatory SCR) serves the "adaptive" function of "allowing the organism to prevent signalled injury to the skin (Dengerink & Taylor, 1971, p. 358). This notion is attractive because it is consistent with general adaptiveness principles in biology, and there is no doubt that there are conditions where increased EDA does serve as an adaptive mechanism. For example, increased EDA appears to aid climbing in monkeys, as noted by Edelberg in another chapter in this book.

However, the question of whether the signal-elicited SCR does, in fact, reduce, the perceived impact of the following noxious event, is an empirically testable issue. A consequence of this view, formulated most explicitly by Perkins (1968) for the signal-elicited SCR, is that there should be a negative correlation, within subjects and over trials, between the magnitude of the anticipatory SCR and the rated impact of the event that follows each SCR. This consequence was first tested and disconfirmed by Furedy (1970), and subsequent studies (Furedy, 1973; Furedy & Doob, 1971; Furedy, Katic, Klajner, & Poulos, 1973) all failed to find any support for this protective-adaptive role of the signal-elicited SCR. Indeed, if the signal-elicited SCR is adaptive in this context, it also follows that signalled shocks should be rated as less intense than unsignalled shocks, and signalled shock should be preferred over unsignalled shocks. As detailed in Furedy (1975), although it is clear that the current Zeitgeist in favor of these notions has led to biassed accounts of the literature in places as prominent as the Annual Review of Psychology" (see Furedy, 1975, pp. 79-80), the evidence generally fails to support these ratings and preference consequences of the adaptiveness position. The evidence, then, for the signal-elicited SCR as a universal protector is quite underwhelming, no matter how attractive this notion may be in general adaptive terms.

## The Conditional SCR as an Epiphenomenon of Cognitive Processing

During the dominancy of S-R theorising, knowledge or awareness of the contingency between the conditional stimulus (CS) and unconditional stimulus (US) in Pavlovian conditioning was considered to be irrelevant or a mere "epiphenomenon" (Furedy, 1973) of the (S-R) conditioning process. As we have elsewhere indicated in more detail (Furedy, 1973; see also Furedy & Riley, 1987), one result of the cognitive paradigm shift of the late sixties was that, in human Pavlovian SCR conditioning, it was the conditional SCR itself that became the epiphenomenon, with S-S learning or awareness of the CS-US contingency being given the super-causal role. The most extreme version of this sort of cognitivism is a chapter by Brewer (1974), but the same spirit underlies, I suggest, the claim that Pavlovian conditioning is "now described as the learning of relations among events" (Rescorla, 1988, p. 151; my emphasis).

There are at least two relatively straightforward consequences of this cognitive-processing, S-S learning position. The first consequence is that the conditional SCR should reflect the contingency difference between a CS that is negatively correlated with the US, and one that is merely uncorrelated with the US, this being the distinction introduced by Rescorla (1967) as one between "explicitly unpaired" and "truly random" CSs. Tests of this first consequence of the S-S position for the human conditional SCR have uniformly disconfirmed it (Furedy, 1971; Furedy & Schiffmann, 1971, 1973; Schiffmann & Furedy, 1972, 1977), although it was also clear that subjects were aware of the contingency differences between the CSs.

Another, even more straightforward, derivable consequence of the S-S learning position is that there should be a positive and high correlation between extent of CS-US contingency awareness and conditional SCR magnitude. In the studies cited immediately above, the obtained correlations were consistently nonsignificant and close to zero. Some investigators suggest that these null correlational results should be dismissed on the ground that correlation does not imply causation. However, a causal explanation (which the cognitive position is) is refuted by the failure to observe the relevant correlations (see also Furedy, 1991, p. 124).

More generally, and as I have argued in more detail elsewhere (Furedy, 1991), it appears that, like most metaphysical positions of which the new cognitivism (like the old S-R position) is a case, contrary evidence has little impact. Rather, the tenets of the new cognitivism have been applied to human SCR Pavlovian conditioning in a quasi-religious way. And the technical advances in computerization have not helped to strengthen the evidential sensitivity of theorising in this area.

There can, indeed, be negative progress not only in theoretical matters, but in more practical ones. For example, anyone familiar with Pavlovian SCR conditioning studies knows that the basic phenomenon itself (CS+>CS-, where CS+ is associated with the US and CS- is the not-so-associated, control stimulus) is not overly robust. Specifically, in a within-subject design, one needs to run at least about 20 subjects to be reasonably sure of obtaining a 5% level of significance. Now it is another tenet of the cognitive approach that the interstimulus interval (ISI) between CS onset and US onset is not critical, since it is the semantic rather than temporal relation between CS and US as events that matters. Also, following a paper by Stewart, Stern, Winokur, & Fredman (1961), it was discovered that if the ISI was extended to 8 seconds in SCR conditioning studies, then it was possible to look at two anticipatory (pre-US) responses, with the second one (second-interval response, or SIR) looking more like the "true" anticipatory response. In the late seventies until quite recently (see Ohman, this book, who has now begun to use a shorter, 3-second ISI), most workers turned to the 8-second ISI on these cognitive grounds. However, the fact is that it is the FIR which provides more robust evidence for conditioning in this 8-second ISI arrangement, with the SIR often providing no significant CS+>CS- effect at all. And, of course, extending the ISI to 8 seconds from the earlier one or half seconds simply weakens the conditioning phenomenon itself. In practical terms, then, Pavlovian conditioning experimenters have bought a cognitive pig in a poke when they went to longer ISIs.

Accordingly, rather than trying to ignore experimental SCR data that do not conform to cognitive-processing, S-S learning notions, it would be more profitable to use these data to gain insight into S-R learning processes that seem, in fact, to occur during human Pavlovian conditioning. The psyche, in other words, probably manifests both cognitive S-S and non- cognitive S-R learning during conditioning.

## The Weak-Stimulus-Elicited SCR as the Sokolovian Neuronal-Model Index.

Attention is an important determinant of behavior, and the concept of the orienting reaction (OR) as introduced by Sokolov (1960) has proved fruitful not only for experimental psychophysiologists but also for students of individual differences in both normal and abnormal subjects. For all these investigators, the SCR has been a frequently employed index of the OR, which, according to Sokolovian theory, habituates to stimulus repetition, and increases (is "reinstated") to stimulus change, provided that the stimuli in question are "weak" (e.g., moderately loud tones and perceivable but not vast changes in illumination, versus loud noises (above 90 db) and electric shocks). The hypothetical mechanism responsible for these SCR decreases and increases to repetition and change, respectively, is the neuronal model which is confirmed by repetition and disconfirmed by change. As I have noted (Furedy, 1989, p. 200), this hypothetical mechanism is cognitive or propositional, because only propositions, having truth value, can be confirmed or disconfirmed; responses cannot. I suggest that part of the reason why the Sokolovian theory has proved so popular is that it is consistent with the cognitive paradigm shift, according to which all behavior is cognitively determined. And in addition to the many experimental studies of SCR ORs, there have also been attempts to use the SCR OR to study brain mechanisms (e.g., Raine, this book).

However, it is a mistake to simply assume that the SCR universally conforms to Sokolovian theoretical notions, no matter how conducive these may be to the current cognitive approach. Even the habituation-to-repetition phenomenon is troublesome, since it does not appear to be restricted to weak stimuli. It is common knowledge among experimenters using loud noises and shocks as USs, that SCR habituation occurs also to these stimuli.

The real can of empirical worms, however, occurs when one considers the evidence on the increase-to-change SCR effect. The basic assumption, here, is that stimulus change is both sufficient and necessary for the SCR-increase phenomenon. Concerning the sufficiency aspect, cross-modal (tone/light or light/tone) change following fifteen repetitions was sufficient to produce the predicted increase in two within-subject comparisons involving samples of 80 subjects each (Furedy, 1968, 1969). However, in the same two samples, a change from twelve repeated alternations (e.g., tone, light, tone, light, ..., tone, light, LIGHT) failed to produce any increase. As to the necessity aspect, this was refuted in a paper by Furedy and Scull (1971), the title of which summarises the results. Specifically, we presented an unsystematically ordered series of cool air puffs and shocks, and found significantly larger responding to trials immediately preceded by a different trial (e.g., shock preceded by puff) than to trials immediately preceded by the same sort of trial (e.g., shock preceded by shock). So, disconfirmatory stimulus change of the cognitive Sokolovian sort is neither sufficient nor necessary for producing an SCR increase.

These generally ignored findings are damaging to Sokolovian theory, but they are relevant also to those who wish to use electrodermal orienting as an individual-differences-related attentional index. Instead of the usual strategy of administering moderate tones, and simply labelling the elicited SCRs as ORs (whereas they may reflect, for example, simple reactivity), it would seem more profitable to actually measure the OR-like properties of these responses, and compare individuals in terms of these properties. Two of the OR-like properties are, as indicated above, habituation (i.e., a gradual[4] decrease over repeated trials) and increase to change. An additional third effect (also reported in Furedy, 1968 and 1969) is a sort of "super" reinstatement effect, wherein the (16th) change trial produces greater electrodermal responding than the initial (1st) repetition trial. This third effect, of course, is consistent with the Sokolovian neuronal model notion, the disconfirmation on the change trial being more salient than on the initial (to-be-repeated) trial. My general point is that rather than taking these attentional effects for granted, it would be more fruitful to actually assess the extent to which they, in fact, occur in the weak-stimulus-elicited SCR. And rather than attempting simply to differentiate individuals in terms of their SCRs to weak stimuli (which may simply be a dimension of reactivity), it would be better to differentiate them in terms of the three attentional, OR-like properties that I have listed in this paragraph. In this way, the EDA is likely to be a more discriminating psychophysiological investigatory tool of the important psychological process of attention.

## LOW-TECH APPROACHES TO PSYCHOLOGICAL PHENOMENA USING EDA

There are some dependent psychophysiological variables like the evoked response potential (ERP) that require technically sophisticated computer hardware and software, but this requirement does not apply to EDA. In this concluding section I shall briefly indicate how a low-tech approach may be useful in elucidating psychological phenomena through psychophysiological experimentation. In my first example, the electrodermal study of deception, the hand-scored SCR is the dependent variable. In the second example, the even lower-tech minute-by-minute-scored SCL turns out to be a valuable marker of the apparent psychological effects of user-hostile programming in a human-computer-interaction experiment.

On the face of it, experimental psychophysiologists would appear to be in a uniquely favored position to contribute to both knowledge and practice regarding deception. In terms of practice, the lack of conscious control over EDA suggests that its measurement should provide an ideal way of detecting deception, on the grounds that while our lips may shield us, our ANS will betray us. And in North America, in particular, this sort of applied psychophysiology has been practiced since the early twenties in the form of the polygraph or "lie detector" (see Ben-Shakhar & Furedy, 1990 for a recent analysis). However, while controversy about the utility of polygraphy persists (see, e.g., Furedy & Heslegrave, 1991a,b, and, especially, Raskin & Kircher, 1991), what has not been disputed is that none of the detection-of-deception experiments reported in such journals as Psychophysiology have, even prima facie, involved manipulating deception as a psychological process. This is because, as detailed in Furedy (1986), neither the so-called "control" question "test" (CQT) nor the more scientifically-based guilty-knowledge-technique (GKT) proposed by Lykken (1959) actually assess deception. Only the recently introduced (Furedy et al., 1988) differentiation-of-deception paradigm (DDP) does this, because only in the DDP does it even make preliminary[5] sense to argue that the only difference between the relevant (experimental) and comparison (control) questions is the presence of deception.

The basic experimental/control contrast, of course, is an elementary but critical conceptual notion in experimentation. So, in the early days of Pavlovian conditioning, studies were presented which showed responding to a CS paired with a US, but there was no attempt to provide a control, comparison stimulus where the only difference between experimental and control stimuli was the association with the US. Although there are still arguments about what the appropriate control for conditioning is in electrodermal work (see, e.g., Furedy, Poulos, & Schiffmann, 1975a, b; Prokasy, 1975a, b), there is agreement about the basic conceptual requirement for the proper control for conditioning. The fact that a parallel process for deception has only begun in the late eighties suggests that the conceptual state of psychophysiological investigations of deception is in a primitive state of development. My guess is that one reason for this state of affairs is that focus on the applied problem of detecting deception has led many to forget the more basic scientific issue of the study or differentiation of deception as a psychological process.

Concerning EDA as a tool for studying human-computer interactions, one of the detrimental effects of computerization in society is the proliferation of user-hostile programmes. For example, in North America, it has been estimated that 80% of VCR owners do not know how to program their machines. At least as variable and difficult is the programming of modern digital watches. Two decades ago there may not have been so many options, but at least it was clear how, if one had one, the alarm could be set and turned off. To-day, if one loses the (often incomprehensible and small-printed) owner's manual, there no one, least of all the jewelers, to turn to. And, of course, the individual has to interact with computers more and more in activities like banking transactions.

As we have recently reported (Muter, Furedy, Vincent, & Pelcowitz, 1992), we assessed the effects of user-hostile programming in a laboratory arrangement where 6-minute bank-teller transaction tasks were presented to subjects. The variable, manipulated within subjects, was whether the programme was user friendly or user-hostile. In addition, to assess whether any differences in physiological responses were due solely to difficulty, we also varied, within subjects, a memorial digit-span task between a relatively easy condition (forward digit span) and a relatively hard condition (backward digit span). Heart rate (HR) was higher during the two bank-teller than during the memorial tasks, but did not vary as a function of task difficulty. On the other hand, average skin conductance level (SCL) uniquely differentiated the user-hostile condition from the other three conditions, which did not differ from each other in terms of SCL. For this experiment we employed very crude, low-tech methods for assessing SCL, simply measuring this function by hand on a minute-by-minute basis. Yet, in this context, it was this low-tech EDA measure that provided the most relevant information. This is not to eschew, in general, the benefits of recent technical advances, but only to argue that, in the end, the focus of the psychophysiologist should be what the measures available tell her or him about psychological process--the psyche of psychophysiology.

## ACKNOWLEDGMENTS

The research described in this chapter was supported by grants from the National Science and Engineering Research and Social Science and Humanities Council of Canada. I am grateful for Wolf Boucsein and Ruediger Baltissen for advice on an earlier version of the writeup, and to participants at the NATO conference for their comments on the oral presentation of the paper on which this chapter is based.

## FOOTNOTES

1 It is interesting to note that at this conference Zoccolotti (this volume) indicated that in a study by Mammucari, Caltagirone, Ekman, Friesen, Gailotti, Pizzamigli, and Zoccolotti (1988), facial expressions which were thoroughly analysed did not differentiate the hedonic tone of movies whereas both the electrodermal skin conductance response (SCR) and cardiac deceleration did. These autonomically-controlled and involuntary physiological changes, then, may be better tools for exploring the emotional aspects of the psyche than facial expressions, even when the latter are measured with considerable technical sophistication. This example illustrates the point (elaborated by another example later in the text) that, in some cases, the psyche of psychophysiology is better investigated by low-tech rather than high-tech tools.

2 Fowles' (1980) adoption of Gray's (1975) three-factor arousal model for EDA is also consistent with Heslegrave's (1982) results, and it is interesting to note that in the extended writeup of his work, (Heslegrave, 1981) argued that deception involved an "inhibitory" form of arousal.

3 There may, of course, be other reasons for preferring the conductance transformation. Specifically, SCR magnitude scores appear to be more normally distributed than SRR magnitude scores. However, these statistical considerations are separate from the

physiological considerations discussed in the text. This difference is further illustrated by the use of further transformations of SCR magnitude scores such as log conductance change, and the further statistical complication that with log transformations a constant has to be added to all scores to resolve problems with zero responding.

4 If all the decrease occurs from the first to the second trial, with asymptotic performance after that, the phenomenon is not really habituation (note that it also does not conform the gradual confirmation or build-up of the neuronal model), but a somewhat different first-trial effect. The SCR usually manifests the more gradual habituation slope, in which case it is possible to compare degrees of habituation not only in terms of first- and last-trial differences, but also in terms of function slopes.

5 The term "preliminary" is used advisedly. A confounding possibility in the DDP is that the deceptively- versus honestly-answered-questions comparison may be confounded by a memorial, retrieval-difficulty effect. That is, deceptive answers may produce bigger SCRs simply because they are more difficult to retrieve than honest ones. This confounding possibility was minimized by instructions in the original DDP study (Furedy et al., 1988), and has, most recently, been assessed and found to be absent by Vincent and Furedy (1992).

## REFERENCES

Ben-Shakhar, G. and Furedy, J.J., 1990, *Theories and Applications in the Detection of Deception: Psychophysiological and Cultural Perspectives*, Springer-Verlag.

Bitterman, M.E., Reed, P., and Krauskopf, J., 1952, The effect of the duration of the unconditioned stimulus upon conditioning and extinction, *American Journal of Psychology*, 65:256-262.

Brewer, W. F., 1974, There is no convincing evidence for operant or classical conditioning in adult humans, in: W.B. Weimer & D.S. Palermo eds., *Cognition and the symbolic process*, Erlbaum, Hillsdale, New Jersey.

Bloch, V., and Bonvallet, M., 1960, Le déclenchement des réponses électrodermales a partir du système réticulaire facilitateur, *Journal de Physiologie*, 51:25-26.

Contrada, R.J., 1992, T-wave amplitude: On the meaning of a psychophysiological index, *Biological Psychology*, 33:249-258.

Davis, C. and Gurevich, M., 1988, Differentiation of deception as a Psychological process: A psychophysiological approach, *Psychophysiology*, 25:683-88.

Dengerink, J.A., and Taylor, S.P., 1971, Multiple responses with differential properties in delayed galvanic skin response conditioning: A review, *Psychophysiology*, 8:348-360.

Edelberg, R., 1967, Electrical properties of the skin, in: C.C. Brown, ed., *Methods in psychophysiology*, 1-53, Williams and Wilkins, Baltimore, MD.

Fowles, D.C., 1980, The three arousal model: Implications of Gray's two-factor learning theory for heart rate, electrodermal activity, and psychopathy, *Psychophysiology*, 17:87-104.

Fowles, D.C., Christie, M.J., Edelberg, R., Grings, W.W., Lykken, D.T., and Venables, P.H., 1981, Publication recommendations for electrodermal measurements, *Psychophysiology*, 18:232-239.

Furedy, J.J., 1968, Human orienting reaction as a function of electrodermal-versus plethysmographic response modes and single versus alternating stimulus series, *Journal of Experimental Psychology*,77:70-78.

Furedy, J.J., 1969, Electrodermal and plethysmographic OR components: Repetition of and change from UCS-CS trials with surrogate UCS, *Canadian Journal of Psychology*, 27:127-135.

Furedy, J.J., 1970, A test of the preparatory-adaptive-response interpretation of aversive classical autonomic conditioning, *Journal of Experimental Psychology*, 84:301-307.

Furedy, J.J., 1971, Explicitly-unpaired and truly-random CS-controls in human classical differential autonomic conditioning, *Psychophysiology*, 8:497-503.

Furedy, J.J., 1973, Some limits on the cognitive control of conditioned autonomic behavior, *Psychophysiology*, 10:108-111.

Furedy, J.J., 1975, An Integrative Progress report on Informational control in humans: Some laboratory findings and methodological claims, *Australian Journal of Psychology*, 27:61-83.

Furedy, J.J., 1983, Operational, analogical, and genuine definitions of psychophysiology, *International Journal of Psychophysiology*, 1:13-19.

Furedy, J.J., 1984, Generalities and specifics in defining psychophysiology: Reply to Stern (1964) and Stern (1984), *Psychophysiology*, 2:2-4.

Furedy, J.J., 1986, Lie Detection as Psychophysiological Differentiation: Some Fine Lines, *Psychophysiology: Systems, Processes, and Applications--A Handbook*, pp. 683-700, in: M. Coles, E. Donchin, and E. Porges eds., Guilford.

Furedy, J.J., 1987, Beyond heart-rate in the cardiac psychophysiological assessment of mental effort: The T-wave amplitude component of the electrocardiogram, *Human Factors*, 29:183-94.

Furedy, J.J., 1989, The post-sixties experimental-psychological study of habituation: Some recalcitrant reflections on the fruits of cognitive psychology, Selected/Revised papers from the *Proceedings of the XXIV International Congress of Psychology*, Vol. 6: *Psychobiology: Issues and Applications*, in: N.W. Bond and D.A.T. Siddle eds., North Holland, NY.

Furedy, J.J., 1991, Some recalcitrant views on the role of noncognitive S-R factors in human Pavlovian autonomic conditioning: Some facts still haunt us, Integrative *Physiological and Behavioral Science*, 26:21-25.

Furedy, J.J. and Doob, A.N., 1971, Autonomic responses and verbal reports in further test of the preparatory-adaptive-response interpretation of reinforcement, *Journal of Experimental Psychology*, 89:258-264.

Furedy, J.J., Katic, M., Klajner, F., and Poulos, C., 1973, Attentional factors and aversiveness ratings in tests of the preparatory adaptive response interpretation of reinforcement, *Canadian Journal of Psychology*, 27:400-413.

Furedy, J.J., and Heslegrave, R.J, 1991a, The forensic use of the polygraph: A psychophysiological analysis of current trends and future prospects, in: *Advances in Psychophysiology*, 4, J.Jennings, M. Coles, and P. Acles eds., Kingsley.

Furedy, J.J., & Heslegrave, R.J., 1991b, A reply to commentators: Some elaborations on the specific-effects orientation's application to the North American CQT polygraph, in: Jennings, et al., *ibid*.

Furedy, J.J., Heslegrave, R.J., and Scher, H., 1992, T-wave amplitude utility revisited: Some physiological and psychophysiological considerations, *Biological Psychology, 33:241-248*.

Furedy, J.J., Poulos, C., and Schiffmann, K., 1975a, Contingency theory and inhibitory conditioning: Some problems of assessment and interpretation, *Psychophysiology*, 12:98-105.

Furedy, J.J., Poulos, C., and Schiffmann, K., 1975b, Logical problems with Prokasy's assessment of contingency relations in classical skin conductance conditioning, *Behavior Research Methods and Instrumentation*, 7:521-523.

Furedy, J.J., Posner, R., and Vincent, A., 1991, Electrodermal differentiation of deception: Memory-difficulty and perceived- accuracy manipulations. *International Journal of Psychophysiology*, 11:91-97.

Furedy, J.J., and Riley, D.M., 1987, Human Pavlovian autonomic conditioning and the cognitive paradigm, in: *Conditioning in Humans*, 1-25, G. Davey ed., Wiley & Sons, Sussex.

Furedy, J.J., & Schiffmann, K., 1971, Test of the propriety of the traditional discriminative control procedure in Pavlovian electrodermal and plethysmographic conditioning. *Journal of Experimental Psychology*, 91,161-164.

Furedy, J.J., and Schiffmann, K., 1973, Concurrent measurement of autonomic and cognitive processes in a test of the traditional discriminative control procedure for Pavlovian electrodermal conditioning, *Journal of Experimental Psychology*, 100:210-217.

Furedy, J.J., and Scull, J., 1971, Orienting-reaction theory and an increase in the human GSR following stimulus change which is unpredictable but not contrary to prediction, *Journal of Experimental Psychology*, 88:292-294.

Gray, J., 1975, *Elements of a Two-Process Theory of Learning*, Academic Press, New York.

Haggard, E. A., 1945, Experimental studies in affective processes: II on the quantification and evaluation of "measured" changes in skin resistance, *Journal of Experimental Psychology*, 35:45-56.

Heslegrave, R.J., 1981, A psychophysiological analysis of the detection of the detection of deception: The role of information, retrieval, novelty and conflict mechanisms, Unpublished Phd Thesis, University of Toronto.

Heslegrave, R.J. 1982, An examination of the psychophysiological mechanisms underlying deception, *Psychophysiology*, 19:298, (abstract).

Lykken, D.T., 1959, The GSR in the detection of guilt, *Journal of Applied Psychology*, 43:385-388.

Mammucari, A., Caltagirone, C., Ekman, P., Friesen, W., Gailotti, G., Pizzamigli, L., and Zoccolotti, P., 1988, Spontaneous facial expression of emotions in brain-damaged patients, *Cortex*, 24:521-533.

Muter, P.M., Furedy, J.J., Vincent, A., and Pelcowitz, T., 1992, User- hostile systems and patterns of psychophysiological activity, *Computers in Human Behavior*, *9:105-111.*

Obrist, P.A., 1976, The Cardiovascular-Behavioral Interaction - As it appears today, *Psychophysiology*, 13:95-107.

Obrist, P.A., 1981, *Cardiovascular Psychophysiology: A Perspective*. Plenum Press, New York.

Ohman, A., Esteves, F., Flykt, A. and Soares, J.J.F., 1993, Gateways to consciousness: emotion, attention, and electrodermal activity (This volume).

Perkins, C.C., 1968, An analysis of the concept of reinforcement, *Psychological Review*, 75:155-172.

Prokasy, W.F., 1975a, Random control procedures in classical skin conductance conditioning, *Behavior Research Methods & Instrumentation*, 7:516-520.

Prokasy, W.F., 1975b, Random controls: A rejoinder. *Behavior Research Methods and Instrumentation*, 7:524-526.

Raine, A. and Lencz, T., 1993, Brain imaging research on electrodermal activity in humans (This volume).

Raskin, D. C., and Kircher, J.C., 1991, Comments on Furedy and Heslegrave: Misconceptions, misdescriptions, and misdirections, in: *Advances in Psychophysiology*, Vol.4, J.R. Jennings, P.K. Ackles, and M.G.H. Coles, eds., JAI Press, Greenwich, Conn.

Rescorla, R.A., 1967, Pavlovian conditioning and its proper control procedures, *Psychological Review*, 74:71-80.

Rescorla, R.A., 1988, Pavlovian conditioning: It's not what you think it is, *American Psychologist*, 43:151-160.

Schiffmann, K., and Furedy, J.J., 1972, Failures of contingency and cognitive factors to affect long-interval differential Pavlovian autonomic conditioning, *Journal of Experimental Psychology*, 96:215- 218.

Schiffmann, K., and Furedy, J.J., 1977, The effect of CS-US contingency variation on GSR and on subjective CS/US relational awareness, *Memory and Cognition*, 5:273-7.

Sokolov, Y.N., 1960, Neuronal models and the orienting reflex, in: *The central nervous system and behavior*, pp. 187-276, M.A.B. Brazier ed., Macy Jr. Foundation, Josiah, New York.

Stern, J.A., 1984, Toward a definition of psychophysiology, *Psychophysiology*, 1:90-91.

Stewart, M., Stern, J.A. Winokur, G., and Fredman, S., 1961, An analysis of conditioning, *Psychological Review*, 68:60-67.

Vincent, A., and Furedy, J.J., 1992, Electrodermal differentiation of deception: Potentially confounding and influencing factors", *International Journal of Psychophysiology*, *13:129-136.*

Zoccolotti, P., Caltagirone, C., Pecchinenda, A. and Troisi, E., 1993, Electrodermal activity in patients with unilateral brain damage (This volume).

# NEURAL CONTROL OF ELECTRODERMAL ACTIVITY:

## SPINAL AND RETICULAR MECHANISMS

Jean-Claude Roy[1], Henrique Sequeira[2,1] and Bernard Delerm[1]

[1]Laboratoire de Neurosciences du Comportement SN4
Université des Sciences et Technologies de Lille
59655 Villeneuve d'Ascq Cedex, France

[2]Département de Psychologie
Fédération Universitaire et Polytechnique de Lille
59016 Lille Cedex, France

## INTRODUCTION

The existence of an electrical current related to sweating on the paws, and evoked by peripheral nerve stimulation, was first discovered in cats by Hermann and Luchsinger (1878), a discovery which preceded by approximately ten years Féré's (1888) well-known description of electrodermal activity (EDA) in humans (see Neuman and Blanton,1970, and Bloch, this volume, for an historical account). Tarchannof (1890) accurately linked skin potential variations in humans with the functioning of the sweat glands. But Darrow (1927) was really the first to clearly demonstrate in humans the close relationship between the activity of the sweat glands and electrodermal activity.

Electrodermal activity is a choice index for the study of central nervous control of autonomic activity, because the sweat glands do not exhibit self-rhythmic activity. In addition, it is classically agreed that the sweat glands are peripherally innervated only by the sympathetic division of the autonomic nervous system (Langley, 1891). It is apparent that EDA is controlled by both excitatory and inhibitory mechanisms which probably act upon spinal autonomic neurons. The purpose of this chapter is to review classical facts regarding the neurophysiological control of EDA by focussing upon results obtained in experimental research with animals. Past findings have been reviewed before (e.g., Darrow, 1936; Wang, 1957, 1958; Bloch, 1965; Venables, 1991) but will be included in this text where relevant. Data published after Wang's reviews (1957, 1958) will be specially detailed. On the other hand, past findings which have failed to be replicated will not be included (for example, results involving the cerebellum and the striatal formations; Wang and Chun, 1967). Cortical and hypothalamo-limbic mechanisms are presented in the next chapter (Sequeira and Roy, this volume), whereas this presentation will focus upon

*Progress in Electrodermal Research,* Edited by
J.-C. Roy *et al.* Plenum Press, New York, 1993

physiological mechanisms of EDA control including the spinal mechanisms and the role of the reticular formations of the brain stem.

We will begin by briefly summarizing the experimental species used in the study of EDA and then delineate the characteristics of EDA in these species. Besides man, electrodermal activity has been studied in rats, cats, and monkeys. EDA recording is difficult with anaesthetized rats, but some researchers have succeeded in producing data with this species (Vernet-Maury, 1970; Yamazaki et al., 1975; Hata et al., 1981; Girardot and Koss, 1984). Yamazaki et al. (1975) performed a comparative study which included one chimpanzee, ten species of monkeys, and two species of prosimiae. As shown in that study, the ape and the monkeys produce monophasic skin potential positive waves, as do humans. But, among monkeys, saimiri produced monophasic negative waves. On the other hand, the prosimiae produced monophasic negative waves, as do rats and carnivorous. Thus, it appears that monkeys would be the ideal experimental species. Unfortunately, their use is limited due to financial and ethical considerations. This being the case, only few experimental studies using monkeys have actually been published. Most experiments have been done on cats because recordings of skin potential responses (SPRs) and skin conductance responses (SCRs) are easily obtained even when the animals are under anaesthesia. In this species, following the stimulation of the peripheral end of a severed nerve, SPR and SCR recordings show similar results as regards latency and evolution of the amplitude (Ba M'Hamed-Bennis, 1984). But, the sodium reabsorption mechanisms are different in cats than they are in humans. That is to say, the sweat from the footpads of cats and rats was found to be hypertonic, indicating no sodium reabsorption. Thus cats are not the suitable species for studying peripheral mechanisms, since the results obtained with this species cannot be extended to man. However, their use does provide certain advantages for neurophysiology, besides accurate stereotaxy; in carnivorous, thermoregulation is controlled by breathing and sweating plays a very small role, if any at all. As stated by Jänig et al. (1983), "there is probably no thermoregulatory sweating in the cat" . Thus, one can hypothesize that in cats, the sweating of the footpad is analogous to "emotional" sweating in human beings. In human beings, sweating increases protection to injury, and increases sensibility (Edelberg, 1972; Fowles, 1986). It also increases grip, as suggested by Darrow (1936). In cats, it seems reasonably established that one of the roles of sweating on paws is also to increase the coefficient of friction between the animal's feet and the substrate (Adams and Hunter, 1969; Adelman et al., 1975).


## SPINAL MECHANISMS

### Sudomotor Neurons

Sudomotor neurons are not specifically distinguished, in the spinal cord, from other sympathetic preganglionic neurons, which are mainly located in the intermediolateral nucleus of the spinal cord (Henry and Calaresu, 1972; Chung and Wurster, 1975; Deuschl and Illert, 1981; Rubin and Purves, 1980; Rao and Bijlani, 1980; Laskey and Polosa, 1988; Cabot, 1990). This nucleus includes part of the layer VII of Rexed and extends laterally into the white matter, in what is called the lateral funicular area. Groups of sympathetic preganglionic neurons are also located dorsolateral to the central canal (see Cabot, 1990, for a review).

In the cat, the sympathetic preganglionic fibers innervating the forepaws leave the spinal cord by the 4th to the 9th thoracic, and those innervating the hindpaws leave from the 12th thoracic to the 3rd lumbar (Langley, 1891, 1922; Patton, 1948).

## Ganglionic Neurons

As such, sweat gland functioning is clearly due to the impulses received from the autonomic neurons located in the spinal ganglions, as shown in Figure 1 (see Janig et al., 1983, and Wallin and Fagius, 1986, for reviews). These sympathetic neurons exhibit a very low level of spontaneous activity. The neurotransmitter involved in the ganglionic relay is acetylcholine, the receptors of which are nicotinic (Langley, 1922). The junction is blocked by hexamethonium, which confirms that the transmission is due to the nicotinic action of acetylcholine (Jänig and Szulczyk, 1981); but this is still a matter of discussion (Koss and Hey, 1988; Walland, 1984a). Jänig et al. (1982) concluded that the α–adrenergic effects depress, but that the β–adrenergic enhance impulse transmission from pre- to post-ganglionic sudomotor neurons. However, the mechanisms by which the catecholamines influence the postganglionic neurons are not known.

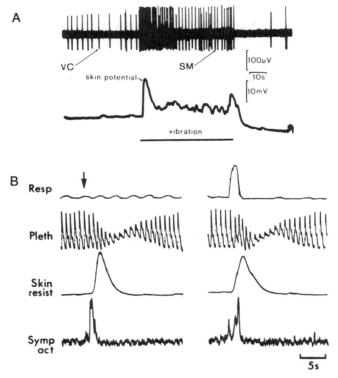

**Figure 1.** A- Activation of sudomotor neurons (SM) and inhibition of vasoconstrictor neurons (VC) by vibrational stimulation. The discharges of the neurons were recorded in postganglionic axons isolated from the medial plantar nerve, in chloralose anaesthetized cat. The skin potential responses were recorded from the pad of the cat's hindpaw.

B- Mean voltage neurogram (Symp act) recorded in median nerve in man. Strong bursts of skin nerve sympathetic activity are elicited by a sudden shout (arrow in the left panel) and deep inspiration (right panel). Tracing from top: respiration, finger pulse plethysmogram, palmar skin resistance, and mean voltage neurogram.

(A: from Jänig and Kümmel, 1981; B: from Wallin and Fagius, 1986; both reproduced with the permission of Elsevier, Amsterdam)

Activation of the sudomotor fibers are nearly invariably accompanied by an inhibition of the cutaneous vaso-constrictor neurons, thus resulting in a peripheral vaso dilatation. The sudomotor response elicited by preganglionic stimulation is abolished by atropine, but the blood flow response is not. These data suggest that postganglionic neurons mediating vasodilatation for the skin of the cat paw are distinct from those that mediate sudomotor secretion (Bell et al., 1985). Jänig and co-workers evaluated conduction speed in the sudomotor fibers of the cat, at 0.77 m/s (Jänig and Kümmel, 1977), or 0.72 m/s, (Jänig and Szulczyk, 1981). These values are probably too low, because the conduction velocities of the sudomotor axons were measured at temperatures of about 30°C, lower than physiological temperatures. In humans, the conduction velocity was evaluated at 1.2-1.4 m/s (Fagius and Wallin, 1980).

Classical studies (Head and Riddoch, 1917; Riddoch, 1917) showed that the sudomotor neurons are influenced by excitatory and inhibitory impulses from the supraspinal centers. In fact, when the spinal cord is severed due to an injury, sweating stops as the individual goes into a state of spinal shock, which may last several days in man during which time the somatic reflexes are equally abolished. Following this period of shock, a state of somatic and autonomic hyper-reflexivity appears in which profuse sweating occurs. The inhibitory impulses were, thus, classically considered as predominating over excitatory commands in normal man. Moreover, after an acute spinal section, an animal preparation must be regarded as being in a state of spinal shock.

## RETICULAR CONTROL

### Excitatory Control

The main supraspinal structure for controlling the EDA appears to be the reticular formation of the brain stem. This structure was shown in the fifties to exert an arousing influence on the cortical hemispheres, as demonstrated by the classical works of Moruzzi and Magoun (1949), of Moruzzi's group in Pisa, and of Dell's group in Paris. In the context of reticular physiology, Bloch and Bonvallet (1960a), and Bloch (1965) demonstrated that SPRs were indices of the reticular activations. Firstly, SPRs are part of the arousal reaction evoked by electrical stimulation of the reticular activating system, or by sensory stimulation. As illustrated in Figure 2, a moderate auditory stimulation evoked an EEG arousal, an increase in the amplitude of a monosynaptic somatic reflex, a rise of blood pressure, together with an electrodermal response.

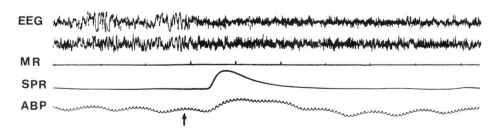

**Figure 2.** Simultaneous effects of an auditory stimulation (arrow) on a drowsy cat: EEG arousal, increase in amplitude of a monosynaptic reflex (shown as RM on Fig.), rise in arterial blood pressure (ABP), and SPR. (from Bloch, 1965, reproduced by permission of Masson, Paris)

A systematic exploration of the brain stem by stereotaxical stimulation, in the cat, led Bloch (1965) to conclude that: "the SPRs can be evoked with low stimulation intensities from the reticular formation lying from the medulla, the pons and the mesencephalon to the posterior hypothalamus" (see Figure 3). These results, have since been largely confirmed (Davison and Koss, 1975). Girardot and Koss (1984) evoked maximal amplitude SPRs in the rat by stimulating the ventral tegmental field. McAllen (1986) was able to trigger SPRs by chemical stimulation of the bulbar reticular formation in the cat, using homocysteic acid to selectively excite cell bodies, thus excluding passing fibers. It was confirmed in the kitten that stimulation of the central tegmental field evokes SPRs, as early as 4 hours after birth (Delerm et al. 1982).

There is no doubt that the reticular formation of the brain stem plays a central role in the nervous control of EDA. After a section at the prebulbar level, thresholds can be up to ten times higher. This is in part explained by the existing bulbar inhibitory mechanisms which will be discussed later. In spinal preparations, SPRs become no longer synchronous in the four paws of the animal (Bloch and Bonvallet, 1959; Ladpli and Wang, 1960). It is still possible to evoke SPRs by cutaneous nociceptive stimulation, or by direct afferent nerve stimulation. However, the thresholds for evoking SPRs are much higher and extremely variable. Thus, the reticular formation is the pace-maker which ensures the synchronicity of spontaneous SPRs. The reticular formation also facilitates SPR reflexes, evoked by peripheral stimulation, by means of tonic descending influences to the spinal autonomic neurons.

Bloch (1965) concluded that electrodermal responses are indices of the activation of the reticulo-cortical system in the sense proposed by Lindsley (1951). These findings have been extended by studying reticular excitability during different stages of vigilance, in which behavioral and electrophysiological (EEG, EMG, EOG) criteria are used to classify the animal's behavior on a scale of vigilance, namely waking, attention and stages of sleep.

## Reticular Thresholds and Vigilance

When a cat is in a drowsy state during acute preparation, stimulation of the reticular formation simultaneously triggers a cortical arousal, a rise in blood pressure, an increase in a somatic motor reflex, and an SPR. Furthermore, the more intense the cortical arousal, the larger the evoked SPR (Bloch and Bonvallet, 1960a). However, it is possible to evoke SPRs with stimulation intensities which do not trigger cortical arousal. The excitability of the reticular formation can be studied by both sensory stimulation and direct electrical stimulation. In their pioneer study, Benoit and Bloch (1960) evaluated the reticular excitability by EEG arousal or by awakening the subject behaviorally. However, one of the drawbacks of the method is waking the cat for each measure. It was shown later that, in most cases, it is possible to evoke SPRs in cats with minimal intensities lower than the awakening thresholds. Using reticular stimulation to evaluate the threshold of evoked SPRs has the advantage of testing central excitability with minimal interference of the sleep-waking cycle. In the study by Roy et al. (1977), the intrareticular excitability was tested in different stages of vigilance, from deep sleep to attentional state. The cats were chronically implanted with EEG, EMG, and eye movement electrodes as well as with one stimulating electrode in the central tegmental field (see Roy et al., 1977, for details). The SPR thresholds were measured during waking, drowsiness, slow wave sleep, and paradoxical sleep (Figure 4). Threshold was defined as the median of the distribution of the percentage of the SPRs evoked for each intensity of stimulation value. As expected, the results showed that thresholds are lowest during the waking state and are even lower when the animals exhibit visual attention to the environment (i.e., visually following moving objects), (Figure 5). It was also found that thresholds gradually rose as the animal fell asleep. The increase in

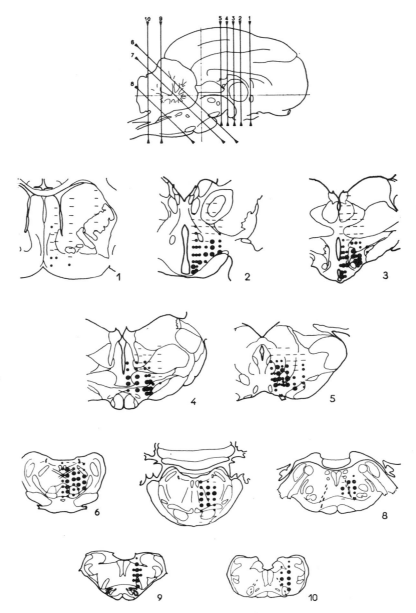

**Figure 3.** Stereotaxical exploration of the brain stem: thresholds of evoking SPRs by electrical stimulation (duration of stimulation: 150 ms; frequency: 300/s; duration of the shocks: 0.1 ms). The sections of the brain are drawn from histological sections, made in the vertical planes of the Horsley-Clarke stereotaxical apparatus (planes 1 to 5 and 9 to 10) and from sections made in a 45° plane (planes 6 to 8).

Large dots:   thresholds between 0,1 and 0,5 V
Middle dots:  thresholds between 0,5 and 1,5 V
Small dots:   thresholds between 1,5 and 3 V
Dashes:       no response

SPRs are evoked with low thresholds from structures which delineate the reticular formation of the brain stem, and the hypothalamus, posterior and anterior. (From Bloch, 1965, reproduced by permission of Masson, Paris).

threshold from waking state to drowsiness was 10%, from waking state to slow wave sleep was 25% and, from waking state to paradoxical sleep was 115% (Figure 6). These findings show a continous measure of the excitability of a subcortical component of the reticulo-cortical system, from a state of attention to paradoxical sleep, with threshold values below cortical arousal.

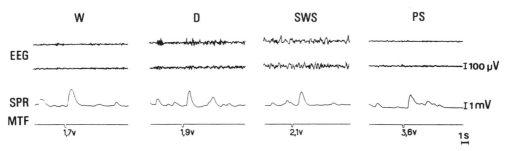

**Figure 4.** Evolution of thresholds of evoking SPRs, as a function of sleep stages in the free-moving cat. SPRs are evoked by mesencephalic central tegmental field (MTF) stimulation. These thresholds increase from waking (W) to drowsiness (D) and slow wave sleep (SWS). The increase is very high when the cat goes into paradoxical sleep (PS). (From Roy et al., 1977, reproduced by permission of Arch. Ital. Biol.).

Spontaneous EDA is significantly lower during sleep in cats, especially during paradoxical sleep (Freixa i Baqué et al., 1981). In man, however, the EDA increases during the first stages (II, III, IV) of the sleep cycle, then decreases sharply during paradoxical sleep (Broughton et al., 1965; Johnson and Lubin, 1966; Freixa i Baqué et al., 1983). No convincing hypothesis has yet been put forward to explain this discrepancy.

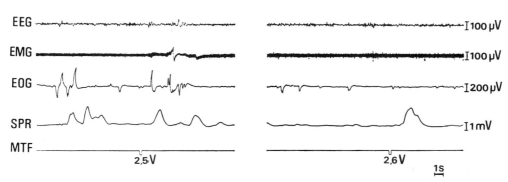

**Figure 5.** Thresholds of evoking SPRs during waking. Left: the animal shows visual attention, as seen from numerous eye movements in the electrooculogram (EOG) and from head movements on the neck electromyogram (EMG). Right: the animal pays no attention. Note that thresholds are higher (2,6 V) in this case. (From Roy et al., 1977, reproduced by permission of Arch. Ital. Biol.).

**Conclusion:** The reticular thresholds of evoked SPRs are extremely sensitive indices of the vigilance state. These thresholds permit delineation of similar central states in terms of reticular excitability. Specifically, it is possible to show that central excitability increases during behavioural attention. These results indicate the existence of a gradual increase in excitability of the reticulo-cortical system from a state of deep sleep to an attentional state. These results are in agreement with some aspects of Lindsley's theory of activation (1951).

The fact that electrodermal responses (EDR) can be triggered with intrareticular thresholds inferior to the overt EEG arousal, and without behaviorally awakening the subject is also of interest. It is well known that human subjects can exhibit large EDRs to significant stimuli they do not overtly discriminate. This phenomenon was termed subception (Lazarus and McCleary, 1951). It has been recently used to show that patients with prosopagnosia (i.e. who have lost the ability to recognize faces) still discriminate between familiar and unfamiliar faces (Tranel et al., 1985; Tranel and Damasio, 1985). Obviously, such a recognition implies a subcortical mechanism, since patients have localized occipito-temporal cortical lesions. It can be hypothesized that reticular mechanisms participate in the autonomic expression of this subliminar perception.

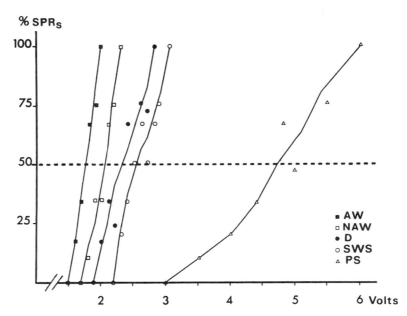

**Figure 6.** Statistical distribution of the thresholds for evoking SPRs as a function of sleep and waking stages ; the mean thresholds are the lowest during attentional waking (AW), then increase during non-attentional waking (NAW), drowsiness (D), slow wave sleep (SWS) ; the increase during paradoxical sleep (PS) is very high. (From Roy et al., 1977, reproduced by permission of Arch. Ital. Biol.).

## Bulbar Inhibitory Control

Wang et al., (1956) observed that the cooling of the medulla on the floor of the 4th ventricle, or a lesion of the medulla by xylocaine injection into the bulbar ventromedial reticular formation facilitated the SPRs evoked by stimulation of a cutaneous nerve in deeply anaesthetized cats. Wang and Brown (1956) also showed that bulbar stimulation inhibited evoked SPRs in deeply anaesthetized cats. SPRs evoked by mesencephalic reticular formation were also inhibited by stimulation of the bulbar ventro-medial reticular formation (Bloch and Bonvallet, 1960b; Yokota et al., 1963; Roy et al., 1974). The nuclei which are responsible for this are the posterior part of the gigantocellular nucleus, the paramedian nucleus, and the anterior part of the ventral reticular nucleus (Roy et al., 1974). In the anaesthetized cat (i.e., where cortical influences are depressed), sensory stimulation (Wang and Hind, 1959) and mesencephalic stimulation (Bloch and Bonvallet, 1960b; Bloch, 1965) which evoke large SPRs are followed by a long period (i.e., about 40 seconds) during which SPRs evoked by any identical stimulus are greatly diminished. Bloch and Bonvallet (1961) and Bloch (1965) concluded that this inhibition was due to the action of the bulbar inhibitory system since the stimulation of the bulbar reticular formation is followed by an identical "refractory period" which, in turn, is suppressed by a novocainisation of the ventromedial bulbar area. All of these mechanisms are functional at birth. Figure 7 illustrates this phenomenon in a chloralose anaesthetized kitten; however, certain characteristics of EDA require post-natal maturation (Delerm et al., 1982).

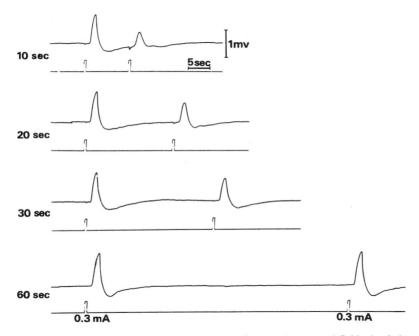

**Figure 7.** Subnormal period of SPRs evoked by mesencephalic central tegmental field stimulation: the two identical stimulus trains are separated by intervals of 10, 20, 30 and 60 s ; the amplitude of the SPR evoked by the second stimulation is 47%, 60%, 77%, and 100% of the control, respectively. (6-day-old kitten, chloralose anaesthetized, 40 mg/kg). (From Delerm et al., 1982, reproduced by permission of Springer Verlag, Berlin).

Complete SPR inhibition can be found under light anaesthesia (for example, 2% halothane, a gazeous anaesthetic; see Figure 8A). When this anaesthesia is temporarily suppressed, the SPR inhibition abruptly diminishes or vanishes (Figure 8B). Different anaesthetic agents have identical effects; therefore a purely pharmacological effect on EDA can be excluded. Thus, it was hypothesized that in non-anaesthetized animals, the bulbar inhibitory mechanism is normally overcome by the excitatory influence of higher systems, most likely the mesencephalic activating system (Mandel and Bach, 1957; Bloch and Bonvallet, 1960b). This is clearly shown by studies of the motor system. In their classical study, Magoun and Rhines (1946) have shown that stimulation of ventro-medial bulbar reticular formation inhibits all motor reflexes in a deeply anaesthetized animal. Niemer and Magoun (1947) demonstrated that these inhibitory effects acted at spinal level. They could not be found, however, on the waking cat after a chronic implantation of electrodes in the bulbar reticular formation (Sprague and Chambers,1954). Furthermore, Mandel and Bach, (1957) obtained motor inhibition during the implantation of the electrodes, under nembutal anaesthesia; after recovery, in the waking cats, no inhibitory effect could be found, but it reappeared after a nembutal injection. Subsequently, most studies on mechanisms of bulbar inhibition on the motor system were done after a transcollicular section which presumably suppress higher excitatory influences. On such a preparation, the stimulation of the bulbar ventro-medial reticular formation inhibits the "decerebration rigidity" (Lundberg and Vykliky, 1963).

In lightly anaesthetized animals, the bulbar SPR inhibition is accompanied by cortical arousal as shown by EEG desynchronisation (Figure 9). Evidence of desynchronisation excludes that the inhibition results from a direct action of the bulbar reticular formation on the mesencephalic excitatory system (Roy et al., 1974). Furthermore, in animals anaesthetized with chloralose, the inhibitory stimulation can be initiated within a time period of 0.5 second after the excitatory stimulation. It is known that in this kind of preparation, half of the 1.2 second latency is due to the peripheral effector. Therefore, it is likely that inhibitory impulses act at a spinal level (probably on sudomotor neurons), rather than at the mesencephalic level (Roy and Bloch, 1968). In some experimental preparations, a post-inhibitory rebound (shown by a large SPR) appears after bulbar stimulation. Yokota et al., (1963) suggested that an inhibitory post synaptic potential (IPSP) developed in the sudomotor neurons during bulbar stimulation and contributed to the initiation of the post-inhibitory rebound after bulbar stimulation.

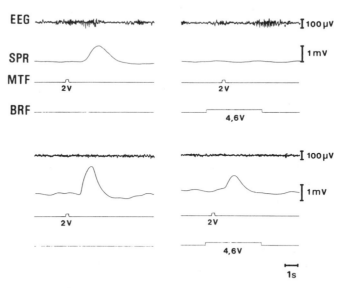

**Figure 8.** Bulbar inhibition of SPRs under anaesthesia.

Upper recordings: The SPR is evoked by the mesencephalic central tegmental field (MTF) stimulation (left). The simultaneous bulbar reticular formation (BRF) stimulation, totally inhibits this response (right). (Halothane, 2%, anaesthetized cat).

Lower recordings: Same procedure, but 30 min after stopping the halothane inhalation. The inhibition (at right) is only partial. (from Roy et al., 1974, reproduced by permission of Elsevier, Amsterdam).

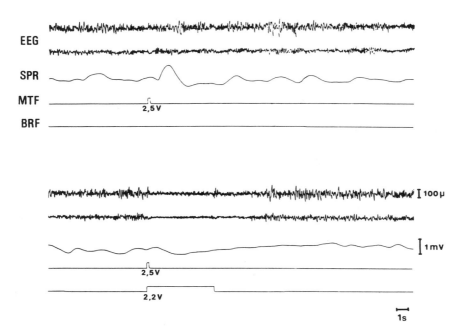

EEG

SPR

MTF        2,5 V

BRF

I 100 µ

I 1mV

2,5 V

2,2 V

1s

**Figure 9.** Dissociation of the effects of bulbar stimulation on the EEG and on SPR.
Upper recordings: The mesencephalic central tegmental field stimulation (MTF) evokes an SPR without EEG arousal.
Lower recordings: The simultaneous bulbar reticular formation (BRF) stimulation inhibits the evoked SPRs and triggers an intense EEG arousal. The cat is lightly anaesthetized with nembutal (5 mg/kg). (From Roy et al., 1974, reproduced by permission of Elsevier, Amsterdam).

The afferent nerve stimulation also inhibits SPRs. In chloralose anaesthetized cats, SPRs are inhibited by vagal afferents (Roy and Denti, 1967; Kumazawa et al.,1968), and by splanchnic nerve afferents, in curarized non-anaesthetized cats. Maximal inhibition was obtained with low frequency of stimulation (5 impulses /s) and then disappeared with stimulation rates higher than 10 /s (Kumazawa and Naotsuka, 1970). Since this inhibition is dependent upon low frequency stimulation, it could be hypothesized that this effect is an indirect one, through the bulbar reticular system.

## RETICULOSPINAL INTEGRATION

### Reticulospinal Pathways

The reticular pathways are numerous and complex; besides rubrospinal pathways, which are classically considered as involved in motor control, the reticular pathways originate from three main areas located in the mesencephalic, the pontine and the bulbar reticular formation. This last area is the main site of origin of the reticulospinal fibers (Torvik and Brodal, 1957; Nyberg-Hansen, 1965).

Reticulospinal fibers originating from the mesencephalon are composed mainly of cells located lateral to the periaqueductal gray matter that course through the anterior funiculus and the lateral funiculus of the spinal cord. The pontine reticulospinal neurons send fibers bilaterally, in both ventrolateral and dorsolateral funiculi, but predominantly in the latter. In the medulla, fibers from the nucleus reticularis gigantocellularis project primarily via the ipsilateral and contralateral ventral funiculi. They terminate mainly in the VI-VIII layers of Rexed, thus including the intermediolateral area of the spinal gray matter where, as mentioned earlier, most of the autonomic neurons are located. Thus, these fibers are probably involved in the control of autonomic activity, including sweating, cardiovascular activities, etc.

Fibers from the nucleus raphe magnus descend through the dorsolateral funiculus, and terminate in the marginal zone and in the substantia gelatinosa of the dorsal horn, and more deeply in laminae V, VI and VII (Basbaum et al., 1978; Holstege and Kuypers, 1987; Matsuyama et al., 1988). The nucleus reticularis magnocellularis projects via the ipsilateral dorsolateral and ventrolateral funiculi. Its projections somehow overlap with those of the raphe magnus. The fibers from periaqueductal gray matter, nucleus raphe magnus and nucleus magnocellularis are thought to be involved in the nociceptive afferents control originating from the brain stem (see Willis, 1988). Recently, a direct pathway has been described, from the caudal raphe nuclei, terminating monosynaptically on the sympathetic preganglionic neurons (Bacon et al., 1990). Furthermore, some of the bulbospinal fibers distribute to the somatic motoneuronal cell group throughout the length of the spinal cord (Kuypers, 1981; Holstege and Kuypers, 1987). In man, the course of descending fibers in the spinal cord has been reconstructed from the clinical studies of traumatic or tumoral lesions. Nathan and Smith (1987) first concluded that the evidence from cord hemisections at cervical and thoracic levels, showed that the descending pathways on each side of the cord supply sudomotor neurons bilaterally. They also concluded that the fibers supplying sudomotor neurons were located lateral to the spinal dorsal horns.

## Neurochemical Aspects

**Catecholamines.** The hypothesis that sweat secretion or electrodermal responses were modulated by catecholamines has been advanced by several researchers (Billigheimer, 1920; Darrow, 1937; Haimovici, 1950). However, the results of systemic injection of catecholamines, or of adrenoreceptor blockers have usually been equivocal (see Edelberg, 1972). The question of peripheral neuroglandular transmission, and especially the problem of the double cholinergic/adrenergic innervation are outside the scope of this paper (see Sato, 1977, 1984; Shields et al., 1987). Several researchers reconsidered, since 1974, the role of catecholamines in the central control of EDA (Koss and Davison, 1976; Koss, 1977; Walland, 1984b; Ito et al., 1988). It was found that intravenous injection of adrenalin inhibits, in dose dependent manner, the SPRs evoked either by central tegmental field stimulation or by direct stimulation of the post-ganglionic fibers (Koss et al., 1976). The injection of angiotensine, a powerful vasoconstrictor agent, has no significant effect on SPRs; this fact rules out the possibility that adrenalin acts through its vascular effects.

It is suggested that this inhibitory effect of adrenalin would involve the $\alpha$-adrenergic receptors (Bernthal and Koss, 1979; Walland, 1981). Several facts support this hypothesis. In the anaesthetized cat, the intravenous administration of the $\alpha$1-adrenoceptor antagonist, prazosin, produced a depression of the centrally evoked SPRs (Ito et al., 1988). The intravenous injection of the $\alpha$2-adrenoceptor agonist, clonidine, depresses the centrally evoked SPRs, in a dose dependent manner (Koss and Hey, 1988). The pretreatment with the $\alpha$2-adrenoceptor antagonist, yohimbine, strongly antagonized the depressive action of both prazosin and clonidine.

Futhermore, the effects of $\alpha$–antagonists on spontaneous EDA have also been studied. Prazosin depresses spontaneous EDA of intact anaesthetized cats, or unanaesthetized cats after a collicular transection, but is without effect on spinal cats. This depressant action is antagonized by yohimbine, or by a previous depletion of the monoamines (Koss et al., 1990). Taken together these results support the hypothesis of a descending inhibitory tone emanating from higher centers and acting at the spinal level. However, a certain number of points remain unclear. Thus, the site of action of clonidine on sudomotor responses is controversial. Walland (1984a, 1984b), concluded that clonidine acted on the sympathetical ganglion, but this conclusion was questioned by Koss and Hey (1988). These authors proposed different sites of action of the clonidine in central nervous system: hypothalamus, ventral medulla, spinal cord. However it must be remembered that clonidine significantly acts at the most peripheral level, on the neuroglandular junction, since it reduces the amplitude of SPRs evoked by stimulation of post-ganglionic fibers (Koss and Hey, 1988).

Finally, one wonders if the powerful inhibitory effects, obtained on EDA from the bulbar reticular formation do depend upon these catecholaminergic controls. In fact, Bernthal and Koss (1984) concluded that two inhibitory sytems acted at spinal level, a catecholaminergic one and a non-catecholaminergic one.

**Neuropeptides.** Sonoda et al., (1986) showed that the periaqueductal gray matter or the nucleus raphe dorsalis stimulation partially inhibited SPRs evoked with high threshold fiber stimulation of the splanchnic nerve, in urethan-chloralose anaesthetized cats. This effect is reversible by naloxone, an antimorphinic substance. These authors suggested the possible involvement of endogenous opioid peptides in the periaqueductal gray matter or nucleus raphe dorsalis stimulation-induced inhibition of SPR. Furthermore the sympathetic neurons in the ventral horn of the spinal cord are known to contain opioid peptide receptors (Hancok, 1982; Krukoff, 1986). They also receive many peptides containing afferent fibers (Anand and Bloom, 1984). We hypothesized that an opioid link could also be involved in bulbar inhibition of EDA ; this hypothesis is based upon the above mentioned findings: i.e. the presence of opioid receptors in the sympathetic preganglionic neurons, and the analogy with the nociceptive analgesic system. It has been shown that the bulbar reticular formation participates in the control of nociceptive afferents. This descending inhibitory control of pain involves opioid substances (see Basbaum and Fields, 1984; Willis,1988; Yaksh, 1987 for reviews). In fact, the structures involved in the bulbar inhibition of SPRs overlap with the ones involved in pain control (Basbaum et al., 1978). In order to test the hypothesis of inhibitory modulation of autonomic activity by opioid peptides, naloxone, an opioid antagonist, was injected intravenously, and its effect assessed on bulbar SPR inhibition.

Cats anaesthetized with chloralose (35 mg/kg) and paralysed with gallamine were used in the experiments. SPRs were evoked by central tegmental field stimulation and inhibited by the simultaneous bulbar reticular stimulation (see Figure 8A). The percentage of inhibition is expressed as the percentage of the mean amplitude of the SPRs evoked during the simultaneous mesencephalic and bulbar stimulations compared to the mean amplitude of the SPRs evoked by mesencephalic reticular stimulation alone. Then an intravenous injection of 1 mg/kg of naloxone was given. The evolution of the inhibition following this injection was expressed as the percentage of SPR inhibition for every three measures, i.e. during every period of six minutes, three control SPRs were compared to three inhibited SPRs.

In 6 of 7 chloralose anaesthetized cats, the intravenous injection of naloxone largely decreased the SPR inhibition. This effect was subject to important individual variations; in some instances the naloxone injection totally suppressed SPR inhibition. This suppression of inhibitory effects generally appeared during the six minutes following the injection, and reached its maximum within 9 minutes. Then the inhibition reappeared gradually. This effect of i.v. naloxone disappeared after approximately 30 minutes. Figure 10 gives the mean value for the seven cats (Traoré, 1992). We can conclude that opioid substances are involved in bulbar SPR inhibition, but cannot conclude that this mechanism takes place at spinal level.

In order to test this last hypothesis, further experiments were done using direct injections of naloxone or of naltrexone, another opioid antagonist, under the dura and above the T4-T9 segments of the spinal cord, corresponding to the command of SPRs on the forepaws. The Yaksh and Rudy (1976) method was adapted for the cat. A catheter was inserted intrathecally allowing different blockers to be injected. The effects were monitored during the bulbar SPR inhibition.

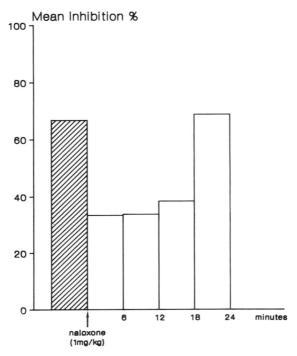

**Figure 10.** Partial suppression of bulbar SPR inhibition by intravenous injection of naloxone (1 mg/kg), in chloralose anaesthetized cat (N=7). (From Traoré, 1992)

The results showed that intrathecally injected naloxone (300 μg) suppressed the bulbar SPR inhibition to approximately 50% of its control value. This effect lasted longer with the intrathecal than with the i.v. injection. (i.e., a mean of 50 minutes for the 5 cats). After this average period of time, SPR inhibition reappeared. When the naloxone solvent was injected alone intrathecally, there was no significant effect on the intensity of the inhibition. Similar results were obtained with naltrexone intrathecally injected.

To conclude, it appears that antimorphinic substances injected at the spinal level partly and reversibly suppressed the bulbar inhibition. Firstly, there is evidence to support the previous hypothesis that the bulbar inhibitory mechanism acts at the spinal level (Roy et al., 1974). Secondly, the antagonistic effect of naloxone and naltrexone does suggest that enkephalin or related peptides are involved in this process.

It is well known that stress increases the opioid level in the organism, especially the plasma level of β–endorphine, to the point of eliciting a "stress induced analgesia". This view is in keeping with the fact that in certain subjects with an anxious personality autonomic activity can be lower than in non anxious subjects. Anxious subjects are usually considered as over-aroused and an increase in EDA usually expected. In fact the studies which examined the relationship between EDA and anxiety led to no decisive conclusions. In recent studies, it was unexpectedly found that non pathological high trait-anxiety subjects showed EDA inhibition compared to low trait-anxiety subjects (Naveteur and Freixa i Baqué, 1987; Naveteur and Roy, 1990).

**Serotonin.** It is known that the antinociception controlling system involves descending serotoninergic fibers (Rivot et al., 1980). These fibers may be responsible for pain inhibitory modulation, possibly through enkephalinergic neurons. Following this, we hypothesized that a serotoninergic mechanism could be involved in reticulo-spinal modulation of autonomic activity. This hypothesis is currently being tested using the above-mentioned experimental procedure.

That is, we first used an antagonist of the serotonin (5-HT) synthesis, the parachlorophenylalanine (PCPA), which prevents the tryptophan hydroxylation (Koe and Weissman, 1966). In the first stage, electrodes were chronically implanted in the mesencephalic central tegmental field and in the bulbar reticular formation. It was verified during narcosis, while the operation was undertaken, that the stimulation of the bulbar reticular formation actually inhibited evoked SPRs. EEG electrodes were also implanted on the cortex, and EMG electrodes into the neck muscles. After complete recovery from surgery, (usually around 10 days), PCPA was injected during 3 consecutive days, at the daily dose of 250 mg/kg. The effectiveness of the 5-HT synthesis-blockade was verified by recording the sleep cycles, since it is classically known that 5-HT depletion suppresses slow wave sleep (Delorme et al., 1966). In fact, slow wave sleep was absent in the PCPA injected cats. In the second stage, animals were anaesthetized again and the SPR inhibition evaluated. The results showed that SPR inhibition was largely diminished after the PCPA injections. In 6 cats, the average control inhibition was 75.6 % before PCPA, and decreased to 44.4 % during the 5-HT blockade.

Furthermore, in an ongoing study, 5-HT-receptor blockers are injected intrathecally above the T4-T9 segments of the spinal cord. Methysergide, a general serotonin receptor blocker was tested first. Recent results showed that, in some though not all cases, the intrathecal injection of methysergide, diminished the bulbar SPR inhibition. In these cases, the bulbar inhibition gradually returned to its previous level. These results are preliminary and, therefore, must be viewed with caution. However, to this point, some data do support the hypothesis of the involvement, in this inhibitory process, of a double neurochemical link, including serotonin and opioid related peptides.

## SUMMARY

The lower control system of EDA is located at the reticular level in the brainstem. At the spinal level, the sudomotor neurons integrate the supraspinal influences. Due to the fact that sweat glands receive only sympathetic innervation, the spinal neurons are considered more as the "final common pathway" for the control of sweating than the ganglionic neurons, which actually are the final control neurons. This is different from the general organization of the autonomic nervous system, which usually carries a double innervation to the peripheral organ. The reticular formation is not seen anymore as a unitary non-specific arousing system. Many nuclei exerting specific excitatory or inhibitory functions have been delineated. They play specific roles in motor and sensory mechanisms. They also play key roles in the autonomic control. An excitatory system has been delineated in the brain stem; reticular activations are linked with cortical arousal, and electrodermal responses are indices of the excitability of the reticulo-cortical system. The intrareticular excitability changes from deep sleep to an attentional state. A powerful EDA inhibitory system has been located in the medial ventral nuclei, at bulbar level. This last autonomic inhibitory system shows some analogy with the pain attenuating system acting from the medulla at spinal level.

Finally, arousal is considered as a basic dimension of emotion (Lang et al. 1990; Öhman et al., this volume). Emotional arousal can probably be partly attributed to the reticular activating system. It is thus of interest to know that EDRs are concomitants of the reticular activation. The arousal component of emotion reflects an energetic dimension of behavior, and thus is a purely quantitative aspect of emotion. The positive or negative value of emotional stimuli probably results from the participation of higher structures of the brain, i.e., the limbic system and the cortex. The limbic and cortical control of EDA will be presented in the next chapter.

## REFERENCES

Adams, T., and Hunter, W.S., 1969, Modification of skin mechanical properties by eccrine sweat gland activity, *J. Appl. Physiol.* 26: 417-419.

Adelman, S., Taylor, C.R., and Heglund, N.C., 1975, Sweating on paws and palms: what is its function ? *Amer. J. Physiol.* 229: 1400-1402.

Anand, P., and Bloom, S.R., 1984, Neuropeptides are selective markers of spinal cord autonomic pathways, *Trends Neurosci.* 7: 267-268.

Ba-M'Hamed-Bennis, S., 1984, *Asymétrie de l'activité électrodermale chez le chat en relation avec la vigilance.* Doctoral Dissertation. Université de Lille I. (UnPub).

Bacon, S.J., Zagon, A., and Smith, A.D., 1990, Electron microscopic evidence of a monosynaptic pathway between cells in the caudal raphe nuclei and sympathetic preganglionic neurons in the rat spinal cord, *Exp. Brain. Res.* 79: 589-602.

Basbaum, A.I., Clanton, C.H., and Fields, H.L., 1978, Three bulbospinal pathways from the rostral medulla of the cat: an autoradiographic study of pain modulating systems, *J. Comp. Neurol.* 178: 209-224.

Basbaum, A.I., and Fields, H.L., 1984, Endogenous pain control systems: brain spinal pathways and endorphin circuitry, *Ann. Rev. Neurosci.* 7: 309-338.

Bell, C., Jänig, W., Kümmel, H., and Xu, H., 1985, Differentiation of vasodilator and sudomotor responses in the cat pad to preganglionic sympathetic stimulation, *J. Physiol.* 364: 93-104.

Benoit, O., and Bloch, V., 1960, Seuils d'excitabilité réticulaire et sommeil profond chez le Chat, *J. Physiol.* (Paris) 52: 17-18.

Bernthal, P.J., and Koss, M.C., 1979, Effects of clonidine and chlorpromazine on a sympathetic-cholinergic reflex, *Eur. J. Pharmacol.* 60: 23-29.

Bernthal, P.J., Koss, M.C., 1984, Evidence for two distinct sympathoinhibitory bulbo-spinal systems, *Neuropharmacology* 23: 31-36.

Billigheimer, E., 1920, Über einen Antagonismus zwischen Pilokarpin und Adrenalin, Naunyn-Schmiedebergs Arch. Exp. Path. Pharmak. 88, 172, cited in Koss et al., 1976.

Bloch, V., 1965, Le contrôle central de l'activité électrodermale, *J. Physiol.* (Paris) 57, suppl.13: 1-132.

Bloch, V., 1993, On the centennial of the discovery of electrodermal activity. In: *Progress in Electrodermal Research*, Roy J.C., Boucsein W., Fowles D.C., and Gruzelier J., eds, Plenum Press, New York.

Bloch, V., and Bonvallet, M., 1959, Contrôle cortico-réticulaire de l'activité électrodermale, (réponse psychogalvanique), *J. Physiol.* (Paris) 51: 405-406.

Bloch, V., and Bonvallet, M., 1960a, Le déclenchement des réponses électrodermales à partir du système réticulaire facilitateur, *J. Physiol.* (Paris) 52: 25-26.

Bloch, V., and Bonvallet, M., 1960b, Le contrôle inhibiteur bulbaire des réponses électrodermales, *C.R. Soc. Biol.* 154: 42-45.

Bloch, V. and M. Bonvallet, 1961, Interactions des formations réticulaires mésencéphalique et bulbaire, *J. Physiol.* (Paris) 53, 280.

Broughton, R.J., Poiré, R., and Tassinari, C.A., 1965, The electrodermogram (Tarchanoff effect) during sleep, *Electroencephal. Clin. Neurophysiol.* 18: 691-708.

Cabot, J.B., 1990, Sympathetic preganglionic neurons: cytoarchitecture, ultrastructure, and biophysical properties. In: *Central Regulation of Autonomic Functions*, Loewy A.D., and Spyer K.M., eds, Oxford University Press, Oxford.

Chung, J.M., and Wurster, R.D., 1975, Sympathetic preganglionic neurons of the cat spinal cord: horseradish peroxidase study, *Brain Res.* 91: 126-131.

Darrow, C.W., 1927, Sensory, secretory, and electrical changes in the skin following bodily excitation, *J. Exp. Psychol.* 10: 197-225.

Darrow, C.W., 1936, The galvanic skin reflex (sweating) and blood pressure as preparatory and facilitative functions, *Psychol. Bull.* 33: 73-94.

Darrow, C.W., 1937, Neural mechanisms controlling the palmar galvanic skin reflex and palmar sweating, *Arch. Neurol. Psych.* 37: 641-663.

Davison, M.A., and Koss, M.C., 1975, Brainstem loci for activation of electrodermal response in the cat, *Amer. J. Physiol.* 229: 930-934.

Delerm, B., Delsaut, M., and Roy, J.C., 1982, Mesencephalic and bulbar reticular control of skin potential responses in kittens, *Exp. Brain Res.* 46: 209-214.

Delorme, F., Froment, J.L., and Jouvet, M., 1966, Suppression du sommeil par la p-chlorometamphétamine et p-chlorophénylalanine, *C.R. Soc. Biol.* 160: 2347-2351.

Deuschl, G., and Illert, M., 1981, Cytoarchitectonic organization of lumbar preganglionic sympathetic neurons in the cat, *J. Autonom. Nerv. Syst.* 3: 193-213.

Edelberg, R., 1972, The electrodermal system. In: *Handbook of Psychophysiology*, Greenfield N.S., and Sternbach R.A., eds, Holt, New York.

Fagius, J. and B.G. Wallin, 1980, Sympathetic reflex latencies and conduction velocities in normal man, *J. Neurol. Sci.* 47, 433.

Féré, C., 1988, Note sur les modifications de la tension électrique dans le corps humain, *C.R. Soc. Biol.* 5: 28-33.

Fowles, D.C., 1986, The eccrine system and electrodermal activity. In: *Psychophysiology: Systems, processes and applications*, Coles M.G.H., Donchin E., and Porges S.G., eds, Elsevier, Amsterdam.

Freixa i Baqué, E., Chevalier, B., Grubar, J.C., Lambert, C., Lancry, A., Leconte, P., Meriaux, H., and Spreux, F., 1983, Spontaneous electrodermal activity during sleep in man: an intra-night study, *Sleep* 6: 77-81.

Freixa i Baqué, E., Delerm, B., and Roy, J.C., 1981, Spontaneous electrodermal activity during sleep and waking in cats, *Psychophysiology* 18: 410-414.

Girardot, M.-N., and Koss, M.C., 1984, A physiological and pharmacological analysis of the electrodermal response in the rat, *Eur. J. Pharmacol.* 98: 185-191.

Haimovici, H., 1950, Evidence for adrenergic sweating in man, *J. Appl. Physiol.* 2: 512-521.

Hancock, M.B., 1982, Leu-enkephalin, substance P, and somatostatin immunohistochemistry combined with the retrograde transport of horseradish peroxidase in sympathetic preganglionic neurons, *J. Autonom. Nerv. Syst.* 6: 263-272.

Hata, T., Kita, R., Yoneda, R., and Tanada, S., 1981, Effects of exogenous stimuli and centrally acting drugs on galvanic skin responses in rats, *Jap. J. Pharmacol.* 31: 23-31.

Head, H., and Riddoch, G., 1917, The automatic bladder, excessive sweating and some other reflex conditions, in gross injuries of the spinal cord, *Brain* 34: 102-254.

Henry, J.L., and Calaresu, F.R., 1972, Topography and numerical distribution of neurons of the thoraco-lumbar intermediolateral nucleus in the cat, *J. Comp. Neurol.* 144: 205-213.

Hermann, L., and Luchsinger, B., 1878, Über die Sekretionsstroeme der Haut, *Archives Gestalt Physiologie* 19: 300-319.

Holstege, G., and Kuypers, H.G.J.M., 1987, Brainstem projections to spinal motoneurons: an update, *Neuroscience* 23: 809-821.

Ito, T., Hey, J.A., and Koss, M.C., 1988, Studies on the mechanism of prazosin induced sympatho-inhibition, *J. Pharmacol.* 158: 225-231.

Jänig, W., Krauspe, R., and Wiedersatz, G., 1982, Transmission of impulses from pre to post-ganglionic vaso-constrictor and sudomotor neurons, *J. Autonom. Nerv. Syst.* 6: 95-100.

Jänig, W., and Kümmel, H., 1977, Functional discrimination of postganglionic neurons to the cat's hindpaw with respect to the skin potentials recorded from the hairless skin, *Pflügers Arch.* 371: 217-225.

Jänig, W., and Kümmel, H., 1981, Organization of the sympathetic innervation supplying the hairless skin of the cat's paw, *J. Autonom. Nerv. Syst.* 3: 215-230.

Jänig, W., Sundlöf, G., and Wallin, B.G., 1983, Discharge patterns of sympathetic neurons supplying skeletal muscle and skin in man and cat, *J. Autonom. Nerv. Syst.* 7: 239-256.

Jänig, W., and Szulczyk, P., 1981, The organization of lumbar preganglionic neurons, *J. Autonom. Nerv. Syst.* 3: 177-191.

Johnson, L.C., and Lubin, A., 1966, Spontaneous electrodermal activity during sleeping and waking, *Psychophysiology* 3: 8-17.

Koe, B.K., and Weissman, A., 1966, Parachlorophenylalanine: a specific depletor of brain serotonin, *J. Pharmacol. Exp. Ther.* 154: 499-516.

Koss, M.C., 1977, Effect of clonidine and chlorpromazine on centrally evoked electrodermal responses and their interaction with yohimbine, *Eur. J. Pharmacol.* 41: 221-224.

Koss, M.C., and Davison, M.A., 1976, The electrodermal response as a model for central sympathetic reactivity: the action of clonidine, *Eur. J. Pharmacol.* 37: 71.

Koss, M.C., Davison, M.A., and Bernthal, P.J., 1976, Epinephrine inhibition of the electrodermal response in the cat, *Psychopharmacology* 50: 149-152.

Koss, M.C., and Hey, J.A., 1988, Clonidine inhibits electrodermal responses by an action on the spinal cord, *Eur. J. Pharmacol.* 148: 397-403.

Koss, M.C., Hey J.A., and Ito, T., 1990, Effect of prazosin on spontaneous sympathetic-cholinergic activity, *Eur. J. Pharmacol.* 182: 381-386.

Krukoff, T.L., 1986, Peptidic inputs to sympathetic preganglionic neurons, *Can. J. Pharmacol.* 65: 1619-1623.

Kumazawa, T., and Naotsuka, T., 1970, Inhibition of galvanic skin response by the splanchnic afferent, *Experientia* 25: 148-149.

Kumazawa, T., T. Naotsuka and K. Takagi, 1968, (in japanese), cited by Kumazawa and Naotsuka, 1970.

Kuypers, H.G.J.M., 1981, Anatomy of the descending pathways. In: *Handbook of Physiology. The Nervous System, vol.II.*, Brookhart J.M., and Mountcastle V.B., eds, Amer.Physiol.Soc., Washington.

Ladpli, R., and Wang, G.H., 1960, Spontaneous variations of skin potentials in footpads of normal, striatal and spinal cats, *J. Neurophysiol.* 23: 448-452.

Lang, P.J., Bradley, M.M., and Cuthbert, B.N., 1990, Emotion, attention and the startle reflex, *Psychol. Rev.* 97: 377-395.

Langley, J.N., 1891, On the course and connections of the secretory fibers supplying the sweat glands of the feet of the cat, *J. Physiol.* (London), 12: 347-374.

Langley, J.N., 1922, The secretion of sweat. Part I, *J. Physiol.* (London) 56: 110-119.

Laskey, W., and Polosa, C., 1988, Characteristics of the sympathetic preganglionic neuron and its synaptic input, *Prog. Neurobiol.* 31: 47-84.

Lazarus, R., and McCleary, R.A., 1951, Autonomic discrimination without awareness: a study of subception, *Psychol. Rev.* 58: 113-122.

Lindsley, D.B., 1951, Emotion. In: *Handbook of Experimental Psychology*, Stevens S.S., ed, John Wiley, New York, pp 473-517.

Lundberg, A., and Vyklicky, L., 1963, Brain stem control of reflex paths to primary afferents, *Acta Physiol. Scand.* 59, suppl.213: 1-91.

Magoun, H.W., and Rhines, R., 1946, An inhibitory mechanism in the bulbar reticular formation, *J. Neurophysiol.* 9: 165-171.

Mandel, A.J., and Bach, L.M.N., 1957, Failure of bulbar inhibitory reticular formation to affect somatic reflex activity in the unanesthetized cat, *Amer J Physiol* 190: 330-332.

Matsuyma, K., Ohta, Y., and Mori, S., 1988, Ascending and descending projections of the nucleus reticularis gigantocellularis in the cat demonstrated by the anterograde neural tracer, Phaseolus vulgaris leucoagglutinin (PHA-L), *Brain Res.* 460: 124-141.

McAllen, R.M., 1986, Action and specificity of ventral medullary vasopressor neurons in the cat. *Neuroscience* 18: 51-59.

Moruzzi, G., and Magoun, H.W., 1949, Brain stem reticular formation and the activation of the EEG, *Electroencephal. Clin. Neurophysiol.* 1: 455-473.

Nathan, P.W., and Smith, M., 1987, The location of descending fibres to sympathetic preganglionic vasomotor and sudomotor neurons in man, *J. Neurol. Neurosurg. Psychiat.* 50: 1253-1262.

Naveteur, J., and Freixa i Baqué, E., 1987, Individual differences in electrodermal activity as a function of subjects anxiety, *Pers. Indiv. Diff.* 8: 615-626.

Naveteur, J., and Roy, J.C., 1990, Electrodermal activity of low and high trait anxiety subjects during a frustrative video game, *J. Psychophysiol.* 4: 221-227.

Neuman, E., and Blanton, R., 1970, The early history of electrodermal research, *Psychophysiology* 6: 453-475.

Niemer, W.T., and Magoun, H.W., 1947, Reticulospinal tracts influencing motor activity, *J. Comp. Neurol.* 87: 367-379.

Nyberg-Hansen, R., 1965, Sites and mode of termination of reticulospinal fibers in the cat. An experimental study with silver impregnation methods, *J. Comp. Neur.* 124: 71-100.

Öhman, A., Esteves, F., Flykt, A., and Soares, J.J.F., 1993, Gateways to consciousness: emotion, attention, and electrodermal activity. In: *Progress in Electrodermal Research*, Roy, J.C., Boucsein, W., Fowles, D.C., and Gruzelier, J., eds, Plenum Press, New York.

Patton, H.D., 1948, Secretory innervation of the cat's foot-pad, *J. Neurophysiol.* 11: 211-227.

Rao, U.C., and Bijlani, V., 1980, The intermediolateral gray column in the spinal cord of macaca mulatta, *J. Autonom. Nerv. Syst.* 2: 259-267.

Riddoch, G., 1917, The reflex functions of the completely-divided spinal cord in man compared with those associated with less severe lesions, *Brain* 40: 264.

Rivot, J.P., Chaouch, A., and Besson, J.M., 1980, Nucleus raphe magnus modulation of response of rat dorsal horn neurons to unmyelinated fibers inputs: partial involvement of serotonergic pathways, *J. Neurophysiol.* 44: 1039-1057.

Roy, J.C., and Bloch, V., 1968, Le lieu de l'action inhibitrice bulbaire sur les réponses électrodermales, *C.R. Soc. Biol.* 162: 1961-1964.

Roy, J.C., Delerm, B., and Granger, L., 1974, L'inhibition bulbaire et l'activité électrodermale chez le chat, *Electroenceph. Clin. Neurophysiol.* 37: 621-632.

Roy, J.C., and Denti, A., 1967, Inhibition des réponses électrodermales par stimulation des fibres afférentes des nerfs vagues, *J. Physiol.* (Paris) 59: 492-493.

Roy, J.C., Leisinger-Trigona, M.C., and Bloch, V., 1977; Seuils réticulaires de déclenchement des réponses électrodermales chez le chat, *Arch. Ital. Biol.* 115: 171-184.

Rubin, E., and Purves, D., 1980, Segmental organization of sympathetic preganglionic neurons in the mammalian spinal cord, *J. Comp. Neurol.* 192: 163-174.

Sato, K., 1977, The physiology, pharmacology, and biochemistry of the eccrine sweat gland. *Rev. Physiol. Biochem. Pharmacol.* 79: 51-131.

Sato, K., 1984, Update on pharmacology of the eccrine sweat gland, *Trends Pharmacol. Sci.* 391-393.

Sequeira, H., and Roy, J.C., 1993, Cortical and hypothalamo-limbic control of electrodermal activity. In: *Progress in Electrodermal Research*, Roy J.C., Boucsein W., Fowles D.C., and Gruzelier J., eds, Plenum Press, New York.

Shields, S.A., Mac Dowell, K.A., Fairchild, S.B., and Campbell, M.L., 1987, Is mediation of sweating cholinergic, adrenergic, or both? A comment on the literature, *Psychophysiology* 24: 312-319.

Sonoda, H., Ikenoue, K., and Yokota, T., 1986, Periaqueductal gray inhibition of viscerointercostal and galvanic skin reflexes, *Brain Res.* 369: 91-102.

Sprague, J.M., and Chambers, W.W., 1954, Control of posture by reticular formation and cerebellum in the intact anesthetized and unanesthetized and in the decerebrated cat, *Amer. J. Physiol.* 176: 52-64.

Tarchanoff, G., 1890, Ueber die galvanische Erscheinungen an der Haut des Menschen bei Reizung der Sinnesorgane und bei verschieden Formen der psychologischen Taetigkeit, *Arch. Ges. Physiol.* 40: 46-55.

Torvik, A., and Brodal, A., 1957, The origin of reticulospinal fibers in the cat, *Anat. Rec.* 128: 113-135.

Tranel, D., and Damasio, A.R., 1985, Knowledge without awareness: an autonomic index of facial recognition by prosopagnosics, *Science* 228: 1453-1454.

Tranel, D., Fowles, D.C., and Damasio, A.R., 1985, Electrodermal discrimination of familiar and unfamiliar faces: a methodology, *Psychophysiology*, 22: 403-408.

Traoré, M., 1992, *Etude des neurotransmetteurs de la régulation inhibitrice de l'activité électrodermale.* Master's Thesis, University of Lille III. (UnPub)·

Venables, P., 1991, Autonomic activity. In: *Windows on the Brain: Neuropsychology Technological Frontiers*, Zappula R.A., Lefever F.F., Jaeger J., and Bilder R., eds, Ann. N.Y. Acad.Sci., vol.620, New York.

Vernet-Maury, E., 1970, Réponses électrodermales chez le rat aux stimulations visuelles, auditives et olfactives, *J. Physiol.* (Paris) 62, 225.

Walland, A., 1981, Inhibition of neurosympathetic sudomotor activity by stimulation of postsynaptic $\alpha2$-adrenoreceptors in the stellate ganglion of the cat, *Arch. Pharmacol.* 316: 857.

Walland, A., 1984a, Clonidine inhibits nicotinic effects in ganglia of the cholinergic sympathetic system, *Eur. J. Pharmacol.* 102: 39-45.

Walland, A., 1984b, Clonidine inhibits electrodermal potentials induced by preganglionic stimulation, *Eur. J. Pharmacol.* 102: 47-53.

Wallin, G., and Fagius, J., 1986, The sympathetic nervous system in man - aspects derived from microelectrode recordings, *Trends Neurosci.* 9: 63-67 (Abstract).

Wang, G.H., 1957, The galvanic skin reflex. A review of old and recent works from a physiologic point of view (part 1), *Amer. J. Physiol.* 36: 295-320.

Wang, G.H., 1958, The galvanic skin reflex: a review of old and recent works from a physiologic point of view (part 2), *Amer. J. Phys. Med.* 37: 35-57.

Wang, G.H., and Brown, V.W., 1956, Suprasegmental inhibition of an autonomic reflex, *J. Neurophysiol.* 19: 564-572.

Wang, G.H., and Chun, R.W.S., 1967, Sweating under different ambiant temperatures in normal, striatal and thalamic cats, *Arch. Ital. Biol.* 105: 379-392.

Wang, G.H., and Hind, J.E., 1959, Supraspinal origin of a post-stimulatory long-lasting inhibition of galvanic skin reflex, *J. Neurophysiol.* 22: 360-366.

Wang, G.H., Stein, P., and Brown, V.W., 1956, Brainstem reticular system and galvanic skin reflex in acute decerebrate cats, *J. Neurophysiol.* 190: 350-355.

Willis, W.D., 1988, Anatomy and physiology of descending control of nociceptive responses of dorsal horn neurons: comprehensive review. In: *Progress in Brain Research, vol.77.*, Fiels H.L., and Besson, J.M., eds, Elsevier, Amsterdam, pp 1-29.

Yaksh, T.L., 1987, Opioid receptor systems and the endorphins: a review of their spinal organization, *J. Neurosurg.* 67: 157-176.

Yaksh, T.L., and Rudy, T.A., 1976, Chronic catheterization of the spinal subarachnoid space, *Physiol. Behav.* 17: 1031-1036.

Yamazaki, K., Tajimi, T., Okuda, K., and Niimi, Y., 1975, Skin potential activity in rats, cats and primates (including man): A phylogenetic point of view. *J. Comp. Physiol. Psychol.* 89: 364-370.

Yokota, T., Sato, A., and Fujimori, B., 1963, Analysis of inhibitory influence of bulbar reticular formation upon sudomotor activity, *Jap. J. Physiol.* 13: 145-154.

# CORTICAL AND HYPOTHALAMO-LIMBIC CONTROL

## OF ELECTRODERMAL RESPONSES

Henrique Sequeira[1,2] and Jean-Claude Roy[2]

[1]Fédération Universitaire et Polytechnique de Lille (FUPL)
Département de Psychologie
59016 Lille Cedex, France

[2]Laboratoire de Neurosciences du Comportement
Université des Sciences et Technologies de Lille (USTL)
59655 Villeneuve d'Ascq Cedex, France

## INTRODUCTION

Hughlings Jackson (1869) was among the first authors to report cortical influences upon the autonomic nervous system. Following Jackson's studies, cardiovascular changes were elicited by stimulation of the frontal cortex (Danilewsky, 1875; Bochefontaine, 1876). At the beginning of this century, some authors (Bechterew, 1905; Karplus and Kreidl, 1909) also obtained an increase of sweating in the foot-pads of the cat, evoked by stimulating the sensorimotor cortex. During the next decades, other reports approached the role of cortical areas in the regulation of autonomic responses (see reviews of Kaada, 1951; Delgado, 1960; Hoff et al., 1963).

The electrodermal activity (EDA) is under the control of the sympathetic branch of the autonomic nervous system and, at central level, the reticular formation is the main center for its command (see Roy et al., this volume). However, one cannot ignore that the hypothalamo-limbic structures play a key role in the control of autonomic activity. But besides the exploration of the hypothalamus and of some limbic and cortical areas not many neurophysiological studies were devoted to the suprareticular control of EDA. Exploratory studies concerning the role of the thalamus and striatal centers, in animals and in humans reported contradictory results (Freeman and Krasno, 1940; Wang and Brown, 1956; Wang, 1964; Bloch, 1965; Sourek, 1965). These studies remain too scarce, and will be not discussed in the present paper.

No recent reviews have been devoted specifically to the cortical and hypothalamo-limbic control of EDA; furthermore, methodological considerations and divergence of results, obtained mainly by stimulation techniques, indicate that such central influences need to be more precisely asserted. Consequently, in this chapter, we will examine the evidence of hypothalamo-limbic and cortical control of electrodermal activity; our analysis will focus on results obtained in experiments with animals (Table I summarizes the experimental conditions and key findings of these experiments). The evidence will be evaluated with respect to the following points: firstly, the participation of the hypothalamus, the limbic structures and the frontal and parietal cortical areas in the control of the EDA; secondly, the pyramidal involvement of the cortical command in the same activity; thirdly, the lateralization of cortical EDA control. We will present data both from literature and from our experimental studies, on the cat. Considering the well-known connections between the hypothalamus and the limbic system (Loewy, 1990), we will present first the findings concerning the hypothalamus, in relation to the limbic control of EDA.

## HYPOTHALAMO-LIMBIC CONTROL OF EDA

### Hypothalamus

Following the classical work of Hess (1954), the hypothalamus is thought to be the main center of autonomic command in the brain. Furthermore, the hypothalamus is known to be centrally implicated in the sympathetic activation of somatic and emotional expressions of behavior (preparedness to "fight and flight reaction", Cannon, 1929). The localisation in the hypothalamus of a "defense area" (Hess and Brugger, 1943) integrating somatic, autonomic and neuroendocrine efferences, confirmed the central role of a such structure in the autonomic activation. As early as 1909, Karplus and Kreidl had demonstrated that stimulating the "tuber cinereum" (medial hypothalamus), in the cat, evoked several autonomic reactions, including a rise in arterial blood pressure and profuse sweating on the pads of all paws. Other early studies have demonstrated hypothalamic participation in the control of sweat gland activity (Wang and Richter, 1928; Hasama, 1929). Such findings were interpreted as indicating that the hypothalamus plays a central role in thermoregulation; thus, it is not surprising to find that the hypothalamus is implicated in the control of the electrodermal activity. In order to support the view that there is such a control, we will review successively results obtained from anterior, medial and posterior hypothalamus (see Table I).

In 1955, Katsumi claimed that the electrical stimulation of anterior nuclei inhibited the evoked skin potential responses (SPRs). Conversely, a lesion of preoptic and other nuclei of the anterior hypothalamus increased the reflexively evoked SPRs. Such an inhibitory function did not receive experimental support in later animal researches. But, in further studies in the cat, Bloch and Bonvallet (1960) elicited SPRs with low thresholds from the ventricular area; Yokota et al. (1963), Celesia and Wang (1964) and Davison and Koss (1975) also evoked SPRs by the stimulation of several nuclei of the anterior hypothalamus. In 1965, Bloch found that it was possible to elicit SPRs from the anterior and postero-lateral hypothalamus with thresholds as low as those of reticular stimulations. However, in the rat, Girardot and Koss (1984) found that the stimulation of the more anterior hypothalamic points rarely evoked SPRs. Available results from humans do not allow a clear excitatory or an inhibitory role in the control of EDA to be attributed to the anterior hypothalamus (Bartfai et al., 1987; Cannon et al., 1988; Schnur et al., 1989).

As previously mentioned, Wang and Richter (1928) first demonstrated an excitatory influence on EDA from the stimulation of the medial hypothalamus in the cat. This result was later reproduced (Langworthy and Richter, 1930; Wang and Lu, 1930; Fujimori et al., 1953; Katsumi, 1955; Celesia and Wang, 1964).

In the cat, Katsumi (1955) reported that the electrical stimulation of the posterior hypothalamus facilitated the reflexively evoked SPRs; the lesion of the same region resulted in a lowering of spontaneous or evoked SPRs amplitude by skin, visual or auditory stimulation. In 1975, Davison and Koss, showed that hypothalamic reactive sites eliciting the greatest SPR amplitude were localized in the rostral border of the posterior hypothalamus. In the rat, Girardot and Koss (1984), Walland (1986) and Koss and Hey (1988) obtained similar results.

Taken together, data from the three hypothalamic regions indicate that the anterior, medial and posterior hypothalamus exert an excitatory influence on the EDA. In classical studies on thermoregulation (Magoun et al., 1938), the sudation was triggered in the paws of cats by thermally stimulating the preoptic and supraoptic areas. Moreover, Wang claimed a *"predominance of the anterior hypothalamus as an excitatory sweat center"* (Wang, 1964, p. 104). Detailed analysis of Wang's work cited here shows some methodological uncertainties, for example, hypothalamic preparations where *"The amount of neural tissue removed from the dorsal thalamus varies from one operation to another"* (p.21). The opposite findings of Katsumi (1955) showing an inhibitory function of the anterior hypothalamus, suggest that further clarification regarding the role of anterior hypothalamus is needed.

Finally, three points should be emphasized: first, in keeping with the work done by most authors, we followed the classical division of anterior, medial and posterior hypothalamus; this anatomical division is not precise enough and, in future animal researches, a stereotaxic exploration of the hypothalamus, nucleus by nucleus, should be carried out; second, it is well known that there are several ascending and descending pathways passing through the hypothalamus (e.g., mesolimbic pathways) and consequently, further studies should use neurochemical methods stimulating specifically the soma of neurons to avoid implicating such "en route" fibers; third, considering this last point and hypothalamic projections to the reticular structures, it is not easy to differentiate between hypothalamic and reticular effects on EDA. Hypothalamo-reticular fibers are known from Ramon y Cajal (1909). The existence of such fibers has been largely confirmed in cats (Beattie et al., 1930; Holstege, 1987) and in rats (Sofroniew and Schrell, 1980; Luiten et al., 1985). Similarly, electrophysiological studies indicate close relations between the hypothalamic and the mesencephalic neurons (Edinger et al., 1977). However, we cannot exclude a direct hypothalamo-spinal control on EDA. Recent data, obtained in rats, cats and monkeys, showed that fibers arising from several hypothalamic nuclei (supraoptic and paraventricular nuclei, dorsal hypothalamus, posterior hypothalamic area, lateral hypothalamic area) project to the intermediolateral nucleus of the spinal cord (Saper et al., 1976; Cechetto and Saper, 1988; Hosoya et al., 1991), where are localized preganglionic sudomotor neurons (Oldfield and MacLachlan, 1981).

To conclude, there is neuroanatomical support in favour of a hypothalamic descending control of EDA by neuronal relays in the brain stem or directly at spinal level. As far as EDA is concerned, it has been hypothesized (Bloch and Bonvallet, 1960) that the posterior hypothalamus is a functional continuum of the mesencephalic reticular formation which corresponds to the classical reticular activating system (RAS). Data presented here are in favour of such a theoretical view.

## Limbic system

The first limbic studies approaching physiological mechanisms related to electrodermal responses showed that, in the cat and in the monkey respectively, the cingulate gyrus participates in the control of sweating (Ward, 1948; Showers and Crosby, 1958); further researches have focussed on the EDA control by specific limbic regions: hippocampus, amygdala and limbic cortex.

Findings with respect to hippocampus are mixed. Yokota et al. (1963), in non anaesthetized curarized cats, obtained an inhibition of SPR amplitude by stimulating the hippocampus. Also, according to Pribram and McGuiness (1975), monkeys with hippocampectomy present a decrease of skin conductance reponses (SCRs) habituation. But Bagshaw et al. (1965) found, also in monkeys, that bilateral lesions of the hippocampus did not influence electrodermal responses. In humans, lesions including the hippocampus did not affect SCRs (Tranel et al., 1990). Finally, in a recent study using Positron Emission Tomography (PET) in schizophrenics, Hazlett et al. (in press) concluded that the hippocampus has an unexpected excitatory role on SCRs.

The amygdala, contrary to the hippocampus, is generally considered to have an excitatory influence on electrodermal activity. In non-anaesthetized cats, the stimulation with strong intensities of the amygdala produced an increase of SPR amplitude (Yokota et al., 1963). Similarly, in lightly anaesthetized cats, Lang et al. (1964) evoked SPRs by the stimulation of the amygdaloid nucleus with weak intensities; the stimulation of the basolateral part of such nucleus gave rise to SPRs of longest duration and shortest latency; furthermore, the stimulation with increased intensity elicited amygdaloid afterdischarges and skin potential level (SPL) variations were then observed. These authors suggested that SPL variations were elicited through reticular activation (Lang et al., 1964). This suggestion is in accordance with knowledge of descending projections from the amygdala to the reticular formation (Hopkins and Holstege, 1978; see Loewy, 1990) and of the control exerted by such structures on EDA. In monkeys, Bagshaw et al. (1965) showed that amygdalectomy diminished the frequency of SPRs to below the level of the most unreactive normal animals; similarly, Bagshaw and Benzies (1968) and Bagshaw and Coppock (1968) found that electrodermal responses were abolished by a bilateral amygdalectomy. These results are in accordance with the classical knowledge that bilateral amygdalectomy induces an apathetic state in animal.

In humans, Dallakyan et al. (1970) reported that the destruction of the amygdala and the medio-basal parts of the temporal lobe had an inhibitory effect on the production of SCRs. Similarly, Raine et al. (1991) using magnetic resonance image (MRI) technique showed that more SCRs, produced by orienting stimuli, were significantly associated with a larger area of left temporal/amygdala regions. However, Tranel and Damasio (1989) and Tranel et al. (1990) stated respectively that patients "*whose entire amygdaloid complex had been destroyed bilaterally*" (p. 381) or showing a "*bilateral mineralization of the amygdala, possibly including the amygdala-hippocampal transition area*" (p. 350) could normally generate SCRs. These studies confirmed results already obtained by Lee et al. (1988) but do not support the idea of an excitatory influence of the amygdala on EDA. Moreover, psychopathological studies, conducted in schizophrenics, support only partially the excitatory role of amygdala (Raine and Lencz, this volume).

The participation of the limbic cortex in eliciting SPRs was clearly shown by Isamat (1961) by direct electrical stimulation of the cortical surface. This work leads to the conclusion that SPRs were most readily evoked by the stimulation of the anterior limbic cortex, around and below the corpus callosum, and the infralimbic cortical areas. However, Kimble et al. (1965) found in the monkey that partial ablation of the anterior cingulate cortex and of the medial frontal cortex, had no effect on EDA. Similarly, an ablation of the anterior region of the limbic cortex did not modify the EDA in the cat (Wilcott, 1967). In these studies, lesions affect structures outside the limbic system and make it difficult to delineate specific limbic electrodermal effects.

Recently, neurochemical techniques were introduced in animal studies in order to identify the role of noradrenergic and dopaminergic pathways, especially the mesolimbic dopamine system, on EDA eliciting (Yamamoto et al., 1984, 1985, 1990). These authors showed that intraventricular administration of 6-hydroxydopamine (6-OHDA, a neurotoxin selectively destroying catecholamine neurons) eliminated habituation of the SCRs to repeated auditory stimuli; the impairement of the habituation was accompanied by a low rate of spontaneous SCRs. Yamamoto et al. (1985) hypothesized that the slow rate of habituation of SCRs, observed in schizophrenia (Gruzelier and Venables, 1973), may be

TABLE I. Main findings of papers on hypothalamo-limbic and cortical control of electrodermal activity (EDA), in animal. Effects on EDA are presented as: (+) excitatory; (-) inhibitory; (=) no effect. Authors are cited in alphabetical order.

| References | Animal | Structure | Anaesthesia | Techniques | Effects |
|---|---|---|---|---|---|
| *Hypothalamus* | | | | | |
| Bloch (1965) | cat | anterior and posterior hypothalamus | curarized, non-anaesthetized | electrical stimulation (S) | ( + ) |
| Bloch & Bonvallet (1960) | cat | anterior hypothalamus | non-anaesthetized | S | ( + ) |
| Celesia & Wang (1964) | cat | anterior and medial hypothalamus | chloralose and urethane | S | ( + ) |
| Davison & Koss (1975) | cat | anterior and posterior hypothalamus | chloralose | S | ( + ) |
| Fujimori et al. (1953) | cat | medial hypothalamus | non-anaesthetized | S | ( + ) |
| Girardot & Koss (1984) | rat | posterior hypothalamus | pentobarbital or chloral hydrate | S | ( + ) |
| | | anterior hypothalamus | | S | ( = ) |
| Katsumi (1955) | cat | posterior hypothalamus | non-anaesthetized | S | ( + ) |
| | | | | lesion | ( - ) |
| | | anterior hypothalamus | non-anaesthetized | S | ( - ) |
| | | | | lesion | ( + ) |
| Koss & Hey (1988) | cat | posterior hypothalamus | pentobarbital | S | ( + ) |
| Langworthy & Richter (1930) | cat | medial hypothalamus | ether | S | ( + ) |
| Walland (1986) | cat | posterior hypothalamus | chloralose or ketamine | S | ( + ) |
| Wang & Richter (1928) | cat | medial hypothalamus | urethane | S | ( + ) |
| Wang & Lu (1930) | cat | medial hypothalamus | ether | S | ( + ) |
| Yokota et al. (1963) | cat | anterior hypothalamus | curarized, non-anaesthetized | S | ( + ) |
| *Limbic System* | | | | | |
| Bagshaw et al. (1965) | monkey | amygdala | chronic | ablation | ( - ) |
| | | hippocampus | monkey | ablation | ( = ) |

(continued)

TABLE I. (Continued)

| | | | | | |
|---|---|---|---|---|---|
| Bagshaw & Benzies (1968) | monkey | amygdala | chronic monkey | ablation | ( = ) |
| Bagshaw & Coppock (1968) | monkey | amygdala | chronic monkey | ablation | ( - ) |
| Isamat (1961) | cat | anterior an inferior limbic cortex | chloralose and urethane | S | ( + ) |
| Kimble et al. (1965) | monkey | cingulate cortex | chronic monkey | ablation | ( - ) |
| Lang et al. (1964) | cat | amygdaloid nucleus | methohexitone | S | ( + ) |
| Wang & Lu (1930) | cat | orbitary gyrus | ether or chloralose | S | ( + ) |
| Wilcott (1967) | cat | anterior limbic region | chronic cat | ablation | ( = ) |
| Yokota et al. (1963) | cat | amygdala | curarized | S | ( + ) |
| | | fornix, hipoccampus | non-anaesthetized | S | ( - ) |

### Other Subcortical Structures

| | | | | | |
|---|---|---|---|---|---|
| Bloch (1965) | cat | thalamus | curarized, | S | ( = ) |
| | | basal ganglia | non-anaesthetized | S | ( = ) |
| | | septum | | S | ( = ) |
| Freeman and Krasno (1940) | cat | caudate nucleus | pentobarbital | S | ( - ) |
| Wang (1964) | cat | thalamus | chloralose or urethane | S | ( + ) |
| Wang and Brown (1956) | cat | cerebellum | chloralose | S | ( - ) |
| | | caudate nucleus | or urethane | S | ( - ) |

### Neocortex

| | | | | | |
|---|---|---|---|---|---|
| Bagshaw et al. (1965) | monkey | lateral prefrontal cortex | chronic monkey | lesion | ( - ) |
| Isamat (1961) | cat | anterior medial cortex | chloralose and urethane | S | ( = ) |
| Langworthy & Richter (1930) | cat | premotor area | decerebrated | S | ( + ) |
| Schwartz (1937) | cat | premotor area | non-anaesthetized | lesion | ( - ) |
| Sequeira-Martinho et al. (1986a) | cat | areas 4,3,2,1,5,7 | curarized, non-anaesthetized | S | ( + ) |
| Spiegel & Hunsicker (1936) | cat | frontal and sygmoid gyri | ether | S | ( + ) |

ed)

TABLE I. (Continued)

| | | | | | |
|---|---|---|---|---|---|
| Wang & Brown (1956) | cat | anterior sigmoid gyrus | chloralose or urethane | S | ( - ) |
| Wang & Lu (1930) | cat | sigmoid gyrus | ether or urethane | S | ( + ) |
| Wang & Mok (1931) | cat | motor cortex | ether or urethane | S | ( + ) |
| Wilcott (1967) | cat | pericruciate area | chronic cat | ablation | ( + ) |
| Wilcott (1969) | cat | premotor area | chronic cat | S | ( + ) |
| Wilcott & Bradley (1970) | cat | premotor area | chronic cat | S | ( - ) |
| Wilcott & Hoel (1973) | cat | anterior sigmoid gyrus | chronic cat | S | ( + ) |

explained by some dysfunction of the catecholaminergic system, particularly the mesolimbic component. In order to determine which catecholamine, the dopamine (DA) or the noradrenaline (NA), is responsible for SCR impairments in experimentally treated animals, these same authors (Yamamoto et al., 1990) destroyed at brain stem level the DA and NA ascending systems, in the cat. Results showed that a selective lesion of the DA system did not elicit any change in the skin conductance activity. By contrast, the destruction of the NA system of the brain eliminated the SCRs to auditory stimuli, decreased the frequency of spontaneous SCRs and lowered the skin conductance level (SCL). These results, obtained by selective pharmacological interventions can contribute to identifying, in animals, neural networks implicated in the impairments of SCRs and have some interest for human studies like those conducted in schizophrenics (Gruzelier and Venables, 1973).

Recent neuroanatomical studies have brought data indicating that limbic influences can be transmitted to spinal preganglionic neurons, either by hypothalamic relays (Price and Amaral, 1981), by reticular structures (Hopkins and Holstege, 1978; see Loewy, 1990) or by direct projections to preganglionic sudomotor neurons (Mizuno et al., 1985; Sandrew et al., 1986). Limbic structures have a complex variety of inputs and outputs and have been implicated in a wide range of reponses integrating autonomic expression of emotions. The close relations of limbic structures with the cerebral cortex (orbital, insular and frontal) and the complexity of descending connections (Loewy, 1990) seem to indicate that limbic influences are integrated under cortical control.

## CORTICAL CONTROL OF EDA

### Reviewed data

As indicated previously, the first studies of the cortical command of sweating were carried out at the beginning of this century and those using direct records of EDA appeared in the twenties (Foà and Peserico, 1923; Dennig, 1924). However, such results, mainly obtained from animal studies, should be evaluated from a methodological point of view. For example, let us consider the use of electrical stimulation techniques: firstly, the localisation of stimulating points is insufficiently described; secondly, the use of high stimulation intensities favored the eliciting of epileptic discharges and the diffusion of the current to subcortical structures and to non neural elements, such as meninges (Bard, 1929). Further studies showed that the stimulation of blood vessels at the cortical surface elicits electrodermal responses with similar thresholds as those of the direct cortical stimulation (Wilcott, 1969). Finally, the use of different types of anaesthesia the action of which is known to modify the cortical activity, complicated the interpretation of results and may explain some differences observed from one experiment to another and sometimes within the same study. From the thirties, a more rigourous approach for eliciting autonomic responses from the cortex was developed (Hoff and Green, 1936; Kaada, 1951). This is true as far as cardiovascular indices are concerned (see Delgado, 1960); unfortunatly, electrodermal studies did not benefit from similar methodological improvements (Langworthy and Richter, 1930; Wang and Lu, 1930).

Cortical studies have been mainly concerned with the identification of excitatory or inhibitory effects of the frontal cortex on EDA. The frontal cortex, mainly the pericruciate area, is the origin of the somatic programs to elaborate directional movements. Darrow (1937) developed the idea of a close association between motor and secretory activity of the extremities. In such hypothesis, the palmar sweating can be considered as a factor of skin protection and a help to perform movements, like grasping. Reinforced by Darrow's hypothesis, the interest for the exploration of the frontal cortex on the control of EDA, increased in the sixties when Luria (1966) developed the idea, confirmed by clinical data, of the frontal lobes having a facilitatory role on orienting activity. From all these studies it can be concluded that frontal lobes have a predominent influence on the control of autonomic responses, particularly, the orbital, insular and prefrontal cortex (Cechetto and Saper, 1990). Studies on frontal control upon the electrodermal system concluded that such control can have excitatory, inhibitory or mixed effects.

An excitatory influence was reported by several studies in the cat (Langworthy and Richter, 1930; Wang and Lu, 1930; Wang and Mok, 1931; Spiegel and Hunsicker, 1936; Schwartz, 1937; Fujimori et al., 1953; Wilcott, 1969) and in the monkey (Fulton, 1949). Other studies concluded also that the prefrontal cortex had an excitatory role on EDA: in monkeys, Bagshaw et al. (1965) reported that SCRs were depressed after lesions of the lateral prefrontal cortex and Grueninger et al. (1965) found that SCRs to orienting stimulus were completely absent, after the bilateral removal of the dorsolateral prefrontal cortex. In humans, with frontal lesions, Luria and Homskaya (1970) reported reduced SCRs to orienting auditory stimuli compared with patients having non-frontal lesions and with normals. Naitoh (1972) reported that lesions of the frontal cortex diminished skin resistance responses and that stimulation of the anterior cingulate frontal cortex evokes SPRs. Raine et al. (1991), using MRI technique in normal human subjects, found significant relationships between the larger area of the prefrontal cortex (left and right) and more electrodermal activity (SCRs). Taken together, these studies strongly support an excitatory influence of the frontal lobes on EDA.

However, other studies found inhibitory effects of the frontal regions on EDA. In fact, the stimulation of the frontal cortex diminishes the amplitude of SPRs evoked either by an auditory stimulus (Wilcott and Bradley, 1970), or by the stimulation of a cutaneous nerve (Wang and Brown, 1956), in the anaesthetized cat. Furthermore, Wilcott (1967), contrary to Schwartz (1937), obtained an increase of SPR amplitude after ablation of premotor and sensorimotor areas in a chronical preparation. Scarce data obtained in humans seemed to show that the ablation of the frontal areas evoked an increase of sweating or EDA, mainly on the contralateral side (Guttman and List, 1928; see Darrow, 1937). Sourek (1965) found, after the removal of the medial and basal parts of the frontal lobe, a *"contralateral increase in SPRs caused by the loss of inhibitory influences of the removed parts of the brain hemisphere"* (p. 62). Such data are in favour of a frontal inhibitory cortical control on EDA.

Other studies reported no changes in EDA after extended cortical lesions. In monkeys, Kimble et al. (1965) did not find any impairment in SCRs following lesions of the medial frontal cortex (such lesions included the anterior cingulate cortex). In humans, no changes in EDA were obtained after a prefrontal lobotomy (Shimizu et al., 1948; Ashby and Basset, 1950). Elithorn et al. (1954), after unilateral prefrontal lobotomy, couldn't draw any clear conclusion in favour of an excitatory or inhibitory function of frontal lobes on EDA control. Finally, Damasio et al. (in press) reports that patients with bilateral lesions of orbital and lower mesial frontal cortex still produce normal SCRs to orienting stimuli.

Several authors reported excitatory effects on the EDA, from electrical stimulation of non-frontal areas, i. e., the posterior cruciate cortex and anterior suprasylvian areas, in the cat (Wang and Lu, 1930; Wang and Mok, 1931; Spiegel and Hunsicker, 1936). However, few stimulation points were explored and the location of such points and the extension of the stimulated areas were usually poorly detailed, as *"two areas adjacent to the motor cortex"* (Langworthy and Richter, 1930, p. 192). In humans, destruction of the mediobasal part of the temporal lobe (but including the amygdala) depressed SCRs (Dallakyan et al., 1970). Raine et al. (1991) concluded that the left temporal cortex (amygdala included) is implicated in the mediation of SCRs to orienting stimulus.

Finally, the cortex appears to exert both inhibitory and excitatory effects on EDA. Studies involving chronical ablations, in animals (Wilcott, 1967) or lesions in humans, concluded that an inhibitory mechanism was lost. It can be hypothesized that such an inhibitory mechanism corresponds to the suppression of cortical inhibitory tonic effects on the reticular formation (Hugelin and Bonvallet, 1957). These cortico-reticular effects, previously shown on motor activity, have been extended to the autonomic control as well (Bloch and Bonvallet, 1959). On the other hand, some old studies found an excitatory effect of cortex stimulation; thus, cortex seems to exert a phasic excitatory control on EDA.

However, methodological problems remain: firstly, some cortical stimulations were delivered after uncontrolled sub-cortical extended lesions (Spiegel and Hunsicker, 1936). Other studies were carried out in non curarized animals and in such cases, recorded electrodermal responses can be influenced by reafferences generated by peripheral muscular activity (Bloch et al., 1965). Secondly, lesion studies, in animals or in humans, lack sufficient precision to delineate the specific effects of one structure (e.g. temporal cortex vs amygdala) or one cortical area (e.g. prefrontal vs premotor or medial prefrontal cortex vs dorsolateral prefrontal cortex). Consequently, cortical influences on EDA should be more precisely asserted. That directed some of our experimental work.

As indicated previously, authors (Darrow, 1937; Edelberg, 1972) hypothesized that EDA is an indicator of cutaneous modifications that are useful for improving tactile acuity during fine motor control of hands. The pyramidal tract is the main pathway responsible for such fine motor control; it has also been reported that stimulation of this pathway could elicit electrodermal responses and other autonomic responses (Langworthy and Richter, 1930; Landau, 1953; Zwirn and Corriol, 1962). Furthermore, the pericruciate area is the main site of origin of pyramidal fibers (Armand and Kuypers,1980; Biedenbach and Devito, 1980; Keizer et al., 1987; Nudo and Masterton, 1990). Thus, we decided to explore the possibility that the pericruciate cortex could generate autonomic efferences together with somatic motor programs. In order to test such a hypothesis we chose to study the influence on the cortical control of EDA of two cortical areas with a high and a low rate of origin of pyramidal fibres, which are respectively the pericruciate and parietal areas. In fact, in the cat, 96 % of pyramidal fibers originate in pericruciate areas (Armand and Kuypers, 1980). These areas correspond, in humans, to precentral (motor area 4 and supplementary motor area 6) and postcentral areas (somatosensory areas 3a-b, 1, 2).

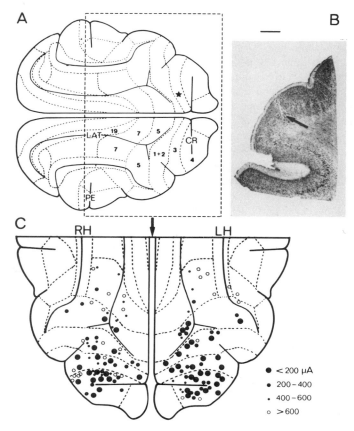

**Figure 1.** Location of stimulating electrodes in the cortex of the cat. A: dorsal view of cerebral hemispheres showing main architectonic subdivisions of pericruciate (areas 4,3,2,1) and anterior parietal (5,7) cerebral cortex on one hemisphere, according to Hassler and Muhs-Clement (1964) and Keizer et al. (1987). B: location of a stimulating electrode in area 3 (arrow); such position is presented in A and indicated as (*); the calibration bar equals 1 mm. C: Distribution of thresholds of intensity to elicit SPRs with cortical stimulations applied to right (RH) and left (LH) hemispheres.

## Experimental data

Experiments were performed in cats, anaesthetized during the surgical procedure with halothane (2 %) and curarized; afterwards, local anaesthesia was applied continuously. SPRs were recorded bilaterally, from the 4 paws. The pericruciate (areas 4,3,2,1; see figure 1) and parietal areas (5,7,19) of the left and right hemispheres were alternatively stimulated, following the architectonic subdivisions of Hassler and Muhs-Clement (1964) and Keizer et al. (1987).

Results showed that the pericruciate and parietal cortex stimulation evoked SPRs from the fours paws and that about 80% of stimulated sites allowed SPRs to be evoked with intensity values inferior to 600 µA. Pericruciate areas allowed SPRs to be elicited more frequently than did anterior parietal areas ($\chi^2(1)=5.46$, P<0.05). The median values of intensity from the pericruciate area 4 (200 μA) is lower than the anterior parietal cortex (300 μA); such a distribution of intensities shows that the stimulation of the pericruciate areas elicited SPRs with significantly lower intensities than the anterior parietal areas. Total results, calculated from five animals and analyzed by ANOVAs for matched groups, show that SPR amplitudes elicited on area 4 were significantly larger than those evoked from parietal areas 5 and 7 (F(1/4)=7.80, p<0.05). Thus, SPRs are more easily elicited on pericruciate areas and thresholds are lower for area 4.

Our results confirm and refine observations reported by several authors (Langworthy and Richter, 1930; Wilcott, 1969; Sequeira-Martinho et al., 1986a). The fact that pericruciate areas present slightly lower thresholds and a higher percentage of points from where SPRs can be elicited is in keeping with the origin of the pyramidal tract but also with cortico-reticular fibres. Relations between the sensorimotor cortex and reticular nuclei, which have a key position in the control of EDA, are demonstrated by neuroanatomical and electrophysiological data. Most of cortico-reticular fibers originate in pericruciate areas (Kuypers, 1958; Berrevoets and Kuypers, 1975) and these areas also contribute massively to pyramidal fibers which send collaterals to reticular structures (Endo et al., 1973; Keizer and Kuypers, 1984; Wiesendanger, 1984). Moreover, monosynaptic influences can be recorded in the bulbar reticular formation by the stimulation of sensorimotor cortex or the pyramidal fibers (Magni and Willis, 1964; Pilyavsky, 1975).

Consequently, descending influences on EDA, from pericruciate areas, can be transmitted to the spinal level, either by pyramidal tracts, or by extrapyramidal pathways. This gives rise to two questions: first, what is the importance of such cortical excitatory effect on EDA? Second, does it reflect the hypothalamic and reticular involvement or is it a corticospinal effect transmitted directly to the spinal cord by the pyramidal tract?

## PYRAMIDAL INVOLVEMENT

In spite of connections between frontal areas and the hypothalamus (Wouterlood et al., 1987), this structure does not seem implicated in the conduction of cortical EDA command. It was shown that the destruction of the hypothalamus had no influence upon SPR amplitude elicited by the stimulation of the pericruciate region (Wang and Lu, 1930; Spiegel and Hunsicker, 1936); such data are not in favour of a cortical control passing through the hypothalamus before reaching the spinal neurons. The anatomical organisation obviously makes it possible for pyramidal fibers to reach, at spinal level, preganglionic sudomotor neurons through the network of interneurones (Nyberg-Hansen and Brodal, 1963; Kostyuk and Vasilenko, 1978; Kuypers, 1981). We can thus hypothesize the existence of a direct cortical control on EDA, transmitted by the pyramidal tract, without the participation of reticular and hypothalamic relays.

Spiegel and Hunsicker (1936) had tried to test this hypothesis by stimulating the motor cortex and carrying out sections of all other descending pathways, except those of the cerebral peduncle, at mesencephalic level. However, these authors spared "...*not only the pyramidal tracts but also the corticopontine systems*" (p. 271). Wang and Lu (1930) and Landau (1953) showed that the direct stimulation of the cerebral peduncle or the pyramidal tract induces SPRs. These experiments did not show specific effects of the pyramidal tract on the command of EDA, since bulbar reticular neurons can be activated by collaterals of the pyramidal tract and can send excitatory command to spinal sudomotor neurons.

In the cat, we carried out a series of experiments and we developed a technique of sectioning, called "*pyramidal preparation*", where all descending pathways except the pyramidal tracts were interrupted at bulbar level (Sequeira-Martinho et al., 1982; Roy et al., 1984; Sequeira-Martinho et al., 1986a). To ensure that the hypothalamo- and reticulo-spinal pathways were completely interrupted, control stimulations of the hypothalamic and

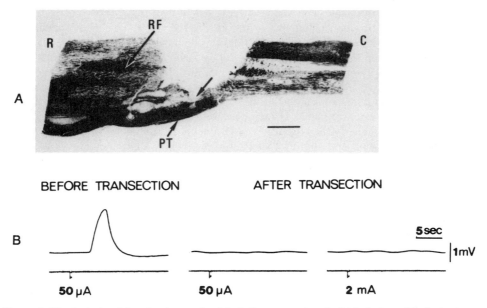

BEFORE TRANSECTION          AFTER TRANSECTION

**Figure 2**: Histological and functional controls of the bulbar transection. A: Sagittal view of the brain stem showing the rostro-caudal (R,C) level and the inferior limit of the bulbar transection (arrow). PT, pyramidal tract; RF, caudal nuclei of the reticular formation; the calibration bar equals 2 mm. B: Stimulation of the reticular formation (Central Tegmental Field, following the atlas of Berman, 1968). Before transection, SPRs could be elicited with very low stimulus intensities; after transection, the stimulation of the same reticular site failed to induce SPR.

reticular structures were delivered before and after the bulbar transection. After sections, no SPR was evoked by either the hypothalamic or the reticular stimulation. An histological control of the extension of the section in the "*pyramidal preparation*" was performed; as expected, in most preparations, only the pyramidal tracts were spared (figure 2).

Results show that after a bulbar transection sparing only the pyramidal tract, the stimulation of the cortex still evoked SPRs from the four paws. However, if we kept the same threshold criteria as before transection (600 µA) SPRs could still be elicited only on the primary motor cortex (area 4). Moreover, results obtained from sites localized in area 4, clearly identified and stimulated with the same intensity as before transection show that the SPRs amplitude diminishes significantly to 60 %. On the other hand, it was difficult to elicit SPRs by the stimulation of a non pericruciate (non pyramidal) area (figure 3). As a complement to cortical stimulations, we stimulated directly, before and after the same transection, the pyramidal tract at low bulbar level (plane P12, following the atlas of Berman, 1968) and that elicited SPRs. But it was observed that the thresholds for evoking SPRs by pyramidal stimulation were generally higher after transection than before. In some preparations, the medulla posterior to the transection was removed; this fact allows us to exclude participation of the reticulospinal neurons localized caudally in this transection.

Results showing that only the stimulation of the pericruciate cortex still evokes SPRs with low thresholds in pyramidal preparations are consistent with the fact that this region is the main site of origin of the the pyramidal tract (Armand and Kuypers, 1980; Nudo and Masterton, 1990). Considering activating effects on EDA exerted by mesencephalic structures, it can be said that the increase of thresholds after the transection is the consequence of the suppression of reticulospinal activation. Such effects could also be explained by the activity of the bulbar reticular inhibiting system, which is under the control of the reticular activating system, in normal preparations (Bloch, 1965; Roy et al., 1974). However, this possibility was suppressed by the ablation of medullary tissue posterior to the transection.

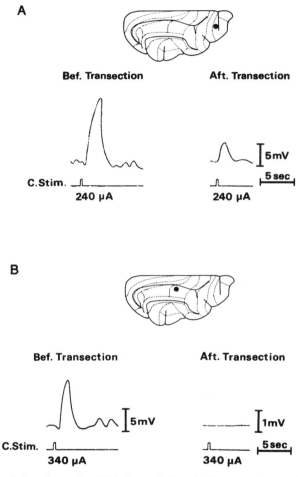

**Figure 3**: Cortical stimulation of areas 4 and 7, before and after a bulbar transection sparing only pyramidal tracts. A: typical SPRs obtained by the stimulation of area 4. After the transection, stimulation with the same intensity as before, still evokes SPRs; however, its amplitude is lower than that obtained in intact preparation. B: stimulation of area 7. After the transection, cortical stimulation of same intensity as before transection failed to induce SPRs.

From these experiments, two main conclusions can be drawn: first, a direct phasic control of EDA can be exerted by the motor cortex through the pyramidal tract and independently of reticulospinal neurons; second, thresholds to eliciting SPRs are higher after the bulbar transection; this fact  favours a reticular amplification of the cortical excitatory effects on EDA, in normal physiological conditions. Our results favour a double mechanism of control of EDA from regions implicated in fine motor activation: a direct effect transmitted by the pyramidal tract and an indirect one by a cortico-reticulo-spinal pathway. Considering the main role of reticular structures on the control of EDA, we believe that the cortico-reticulo-spinal circuit is predominant in normal conditions; cortical volleys transmitted by the pyramidal tract can be implicated in final adjustments upon preganglionic sudomotor neurons in order to facilitate cutaneous adaptations.

## LATERALIZATION OF CORTICAL EDA CONTROL ?

Bilateral EDA has become a much used parameter in research dealing with hemispheric asymmetry in humans. In fact, in the last twenty years, a growing number of authors have postulated a possible lateralization of EDA consecutive to the preferential activating of one or other of the brain hemispheres. EDA bilateral measures were used as an index of hemispheric differences in cognitive function and in research on psychopathology including schizophrenia, depression and unilateral neglect manifestations (Gruzelier and Venables, 1973; Heilman et al., 1978; Myslobodsky and Horesh, 1978; Lacroix and Comper, 1979). Results obtained in humans and reviewed by Freixa i Baqué et al. (1984) and Hugdahl (1984) provided an equivocal picture about the EDA asymmetry. Four years later, Hugdhal (1988) reviewed nine experimental works using non-invasive methods to stimulate hemispheres and argued that the analysis of overall data might be in favour of a neural model of contralateral inhibitory hemispheric influences. In fact, contrary to the known contralateral excitatory pattern of somatomotor response control, results concerning cortical command of EDA were mostly interpreted, since Sourek (1965), in terms of ipsilateral or contralateral inhibiton.

It seems thus relevant to explore neurophysiological mechanisms underlying a lateralized hemispheric control of EDA, in animals. Old animal data obtained by lesion and stimulating methods are inconclusive on the lateralization of the EDA control. In fact, such studies found, either a predominance of contralateral responses (Schwartz, 1937; Wilcott, 1967), or an absence of differences between ipsilateral and contralateral electrodermal responses (Landau, 1953; Wang and Brown, 1956; Bloch, 1965; Wilcott and Bradley, 1970). Knowing that the stimulation of the pericruciate cortical area, the main source of lateralized somatomotor responses, and of the pyramidal tract, elicits electrodermal responses, we considered that the stimulation of the pericruciate cortical area and of the pyramidal tract is an optimal situation for eliciting lateralized electrodermal responses. Consequently, experiments were carried out in order to answer the question: is the corticospinal EDA control lateralized, and if so, is the control ipsilateral or contralateral?

Ten cats were submitted to electric stimulations in area 4 of the left and right hemisphere alternatively (Figure 4). In another eight animals, the right and the left pyramidal tract were stimulated 3 mm rostrally to the plane of a bulbar transection which spared only the pyramidal tract; consequently, only lateralized effets elicited by the pyramidal stimulation were transmitted to the spinal level. SPRs were recorded bilaterally from the four foot pads.

Cortical and pyramidal stimulations evoked bilateral SPRs of different amplitudes; the direction of this difference remained constant whichever side was stimulated. Thus, SPRs amplitude does not seem dependent on lateralization of the pyramidal tracts. In intact preparations, EDA command, elicited by lateralized hemispheric stimulation, can be transmitted by collaterals to bilateral reticular structures; in such a case, the lateralization of cortical information would be lost through the reticular network which transmits information to ipsi- and contralateral sudomotor neurones of the spinal cord. Because of the pyramidal decussation, most pyramidal fibers were crossed; consequently, we expected higher amplitudes in the side opposite to the pyramidal stimulation, which was delivered above the decussation. Surprisingly, bilateral SPR amplitude differences have the same direction, as in the case of cortical stimulations. However, in this situation, we cannot exclude the diffusion of descending influences to the other side of the spinal cord through ipsilateral pyramidal fibers.

Finally, in order to eliminate spinal diffusion due to the stimulation of ipsilateral pyramidal fibers, we combined, in four cats, a bulbar transection sparing only pyramidal

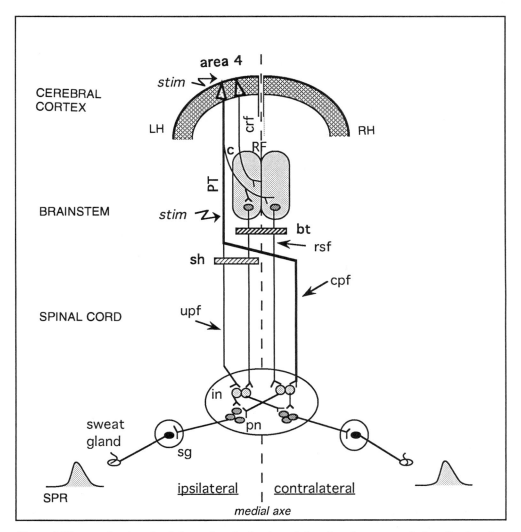

**Figure 4.** Diagram showing stimulation and section levels carried out in order to assess the lateralization of the corticospinal control of bilateral EDA. bt, bulbar transection; c, pyramidal collaterals; cpf, crossed pyramidal fibers; crf, cortico-reticular fibers; in, interneurons network; LH, left hemisphere; pn: preganglionic sympathetic neurones; PT: pyramidal tract; RF: reticular formation; RH: right hemisphere; rsf, reticulo-spinal fibers; sg, sympathetic ganglion; sh, spinal hemisection; stim, stimulation; upf, uncrossed pyramidal fibers. Ipsilateral or contralateral: recording side in relation to the central site of stimulation.

tracts, with a hemisection of the spinal cord at C1 level. By this means reticulospinal fibers were eliminated and contralateral pyramidal fibers were exclusively stimulated. Results show that the stimulation of such fibers still elicits SPRs in four paws; calculations did not show any lateralized effect of SPR amplitude. It can be concluded that, in the cat, lateralized hemispheric influences elicited by the stimulation of the primary motor area do not induce lateralized EDA; a bilateral distribution of the nervous command coming from the sensorimotor cortex is carried out to both sides of the spinal cord. Oldfield and McLachlan (1981) showed that preganglionic neurons have dendritic ramifications that extend laterally as far as the contralateral side; this bilateral distribution favours certainly the spinal diffusion of supraspinal signals. These data are not compatible with the hypothesis of predominance of a lateralized central influence. Consequently, bilateral differences of EDA can be interpreted in terms of peripheral factors, as discussed elsewhere (Sequeira-Martinho et al., 1986b). The influence of such factors, as skin temperature, could indeed determine a specific configuration of bilateral differences, independently of a lateralized hemispheric predominance of EDA command.

## SUMMARY AND CONCLUSIONS

The literature about animal studies on hypothalamo-limbic and cortical control on EDA was reviewed. There is neuroanatomical and functional support of an excitatory hypothalamic descending control of EDA by neuronal relays in the brain stem or directly at spinal level. Limbic influences, either inhibitory or excitatory, are probably integrated under cortical control and can be transmitted to spinal level, either by hypothalamic relays, by reticular structures or by direct projections to preganglionic sudomotor neurons. Reviewed data also shows that the cortex exerts both inhibitory and excitatory effects on EDA; however, several methodological problems indicate that cortical influences on EDA need to be more precisely asserted.

Different authors (Darrow, 1937; Edelberg, 1972; Jänig, 1990) hypothesized that the EDA can be an indicator of cutaneous modifications that contribute to improve tactile acuity during fine motor control; within the theoretical frame of somato-autonomic interactions, we explored, in the cat, the contribution of motor areas to the EDA control. We concluded that a double system of EDA command originates in the motor cortex: a cortico-reticulo-spinal circuit and a direct corticospinal control acting by means of the pyramidal tract on the spinal network of preganglionic sudomotor neurons. We hypothesize that such corticospinal control contributes to final autonomic adjustments, particularly during grasping movements.

The lateralization of EDA was also explored following the preferential activating of one or other of the brain hemispheres. In fact, previous data obtained in humans and in animals provide an equivocal picture of cortical influences on EDA asymmetry. In our experimental work in the cat, we found that the stimulation of area 4, which is the main origin of lateralized descending pathways, the pyramidal tracts, elicits bilateral SPRs whose amplitude difference direction remains constant whichever side is stimulated. Hemisection of the spinal cord did not modify bilateral differences in SPR eliciting. Such results are not in favour of a lateralized hemispheric control of EDA, and lead us to consider a possible influence of peripheral factors in EDA asymmetry, at least in the cat.

Experimental data presented in this paper throws some light on the cortical control of EDA and on the mechanism of autonomic adjustments related to fine motor expressions; somato-autonomic efferences are probably initiated by common programs in premotor and motor cortical areas. Such studies may help to understand better somato-autonomic interactions and their clinical implications.

# REFERENCES

Armand, J., and Kuypers, H.G.J.M., 1980, Cells of origin of crossed and uncrossed corticospinal fibers in the cat, *Exp. Brain Res.* 40: 23-34.

Ashby W.R., and Basset, M., 1950, The effect of prefrontal leucotomy on the psychogalvanic response, *J. Ment. Sci.* 96: 458-469.

Bagshaw, M.H., and Benzies, S., 1968, Multiple measures of the orienting reaction and their dissociation after amygdalectomy in monkeys, *Exp. Neurol.* 20: 175-187.

Bagshaw, M.H., Kimble, D.P., and Pribram, K.H., 1965, The GSR of monkeys during orienting and habituation and after ablation of the amygdala, hippocampus, and inferotemporal cortex, *Neuropsychologia* 3: 111-119.

Bagshaw, M.H., and Coppock, H.W. (1968), Galvanic skin response conditioning deficit in amygdalectomized monkeys, *Exp. Neurol.* 20: 188-196.

Bard, P., 1929, The central representation of the sympathetic system, *Arch. Neurol. Psychiat.* 22: 230-246.

Bartfai, A., Levander, S.E., Nyback, H., and Schalling, D., 1987, Skin conductance nonresponding and non-habituation in schizophrenic patients, *Acta Psychiat. Scand.*, 75: 321-329.

Beattie, J., Brow, G.R., and Long, C.N.H., 1930, Physiological and anatomical evidence for the existence of nerve tracts connecting the hypothalamus with spinal sympathetic centers, *Proc. Roy. Soc.* (London) B 106: 253-275.

Bechterew, W.V., 1905, Der Einfluss der Hirnrinde auf die Thränen Schweiss und Harnabsonderung, *Arch. f. Anat. u. Physiol.*, 297: 297-305, cited by Darrow, 1937.

Berman, A.L., 1968, *"The Brain Stem of the Cat. A Cytoarchitectonic Atlas with Stereotaxic Coordinates"*, The university of Wisconsin Press, Madison.

Berrevoets, C.E., and Kuypers, H.G.J.M., 1975, Pericruciate cortical projecting to brain stem reticular formation, dorsal column nuclei and spinal cord in the cat, *Neurosci. Lett.* 1: 257-262.

Biedenbach, M.A., and DeVito, J.L., 1980, Origin of the pyramidal tract determined with horseradish peroxydase, *Brain Res.* 193: 1-17.

Bloch, V., 1965, Le contrôle central de l'activité électrodermale, *J. Physiol.* (Paris) 57, Suppl. 13: 1-132.

Bloch, V., and Bonvallet, M., 1959, Contrôle cortico-réticulaire de l'activité électrodermale, *J. Physiol.*, (Paris), 51: 405-406.

Bloch, V., and Bonvallet, M., 1960, Le déclenchement des réponses électrodermales à partir du système réticulaire facilitateur. *J. Physiol.* (Paris) 52: 25-26.

Bloch, V., Valat, M., and Roy, J.C., 1965, Influences des afférences musculaires sur le tonus réticulaire, *J. Physiol.* (Paris), 57: 561-562.

Bochefontaine, L.T., 1876, Etude expérimentale de l'influence exercée par la faradisation de l'écorce grise du cerveau sur quelques fonctions de la vie organique, *Arch. Physiol. Norm. Pathol.* 2: 140-172.

Cannon, T.D., Fuhrmann, M., Mednick, S.A., Machon, R.A., Parnas, J., and Schulsinger, F., 1988, Third ventricle enlargement and reduced electrodermal reponsiveness, *Psychophysiology*, 25: 153-156.

Cannon, W.B., 1929, *Bodily Changes in Pain, Fear and Rage*, Appleton, New York.

Cechetto, D.F., and Saper, C.B., 1988, Neurochemical organization of the hypothalamic projection to the spinal cord in the rat, *J. Comp. Neurol.* 272: 579-604.

Cechetto, D.F. and Saper, C.B., 1990, Role of the Cortex in autonomic function, *in: Central Regulation of Autonomic Functions*, Loewy, A.D., Spyer, K.M., eds, Oxford University Press, New York.

Celesia, G.G., and Wang, G.H., 1964, Sudomotor activity induced by single shock stimulation of the hypothalamus in anesthetized cats, *Arch. Ital. Biol.* 102: 587-598.

Dallakyan, I.G., Latash, L.P., and Popova, L.T., 1970, Certain regular relationships between the expressivity of the galvanic skin responses of the EEG in local lesions of the limbic (rhinencephalic) structures of the human brain, *Dokl. Akad. Nauk.*, 190: 991-999.

Damasio, A.R., Tranel, D. and Damasio, H., in press, Somatic markers and the guidance of behavior: theory and preliminary testing, *in: Frontal Lobe Function Injury*, H. Levin, H. Eisenberg and A. Benton, eds., Oxford University Press, New York, cited by Raine and Lencz, this volume.

Danilewsky, B., 1875, Experimentelle Beiträge zur Physiologie des Gehirns, *Pflüg. Arch. Ges. Physiol.,* 11: 128-138, cited by Hoff et al., 1963.

Darrow, C.W., 1937, Neural mechanisms controlling the palmar galvanic skin reflex and palmar sweating, *Arch. Neurol. Psych.* 37: 641-663.

Davison, M.A. and Koss, M.C., 1975, Brainstem loci for activation of electrodermal response in the cat, *Amer. J. Physiol.* 229: 930-934.

Delgado, J.M.R., 1960, Circulatory effects of cortical stimulation, *Physiol. Rev.* 40 (Suppl. 4): 146-171.

Dennig, H., 1924, Die Bahn des psychogalvanischen Reflexes in Zentralnervensystem, *Z. Ges. Neurol. Psychiat.* 92: 373-377, cited by Darrow, 1937.

Edelberg, R., 1972, The electrodermal system, *in: Handbook of Psychophysiology*, N.S. Greenfield and R.A. Sternbach, eds., Holt, New York.

Edinger, H.M., Kramer, S.Z., and Siegel, A., 1977, Effect of hypothalamic stimulation on mesencephalic neurons, *Exp. Neurol.* 54: 91-103.

Elithorn, A., Piercy, M.F., and Crosskey, M.A., 1954, Autonomic change after unilateral leucotomy, *J. Neurol. Neurosurg. Psychiat.* 17: 139-144.

Endo, K., Araki, T., and Yagi, N., 1973, The distribution and pattern of axon branching of pyramidal tract cells, *Brain Res.* 57: 484-491.

Foà, C., and Peserico, E., 1923, Le vie del riflesso neurogalvanico, *Arch. Fisiol.* 21(2): 119-130, cited by Wang, 1964.

Freeman, G.L., and Krasno, L., 1940, Inhibitory functions of the corpus striatum, *Arch. Neurol. Psychiat.* 44: 323-327.

Freixa i Baqué, E., Catteau, M.-C., Miossec, Y., and Roy, J.C., 1984, Asymmetry of electrodermal activity: a review, *Biol. Psychol.* 18: 219-239.

Fujimori, B., Otsubo, T., Homma, I., and Shiroiwa., T., 1953, GSR by the cerebral stimulation, *Iryo (Therapy)* 7: 425-431.

Fulton, J.F., 1949, Cerebral cortex: autonomic representation in precentral motor cortex, *in: Physiology of the Nervous System,* J.F. Fulton, ed., Oxford University Press, New York.

Girardot, M.-N., and Koss, M.C., 1984, A physiological and pharmacological analysis of the electrodermal response in the rat, *Eur. J. Pharmacol.* 98: 185-191.

Grueninger, W.E., Kimble, D.P., Grueninger, J., and Levine, S., 1965, GSR and corticosteroid response in monkeys with frontal ablations, *Neuropsychologia* 3: 205-216.

Gruzelier, J.H., and Venables, P.H., 1973, Skin conductance responses to tones with and without attentional significance in schizophrenic and non-schizophrenic psychiatric patients, *Neuropsychologia* 11: 221-230.

Guttman, L., and List, C.F., 1928, Die nervosen Leitungsbahnen der Schweissekretion beim Menschen, *Deut. Zeit. Nervenheilkunde* 107: 61-71.

Hasama, B., 1929, Pharmakologische und physiologische Studien über die Schweisszentren: II. über den Einfluss der direkten, mechanischen thermischen und elektrischen Reizung zuf die Schweiss-sowie Warmezentren, *Arch. Exp. Pathol. Pharm.* 146: 129-161, cited by Darrow, 1937.

Hassler, R., and Muhs-Clement, K., 1964, Architektonischer aufbau des sensormotorischen und parietalen Cortex der Katze, *J. Hirnforsch* 6: 377-420.

Hazlett, E., Dawson, M., Buchsbaum, M.S. and Nuechterlein, K., in press, Reduced regional brain glucose metabolism assessed by PET in electrodermal non responder schizophrenics: a pilot study, *J. Abn. Psych.,* cited by Raine and Lencz, this volume.

Heilman, K.M., Schwartz, H.D., and Watson, R.T., 1978, Hypoarousal in patients with the neglect syndrome and emotional indifference, *Neurology* 28: 229-232.

Hess, W.R., 1954, *Diencephalon, Autonomic and Extrapyramidal Functions,* Grune and Stratton, New York.

Hess, W.R., and Brugger, M., 1943, Das subkorticale Zentrum der affektiven-Abwehrreaktion, *Helv. Physiol. Acta* 1:33-52.

Hoff, E.C., Green, H.D., 1936, Cardiovascular reactions induced by electrical stimulation of the cerebral cortex, *Amer. J. Physiol.* 117: 411-422.

Hoff, E.C., Kell, J.F., and Carroll, M.N., 1963, Effects of cortical stimulation and lesions on cardiovascular function, *Physiol. Rev.* 43: 68-114.

Holstege, G., 1987, Some anatomical observations on the projections from the hypothalamus to brainstem and spinal cord: an HRP and autoradiographic tracing study in the cat, *J. Comp. Neurol.* 260: 98-126.

Hopkins, D.A., and Holstege, G., 1978, Amygdaloid projections to the mesencephalon, pons and medulla oblongata in the cat, *Exp. Brain Res.* 32, 529-547.

Hosoya, Y., Sugiura, Y., Okado, N., Loewy, A.D., and Kohno, K., 1991, Descending input from the hypothalamic paraventricular nucleus to sympathetic preganglionic neurons in the rat, *Exp. Brain. Res.* 85: 10-20.

Hugdahl, K., 1984, Hemispheric asymmetry and bilateral electrodermal recordings: a review of evidence, *Psychophysiology* 21: 371-393.

Hugdahl, K., 1988, Bilateral electrodermal asymmetry: past hopes and future prospects, *Intern. J. Neurosci.* 39: 33-44.

Hugelin, A., and Bonvallet, M., 1957, Etude expérimentale des interelations réticulo-corticales. Proposition d'une théorie de l'asservissement réticulaire à un système diffus cortical, *J. Physiol.* (Paris) 49: 1201-1223.

Isamat, F., 1961, Galvanic skin responses from stimulation of limbic cortex, *J. Neurophysiol.* 24: 176-181.

Jackson, J.H., 1869, On the anatomical and physiological localization of movements in the brain, *in: Selected writings of John Hughlings Jackson,* J. Taylor, ed., Hodder & Stoughton, London.

Jänig, W., 1990, Functions of the sympathetic innervation of the skin, *in: Central regulation of atutonomic functions,* A.D. Loewy and K.M. Spyer, eds., Oxford University Press, New York.

Kaada, B.R., 1951, Somato-motor, autonomic and electrocorticographic responses to electrical stimulation of "rhinencephalic" and other structures in primates, cat and dog, *Act. Physiol. Scand.* 24, Suppl. 83: 1-285.

Karplus, J.P., and Kreidl, A., 1909, Gehirn und sympathicus, *Pflüg. Arch. Ges. Physiol.* 129: 138-144, cited by Wang, 1964.

Katsumi, M., 1955, Experimental study on the central mechanism of psychogalvanic skin response. I. Relation between psychogalvanic response and hypothalamus, *Med. J. Osaka Univ.* 6: 649-668.

Keizer, K., and Kuypers, H.G.J.M., 1984, Distribution of corticospinal neurons with collaterals to lower brainstem reticular formation in the cat, *Exp. Brain Res.* 54: 107-120.

Keizer, K., Kuypers, H.G.J.M., and Ronday, H.K., 1987, Branching cortical neurons in cat which project to the colliculi and to the pons: a retrograde fluorescent double-labeling study, *Exp Brain Res.* 67: 1-15.

Kimble, D.P., Bagshaw, M.H., and Pribram, K.H., 1965, The GSR of monkeys during orienting and habituation after selective partial ablations of the cingulate and frontal cortex, *Neuropsychologia* 3: 121-128.

Koss, M.C., and Hey, J.A., 1988, Clonidine inhibits electrodermal responses by an action on the spinal cord, *Europ. J. Pharmacol.* 148: 397-403.

Kostyuk, P.G., and Vasilenko, D.A., 1978, Propriospinal neurones as a relay system for transmission of corticospinal influences, *J. Physiol.* (Paris) 74: 247-250.

Kuypers, H.G.J.M., 1958, An anatomical analysis of cortico-bulbar connections to the pons and lower brain stem in the cat, *J. Anat.* 92: 198-218.

Kuypers, H.G.J.M., 1981, Anatomy of descending pathways, *in: Handbook of Physiology, sect I: The nervous system,* J.M. Brookhart, V.B. Mountcastle, V.B. Brooks and S.R. Geiger, eds., Williams and Wilkins, Baltimore.

Lacroix, J.M., and Comper, P., 1979, Lateralization in the electrodermal system as a function of cognitve/ hemispheric manipulations, *Psychophysiology* 16: 116-129.

Landau, W.M., 1953, Autonomic responses mediated via the corticospinal tract, *J. Neurophysiol.* 16: 299-312.

Lang, A.H., Tuovinen, T., and Valleala, P., 1964, Amygdaloid afterdischarge and galvanic skin response, *Electroenceph. Clin. Neurophysiol.* 16: 366-374.

Langworthy, O.R., Richter, C.P., 1930, The influence of efferent cerebral pathways upon the sympathetic nervous system, *Brain* 53: 178-193.

Lee, G.P., Arena, J.G., Meador, K.J., Smith, J.R., Loring, D.W., and Flanigan, H.F., 1988, Changes in autonomic responsiveness following amygdalectomy in humans, *Neuropsychiat. Neuropsychol. Behav. Neurol.* 1:119-130.

Loewy, A.D., 1990, Central autonomic pathways, *in: Central Regulation and Autonomic Functions.* A.D. Loewy, K.M. Spyer, eds, Oxford University Press, New York.

Luiten, P.G.M., Horst, G.J., Karst, H., and Steffens, A.B., 1985, The course of paraventricular hypothalamic efferents to autonomic structures in medulla and spinal cord, *Brain Res.* 329: 374-378.

Luria, A.R., 1966, *Higher cortical functions in man,* Basic Books, New York.

Luria, A.R., and Homskaya, E.D., 1970, Frontal lobe and the regulation of arousal processes, *in: Attention: Contemporary Theory and research*, Mostofsky, ed., Appleton Century Crofts, New York.

Magni , F., and Willis, W.D., 1964, Cortical control of brain stem reticular neurons, *Arch. Ital. Biol.,* 102: 418-433.

Magoun, H.W., Ranson, S.W., and Hetherington, A., 1938, Descending-connections from the hypothalamus, *Arch. Neurol. Psych.,* 39: 1127-1149.

Mizuno, N., Takashi, O., Satoda, T., and Matsushima, R., 1985, Amygdalospinal projections in the macaque monkey, *Neurosci. Lett.,* 53: 327-330.

Myslobodsky, M.S., and Horesh, N., 1978, Bilateral electrodermal activity in depressive patients, *Biol. Psychol.,* 6: 111-120.

Naitoh, P., 1972, The effect of alcohol on the autonomic nervous system of humans: psychophysiological approach, *in: The biology of Alcoolism", Vol. 2: Physiology and Behavior,* Plenum Press, New York.

Nudo, R.J., and Masterton, R.B., 1990, Descending pathways to the spinal cord, III: Sites of origin of the corticospinal tract, *J. Comp. Neurol.* 296: 559-584.

Nyberg-Hansen, R., and Brodal, A., 1963, Sites of termination of corticospinal fibers in the cat. An experimental study with silver impregnation methods, *J. Comp. Neurol.* 120: 369-391.

Oldfield, B.J., and McMachlan, E.M., 1981, An analysis of the sympathetic preganglionic neurons projecting from the upper thoracic spinal roots of the cat, *J. Comp. Neurol.* 196: 329-345.

Pilyavsky, A.I., 1975, Characteristics of fast and slow cortico-bulbar fibre projections to reticulo-spinal neurones, *Brain Res.* 85: 49-52.

Pribram, K.H., and McGuinness, D., 1975, Arousal, activation, and effort in the control of attention, *Psychol. Rev.* 82: 116-140.

Price, J.L., and Amaral, D.G., 1981, An autoradiographic study of the projections of the central nucleus of the monkey amygdala, *J. Neurosc.* 1: 1242-1259.

Raine, A., and Lencz,T., 1993, Brain imaging research on electrodermal activity in humans, *in: Progress in Electrodermal Research*, J.C. Roy, W. Boucsein, D.C. Fowles and J. Gruzelier, eds., Plenum, New York.

Raine, A., Reynolds, G.P., and Sheard, C., 1991, Neuroanatomical correlates of skin conductance orienting in normal humans: a magnetic imaging study. *Psychophysiology* 28: 548-558.

Ramon y Cajal., S.,1909, *Histologie du Système Nerveux de l'Homme et des Vertébrés.* A. Maloine, Paris.

Roy, J.C., Delerm, B., and Granger, L., 1974, L'inhibition bulbaire de l'activité électrodermale chez le chat, *Electroenceph. Clin. Neurophysiol.* 37: 621-632.

Roy, J.C., Sequeira, H., and Delerm, B., 1993, Neural control of electrodermal activity: spinal and reticular mechanisms, *in: Progress in Electrodermal Research,* J.C. Roy, W. Boucsein, D.C. Fowles and J. Gruzelier, eds., Plenum, New York.

Roy, J.C., Sequeira-Martinho, H., and Brochard, J., 1984, Pyramidal control of skin potential responses in the cat, *Exp. Brain Res.,* 54: 283-288.

Sandrew, B.B., Edwards, D.L., Poletti, C.E., and Foote, W.E., 1986, Amygdalospinal projections in the cat, *Brain Res.,* 373: 235-239.

Saper, C.B., Loewy, A.D., Swanson, L.W., and Cowan, W.M., 1976, Direct hypothalamo-autonomic connections, *Brain Res.* 117: 305-312.

Schnur, D.B., Bernstein, A.S., Mukherjee, S., Loh, J., Degreef, G. and Piedel, J., 1989, The autonomic orienting response and CT scan findings in schizophrenia, *Schizoph. Res.* 2: 449-455.

Schwartz, H.G., 1937, Effect of experimental lesions of the cortex on the "psychogalvanic reflex" in the cat, *Arch. Neurol. Psych.* 38: 308-320.

Sequeira-Martinho, H., Roy, J.C., and Brochard, 1982, Participation du faisceau pyramidal à la commande d'une réponse végétative, la réponse électrodermale, chez le chat, *C.R. Ac. Sci.* (Paris) 294: 271-274.

Sequeira-Martinho, H., Roy, J.C., and S. Ba-M'Hamed-Bennis, 1986a, Corticospinal control of electrodermal activity in the cat, *J. Auton. Nerv. Syst.* (suppl): 567-570.

Sequeira-Martinho, H., Roy, J.C., and S. Ba-M'Hamed-Bennis, 1986b, Cortical and pyramidal stimulation elicit nonlateralized skin potential responses in the cat, *Biol. Psychol.* 23: 85-86.

Shimizu, S., Nagasaki, N., and Aoyama, H., 1948, The galvanic skin reaction by the prefrontal lobotomy and nucleotomia lentiformis, *Fol. Psych. Neurol. Jap.* 3: 196-197.

Showers, M.J.C., and Crosby, E.C., 1958, Somatic and visceral responses from the cingulate gyrus, *Neurology* 8: 561-565, Cited by Isamat, 1961.

Sofroniew, M. V., and Schrell, U., 1980, Hypothalamic neurons projecting to the rat caudal medulla oblongata, examined by immunoperoxidase staining of retrogradely transported horseradish peroxidase, *Neurosci. Lett.* 19: 257-263.

Sourek, K., 1965, *The Nervous Control of Skin Potentials in Man.* Nakladatelstvi Ceskoslovenske Akademie Ved, Praha.

Spiegel, E.A., and Hunsicker, W.C., 1936, The conduction of cortical impulses to the autonomic system, *J. Nerv. Ment. Dis.* 83: 252-274.

Tranel, D., Bradley, T., and Hyman, T., 1990, Neuropsychological correlates of bilateral amygdala damage, *Arch. Neurol.* 47: 349-355.

Tranel, D., and Damasio, H., 1989, Intact electrodermal skin conductance responses after bilateral amygdala damage, *Neuropsychologia* 27: 381-390.

Walland, A., 1986, Spinal facilitation in cholinergic-sympathetic efferents by desipramine, *Naunyn-Schmiedeberg's Arch. Pharmacol.* 334: 352-356.

Wang, G.H., 1964, *The neural Control of Sweating.* University of Wisconsin Press, Wisconsin.

Wang, G.H., and Brown, V.W., 1956, Suprasegmental inhibition of an autonomic reflex. *J. Neurophysiol.* 19: 564-572.

Wang, G.H., and Lu, T.W., 1930, Galvanic skin reflex induced in the cat by stimulation of the motor area of the cerebral cortex, *Chin. J. Physiol.* 3: 303-324.

Wang, G.H., and Mok, K.H., 1931, The effect of hemisection of the cervical spinal cord on the galvanic skin response induced by cortical stimulation, *Chin. J. Physiol.* 5: 141-148.

Wang, G.H., and Richter, C.P., 1928, Action currents from the pad of the cat's foot produced by stimulation of the tuber cinereum, *Chin. J. Physiol.* 2: 279-284.

Ward, A., Jr., 1948, The cingular gyrus: area 24, *J. Neurophysiol.* 110: 130-23, cited by Wang, 1964.

Wiesendanger, M., 1984, Pyramidal tract function and the clinical "pyramidal syndrome", *Hum. Neurobiol.* 2: 227-234.

Wilcott, R.C., 1967, Cortical control of skin potential, skin resistance and sweating. *Psychophysiology* 4: 500.

Wilcott, R.C., 1969, Electrical stimulation of the anterior cortex and skin-potential responses in the cat, *J. Comp. Physiol. Psychol.* 69: 465-472.

Wilcott, R.C., and Bradley, H.H., 1970, Low-frequency electrical stimulation of the cats anterior cortex and inhibition of skin potential responses, *J. Comp. Physiol. Psychol.* 72: 351-355.

Wilcott, R.C., and Hoel, C.E., 1973, Arousal response to electrical stimulation of the cerebral cortex in cats, *J. Comp. Physiol. Psychol.* 85: 413-420.

Wooterlood, F.G., Steinbusch, H.W.M., Luiten, P.G.M., and Bol, J.G.J.M., 1987, Projection from the prefrontal cortex to histaminergic cell groups in the posterior hypothalamic region of the rat. anterograde tracing with Phaseolus vulgaris leucoagglutinin combined with immunocytochemestry of histidine decarboxylase, *Brain Res.* 406: 330-336.

Yamamoto, K., Arai, H., and Nakayama, S., 1990, Skin Conductance Response after 6-hydroxydopamine lesion of central noradrenaline system in cats, *Biol. Psychiat.* 28: 151-161.

Yamamoto, K., Hagino, K., Moroji, T., and Ishii, T., 1984, Habituation failure of skin conductance response after intraventricular administration of 6-hydroxy-dopamine in cats, *Experientia* 40: 344-345.

Yamamoto, K., Kiyosumi, H., Yamaguchi, K., and Moroji, T., 1985, Two types of changes in skin conductance activity after intraventricularr administration of 6-hydroxydopamine in rats, *Prog. Neuro-Psychopharm. Biol. Psychiat.* 9: 245-250.

Yokota, T., Sato, A., and Fujimori, B., 1963, Inhibition of sympathetic activity by stimulation of limbic system, *Jap. J. Physiol.* 13: 137-143.

Zwirn, P., and Corriol, J., 1962, Fibres corticopyramidales dilatatrices des membres, *Arch. Sci. Physiol.* 16: 325-345.

# BRAIN IMAGING RESEARCH ON ELECTRODERMAL

# ACTIVITY IN HUMANS

Adrian Raine and Todd Lencz

Department of Psychology
University of Southern California
Los Angeles, CA 90089-1061

## INTRODUCTION

This chapter reviews those studies conducted to date which have attempted to use brain imaging techniques to help identify the neuroanatomical and neurophysiological basis of skin conductance (SC) activity in humans. Methodological issues in the use of brain imaging as applied to electrodermal activity will be identified, and methodological issues in the recording of electrodermal activity will also be discussed in the context of findings from imaging studies. The potential value of using cluster analysis to seek categorical as opposed to continuous relationships between imaging and SC variables will be illustrated in a study which also attempts to demonstrate how more basic science research into brain mechanisms underlying SC activity can importantly inform clinical issues. Finally, conceptual and methodological issues in brain imaging - SC research will be discussed, and recommendations for future research in this area will be made. Because most studies have focussed on orienting activity, the focus of this review will be specifically on SC orienting.

One important distinction to be made at the outset is that there are two basic types of brain imaging techniques, yielding two kinds of information: (a) information on brain function and (b) information on brain structure. To date, most studies have focussed on the latter type of imaging. The only functional brain imaging technique that has been used in the study of SC orienting is PET, while the two main structural brain imaging techniques consist of CT and MRI.

## NEUROANATOMY OF SC: ANTECEDENTS TO NEUROIMAGING

Prior to the development of modern neuroimaging technology, the neuroanatomical basis of skin conductance orienting was examined by means of brain lesion and stimulation studies in animals, as well as studies of brain-injured human patients. A detailed review of the animal literature may be found in Roy (this volume) and Sequeira and Roy (this volume). These studies have converged on several significant brain regions involved in the SC response, ranging from the subcortical regions to the limbic system and the neocortex.

*Progress in Electrodermal Research,* Edited by
J.-C. Roy *et al.* Plenum Press, New York, 1993

These studies have helped direct the subsequent investigations of researchers utilizing brain imaging techniques. Specific brain regions implicated in these studies include:

(1) Pons: Darrow (1937) cited several findings in support of the notion that the tegmental region of the pons may constitute an important non-hypothalamic excitatory center for palmar sweating. The nucleus reticularis pontis oralis (rostral pons) plays a critical role in EEG desychronization (Thompson, 1967), indicating that this area is involved in orienting activity. Furthermore, the reticular formation of the pons occupies a position in the central tegmentum (posterior pons), and stimulation of the brainstem reticular activating system has an excitatory effect on SC activity in animals (Bloch and Bonvallet, 1960).

(2) Hypothalamus : Traditionally, the anterior hypothalamus has been viewed by most reviewers as having an excitatory influence on SC activity, while the posterior hypothalamus has been considered to be an inhibitory center (Wang, 1964; Edelberg, 1972; Venables and Christie, 1973; Bloch and Bonvallet, 1960), although Sequeira and Roy (this volume) convincingly argue that both the posterior and medial hypothalamus also acts as an excitatory center in animals. As we shall see, neuroimaging studies have examined enlargement of the third ventricle as an indirect index of tissue loss to the excitatory anterior hypothalamus. Thus, enlargement of the third ventricle would be predicted to result in reduced SC orienting.

(3) Temporal lobe / amygdala / hippocampus: The mesial aspects of the temporal lobe have long been associated with orienting in monkeys (Schwartzbaum, Wilson and Morrissette, 1961). In humans, Gruzelier and Venables (1972) suggested that the amygdala appears to play an important excitatory role in electrodermal orienting. Lesions of the amygdala in monkeys abolish SC orienting (Bagshaw et al. 1965), a finding replicated by Bagshaw and Benzies (1968). Furthermore, stimulation of the amygdala in cats is known to produce changes in skin potential levels (Lang, Tuovinen, and Valleala 1964). In humans destruction of the medio-basal aspect of the temporal lobe (particularly the amygdala) has been reported to result in decrements in the SC response (Dallakyan, Latash, and Popova, 1970).

Work with animals has implicated the hippocampus as having an inhibitory influence on SC orienting. Stimulation of the hippocampus in anesthetized cats results in inhibition of SC responses (Yokata et al. 1963), while Bagshaw et al. (1965) observed that bilateral hippocampal lesions in monkeys did not affect SC orienting responses. Theorizings by Gruzelier and Venables (1972), and a review by Edelberg (1972), have also suggested a possible inhibitory role of the hippocampus.

(4) Prefrontal area: Bagshaw et al. (1965) showed that ablation of lateral frontal cortex in monkeys resulted in reduced SC orienting, while Grueninger et al. (1965) found an abolition of SC orienting after dorsolateral prefrontal lesions. In human patients, Luria and Homskaya (1970) showed that frontal lesion patients had reduced SC orienting. These studies indicate an excitatory influence of pre-frontal, and particularly lateral prefrontal, area on SC orienting.

However, findings with respect to medial frontal cortex, orbito-mesial frontal cortex, and the cingulate gyrus are mixed. For example, Kimble, Bagshaw and Pribram (1965) did not observe any impairment in SCRs in monkeys following lesions of medial frontal cortex (including the anterior cingulate cortex), and similarly Isamat (1961) failed to obtain SCRs after stimulating regions of medial cortex (see Venables and Christie, 1973). More recently, Damasio et al. (in press) reported smaller orienting to target stimuli in a passive attend condition in patients with orbito-mesial lesions but also found that patients with bilateral orbital and lower mesial frontal lesions give normal SCRs to what they term "orienting" stimuli (viz., an unexpected loud hand clap).

# POSITRON EMISSION TOMOGRAPHY (PET) AND SC

After this brief overview of the range of brain structures that have traditionally been linked to skin conductance, we now turn to the imaging literature. As noted above, brain imaging can be used to assess either the neurophysiological functioning of the brain or its neuroanatomical structure. We begin with a discussion of the single brain imaging study utilizing functional neuroimaging techniques, specifically positron emission tomography (PET).

## PET Methodology

This functional imaging technique is used to measure the metabolic activity of different regions of the brain by radioactively tagging glucose in order to observe which brain areas are utilizing more energy. Typically, a cyclotron is used to manufacture a short-lived isotope such as fluorine-18; the relatively short half-life of this positron emitter (approximately 110 minutes) helps keep the dose of radiation to the patient relatively low. Radiation in PET is about half of the exposure received in CT. The isotope is then "tagged" or integrated with an analogue of glucose-2-deoxyglucose. This compound (fluorodeoxyglucose or FDG) is then injected into the subject just after the start of a psychological task (e.g Wisconsin card sorting or continuous performance task). A series of blood samples are then taken from the subject to measure glucose and deoxyglucose. Since glucose is the only source of energy used by the brain, the flourine is quickly transported to the brain, where the most active regions receive the largest quantities. After about 30 minutes the deoxyglucose uptake is largely completed, so that the radioactivity is "fixed" in the brain at this point, remaining relatively stable for the following hour when the brain's metabolic rate is imaged (Buchsbaum, 1987).

The subject is then taken to the PET scanner. Positrons emitted by the decay of the isotope interact with electrons to emit two gamma photons which travel in opposite directions. Crystals which detect these photons are positioned around the head, and the origin of the gamma rays can be mapped by a computer to eventually produce a picture of the brain. Because more gamma rays are released by regions of higher metabolic activity, the neural activity in different parts of the brain can be visualized. Because radioactivity mostly fixed by the end of the challenge task, measures obtained during scanning reflect glucose metabolism at the time of the earlier task rather than at the time of the actual scanning sequence.

There are a number of advantages of PET imaging. First, it provides a direct measurement of brain glucose metabolism, and therefore of brain activity which can be localized to specific regions. Second, the spatial resolution is reasonably good, i.e. PET scanners with a resolution of 10 mm can image structures such as the caudate nucleus, and more recent scanners are able to provide even better resolution than this. Such resolution is better than other functional methods, but not as good as MRI. Another advantage of PET is that a hypothesized dysfunction to a specific brain region can be tested by "challenging" this brain region with a neuropsychological task thought to involve this region, and measuring glucose metabolism at this brain site relative to other brain sites. Finally, PET can now be used to measure neurotransmitter functions. The relative disadvantages of PET are: (a) its cost (approximately $3,000 / subject); (b) exposure of the subject to radioactivity (though this is less than exposure from a CT); (c) logistic difficulties sometimes involved by the availability of a cyclotron for production of the isotope; (d) poor temporal resolution, i.e. activity levels are averaged over the 30-minute uptake period. However, recent developments using oxygen 15 with a half-life of only two minutes allow for an increase in temporal resolution.

## PET and SC Orienting

To date there has been only one study of the relationship between SC and PET. Preliminary findings from this study were reported by Dawson (1990), while more detailed findings were reported by Hazlett et al. (in press). Subjects were six unmedicated schizophrenics. Three of these were found to be SC nonresponders while three were found to be responders. Six normal controls matched to the schizophrenics on age and sex on whom PET measures were available were also included, although no SC data were obtained on these subjects.

Results indicated that SC responder schizophrenics relative to nonresponders had significantly higher absolute glucose metabolism in a number of brain areas selected for analysis. These areas consisted of prefrontal cortex (lateral middle gyrus and medial superior gyrus), four regions of the thalamus, and two regions of the hippocampus. Mean values for the normal controls fell in between these two groups. Values for the amygdala did not significantly differ between the schizophrenic responders and nonresponders.

Total brain metabolic rate was found to be 20% lower in the nonresponders relative to responders. To correct for this global brain effect, analyses were conducted on relative metabolic rates. Fewer brain areas produced statistically significant results, although the pattern of findings remained the same. One difference was that responders were found to have higher metabolic rates in the right but not left amygdala. Groups were not found to differ on performance on the CPT, with mean values being almost identical.

## Evaluation of PET-SC Relationships

There are three key findings from this important pilot study. First, nonresponders had significantly less glucose uptake in the prefrontal cortex and the thalamus, supporting previous findings that these areas have important excitatory influences on SC activity (Wang, 1964; Venables and Christie, 1973; Edelberg, 1972). Second, the hippocampus was unexpectedly found to play an excitatory role with respect to SC orienting, insofar as the SC responders had significantly higher glucose utilization compared to nonresponders. Previous data and theory (Yokata et al. 1963; Bagshaw et al. 1965; Gruzelier and Venables 1972; Edelberg 1972) suggested a possible inhibitory role of the hippocampus. Third, and perhaps more surprising, there was only partial evidence supporting the amygdala as having an excitatory influence on SC orienting.

Negative findings must, however, be treated with caution for two reasons. First, because the sample size was very small, Type II errors become problematic. Second, the pattern of findings that emerge from PET studies of SC may well be a function of the type of challenge task used. Buchsbaum et al. (1990) have found that the degraded stimulus version of the CPT activates bilateral frontal as well as right temporal and parietal brain areas. Consequently, while the CPT may be an excellent challenge task with respect to the frontal lobes, it may be less ideal for assessing the amygdala and midbrain structures. This consideration might well explain why the right but not left amygdala was significantly associated with group differences in SC orienting, since the CPT activates right but not left temporal brain areas (Buchsbaum et al. 1990).

The study by Hazlett et al. (in press), while preliminary, provides an important basis on which future functional brain imaging studies of SC orienting may build. The use of unmedicated schizophrenics is a notable strength. As a pilot study, it gives strong initial support for the excitatory role of prefrontal cortex and the thalamus in SC orienting, at least in schizophrenic groups. Finally, it is interesting to note that in this study, the nonresponder schizophrenics did not differ from the responder schizophrenics in their scores on the CPT. The study points to the complexities of the chain of neural processes involved in CPT performance, and reminds us that abnormalities may be produced by a breakdown at one of several different places along that chain. This reasoning can be extended to the chain of neural processes underlying the skin conductance orienting response.

## CT STUDIES OF EDA

Computerized tomography (CT) is the older of the two structural imaging techniques, and almost all of the studies to date have utilized this technology. Before examining the findings of these studies, a discussion of the nature of the technology is important, so that the strengths and weaknesses of this approach can be seen.

### CT Methodology

CT was introduced in 1973 and as such is the oldest of the modern brain imaging techniques. In CT, standard X-rays are passed through the brain from one side of the head, and the amount of radiation which is not absorbed by intervening tissue is measured by radiation sensors within the CT scanner. The X-ray source is then moved across the subject's head and the process repeated on 160 locations. The X-ray source is then rotated $1^0$ and the procedure repeated throughout $180^0$. A computer is then used to digitize the data stored by the radiation sensors; this data matrix can then be used to reconstruct the subject's brain in the transverse (horizontal) plane. Effectively therefore, CT can be viewed as a three-dimensional X-ray.

CT has a number of disadvantages, including the facts that the subject is exposed to X-rays, spatial resolution of internal brain structures (e.g., the hippocampus) is poor, and images are affected by spectral shift artifact which distorts the signals at the skull boundary. Set against these disadvantages, CT is an inexpensive technique relative to other imaging procedures, and not surprisingly, most of the imaging research on SC has been conducted using this technique. Furthermore, CT provides a good image of the overall brain in the transverse plane and also of the lateral ventricles, with a ventricle / brain ratio (VBR) being one of the more commonly derived indices used in research on disordered groups.

### Findings from CT Studies

As stated above, CT studies make up the bulk of the currently small literature on brain imaging studies of SC activity, constituting seven of the nine brain imaging studies. Key features and the main results of these seven studies are listed in Table 1. This table illustrates a number of general points on this literature. First, it can be seen that all of these studies have taken place in the past 10 years, illustrating the fact that brain imaging and SC activity represents a new and emerging research area. Second, all of these studies have utilized subjects with schizophrenia, with schizophreniform disorder, or at risk for schizophrenia. Katsanis et al. (1991) also employed patients with affective disorders in addition to schizophrenics and schizophreniform patients. As such, it must be remembered that these data are based on subjects with diseased brains, and findings from such populations may or may not extrapolate to more normal populations. While this represents a limitation, the converse is that these studies are useful for illuminating the neuroanatomical basis of SC abnormalities in schizophrenia.

Third, while a number of different anatomical measures are typically derived from CT studies, it can be seen from the column entitled "key structures" that the ratio between area of the lateral ventricles and whole brain area or VBR (ventricle to brain ratio)

**Table 1.** Key findings of computerized tomography (CT) studies of skin conductance (SC) activity. SZ = schizophrenics. R = responders. NR = nonresponders. HAB = Habituators. NHAB = Nonhabituators. VBR = ventricle / brain ratio for lateral ventricles. 3V = third ventricle. FH = frontal horn. PF = prefrontal. P-O = parietal - occipital. FH BR = frontal horn / brain ratio. SCOR = SC orienting response. RT = reaction time. T2 = secondary reaction time. SCL = SC level. NSF = non-specific fluctuations.

| | SUBJECTS | N | STRUCTURES | KEY FINDINGS |
|---|---|---|---|---|
| Zahn et al. (1982) | SZ Atrophy<br>SZ Normal | 8<br>20 | Sulci/Fissures | Smaller SCORs, Slower RT and T2 in SZ atrophy group |
| Alm et al. (1984) | SZ R<br>SZ NR | 12<br>22 | VBR | N.S.D. |
| Bartfai et al. (1987) | SZ NR<br>SZ HAB<br>SZ NHAB | 6<br>7<br>5 | 3V width<br>FH width<br>Sulci | Trend: Wide 3V in SZ nonhabituators<br>N.S.D.<br>N.S.D. |
| Cannon et al. (1988) | SZ High Risk | 34 | 3V width<br>VBR | Wide 3V corr. with reduced SCOR amplitude<br>N.S.D. |
| Schnur et al. (1989) | SZ R<br>SZ NR | 9<br>15 | 3V width<br>VBR<br>PF sulci<br>P-O sulci | Wide 3V in SZ responders<br>N.S.D.<br>N.S.D.<br>N.S.D. |
| Katsanis et al. (1991) | SZ<br>Affective<br>Schizophreniform | 36<br>33<br>19 | VBR | N.S.D. in SCL, NSF, #SCOR. |
| Katsanis & Iacono (1992) | SZ | 65 | VBR<br>3V Width<br>FH BR<br>Sulcal width | N.S.D. SCL, NSF, Habituation rate<br>N.S.D. "  "  "  "<br>N.S.D. "  "  "  "<br>N.S.D. "  "  "  " |

represents that structure most commonly assessed, having been taken in 5 of the seven studies. Width of the third ventricle has been measured in 4 of the studies. Ventricular enlargement is the most commonly utilized brain measure in CT studies due to the fact that CT images do not have the resolution to differentiate grey from white matter within the cortex. Brain-CSF differentiation is relatively clear, however, and the ventricles are large enough to be measured with good reliability. If ventricular enlargement is discovered, it is then necessary to infer which structures are implicated as the cause of the enlargement. These structures are typically thought to the thalamus and the hypothalamus.

Generalized cortical atrophy has been assessed in CT studies in two ways. One such method consists of measuring the width of brain sulci. Such measures are generally qualitative clinical ratings made on a three-point scale, assessing the extent to which the sulci can be visualized. Sulci that are larger are more easily visualized, indicating brain atrophy. Similarly, linear measures are taken to assess the width of the inter-hemispheric fissure: the greater the width, the greater the degree of cortical atrophy. Some studies also take more specific measures in an attempt to obtain some degree of localization. For example, Katsanis and Iacono (1992) have measured a frontal horn / brain ratio; a larger ratio would potentially indicate atrophy to frontal white matter. Similarly, Schnur et al. (1989) measured sulcal prominence of the parieto-occipital lobes, assessing the extent of posterior cortical atrophy.

Brain - SC relationships have been assessed in three ways. Most commonly, schizophrenics are divided into SC responders or nonresponders based on responsivity to orienting stimuli in order to determine whether these groups differ on brain structural measures; one study (Bartfai et al. 1987) additionally divides responders into habituators and non-habituators. A second method consists of dividing schizophrenics into those with and without brain atrophy and looking for group differences in SC activity (Zahn et al. 1982; Katsanis et al. 1991; Katsanis & Iacono, 1992). Third, some studies assess correlations between SC activity and brain structural measures for the whole patient group (Cannon et al. 1988).

The findings from Table 1 can be summarized as follows: (1) No significant relationships have been observed between enlargement of the lateral ventricles and SC orienting. (2) Cortical atrophy, as determined by sulcal prominence was not significantly related to SC activity, with the exception of one study (Zahn et al. 1982). (3) Results for the third ventricle are mixed. One study (Cannon et al. 1988) finds increased width of the third ventricle to be associated with reduced SC orienting. However, Schnur et al. (1989) found exactly the opposite result, i.e., increased third ventricle width was associated with increased SC orienting. In support of this latter finding, Bartfai et al. (1987) found a trend (p < .10) for larger third ventricles to be associated with SC responding.

There are a number of possible explanations for the conflicting findings regarding the third ventricle. First, Schnur et al. (1989) defined nonresponding using both SC and finger pulse volume measures (which the authors indicate may more reliably index a central orienting deficit), whereas Cannon et al. (1988) and other studies only used SC as a measure of orienting. However, this difference cannot account for differences in findings between Cannon et al. (1988) and Bartfai et al. (1987), both of which measured orienting using SC only. Further, it is unlikely that the addition of finger pulse volume orienting would result in radically different results from using SC alone since approximately 80% of schizophrenic SC nonresponders are also finger pulse volume nonresponders.

Second, the two studies finding a positive correlation between the third ventricle and SC employed schizophrenic patients whereas the study by Cannon et al (1988) used a population at risk for schizophrenia (children of schizophrenics). In addition, the Cannon et al. study was prospective in nature, with SC measured at age 15 related to enlarged third ventricles measured at age 33, whereas the other two studies measured SC and CT concurrently. Finally, Schnur et al. (1989) divided subjects into responders and nonresponders whereas Cannon et al. (1988) derived correlations between CT and SC measures in the total sample.

Although the findings of Cannon et al. (1988) conflict with those of two other studies in the direction of the observed effect, the findings of this study are supported in two ways. First, the findings of Cannon et al. (1988) make neuroanatomical sense, based on the traditional view of the role of the anterior hypothalamus. Enlargement of the third ventricle would be expected to be associated with tissue loss in the anterior hypothalamus which surrounds the base of the third ventricle (Barr, 1979). Because the anterior hypothalamus has been viewed as having an excitatory influence on SC activity (Wang, 1964; Edelberg, 1972; Venables and Christie, 1973; Bloch and Bonvallet, 1960), enlargement of the third ventricle (and associated tissue loss to the excitatory anterior hypothalamus) would be consistent with reduced SC orienting. Second, Cannon et al. (1992) have also found that enlargement of the third ventricle in this sample is also associated with reduced resting heart rate level. Since heart rate and SC are essentially uncorrelated, this can be viewed as providing some independent support for the notion that the periventricular structures associated with the third ventricle, such as anterior hypothalamus, may have excitatory influences on autonomic activity.

### Limitations of CT Studies

The seven CT studies listed in Table 1 have provided very important data on the neuroanatomical basis of SC in humans. At the same time, results from these studies have generally been disappointing. Reasons for these generally negative findings may be due to inherent limitations in CT methodology. The major limitation of CT is that grey / white differentiation is poor relative to MRI. Gray matter structures such as the hippocampus cannot be clearly distinguished on CT, so the measures derived from CT are relatively global and non-specific. Slice thickness in CT studies is usually 10mm, resulting in significant "partial volume effect," that is, a particular gyrus might fill only 3mm or 5mm of a given slice, thus appearing hazy on the image or as a region of partial signal intensity. The partial volume effect makes it particularly difficult to clearly differentiate and assess sulci, which is a commonly used measure in CT studies. Furthermore, imaging is restricted to the transverse plane which limits the structures which can be reasonably assessed.

## MAGNETIC RESONANCE IMAGING (MRI) AND SC

### Technological Advantages

Most of the limitations of CT scanning outlined above are overcome by MRI, which has a substantially higher signal-to-noise ratio compared to CT. This imaging procedure involves the yoking together of magnetism and radiofrequency radiation. Initially, a high-strength magnetic field is used to align atomic nuclei in the brain (these nuclei are otherwise randomly oriented). The second stage consists of applying a radio frequency (RF) signal at right angles to the magnetic field, moving some of the nuclei out of alignment with the magnetic field. The third stage consists of turning off this RF pulse; the nuclei then return to their initial alignment, and in doing so a voltage is induced in the electrical field (termed "magnetic resonance"); this voltage change is then detected and measured by a coil of wire around the tissue.

The bulk of the MRI signal derives from hydrogen because the best magnetic signal to noise ratio is found for hydrogen protons. Hydrogen is the most common element in biological tissue, in the form of water. Because the different types of tissue in the brain (white matter, gray matter, CSF, blood, and diseased tissue) all differ in terms of their water content, these tissues have different responses to the RF pulse, and excellent visualization and differentiation of structures can be produced. Different types of scanning sequences can be utilized depending on the investigator's purposes. For example, T1-weighted images produce very good differentiation of gray matter (neurons) and white matter (axons), while a T2-weighted scan will allow optimal visualization of diseased tissue (e.g., tumors).

The key advantages to MRI include: (a) visualization of many anatomical structures are much superior to CT (b) there is no exposure to radiation (c) the brain can be imaged in all three planes (d) there is no significant bone artifact (e) recent advances in MRI acquisition and computer software allow the brain to be displayed in three dimensions, and cut in any plane (f) slice thicknesses as low as 1 mm are now possible, resulting in a major reduction of partial volume effect (g) faster scanning techniques are bringing about a major reduction in scan time and consequently a reduction in "aliassing" artifact due to movement. Key disadvantages are that the technique cannot be used with patients with pacemakers, aneurysm clips, or ferromagnetic implants, and it is also relatively costly (approximately $1,000 / subject). Perhaps due to its relative recency, there has only been one MRI study of SC to date.

## MRI Findings on SC Orienting: Background and Methodology

Raine et al. (1991) tested hypotheses of the neuroanatomy of SC orienting in a group of 17 normal subjects by relating individual differences in SC orienting to individual differences in selected neuroanatomical areas. Based on previous animal and human studies described earlier in this chapter, it was hypothesized that significant positive correlations would exist between SC responding and size of pons and the temporal/amygdala area. Additionally, it was anticipated that prefrontal area measured from a coronal cut (including dorsolateral and orbito-frontal area) would be positively correlated with SC orienting, whereas medial prefrontal area (measured from a mid-sagittal cut) would not be related to SC orienting. As indicated earlier, findings on the third ventricle from CT studies have been mixed. Consequently, no firm predictions were generated for this structure.

In addition to these areas, medial prefrontal, posterior (non-prefrontal) cortex, and area of the cerebellum were also taken as control measures with the expectation that they would not relate to SC orienting. Non-prefrontal areas within the frontal lobe, such as area 6 (pre-motor cortex), appear to play both an excitatory and inhibitory role with respect to electrodermal activity (Edelberg, 1972). No clear relationships have been observed for posterior cortical areas in humans. The cerebellum was taken as a control measure for the pons, because removal of the cerebellum has no effect on SC activity in cats (Wang, 1964), and because it is approximately of the same phylogenetic age as the pons. Full details of scanning sequence, delineation of targeted brain structures, and scoring procedures may be found in Raine et al. (1991).

## MRI Findings

Significant positive correlations ranging from .44 to .60 were found between left and right prefrontal area measures from the coronal cut and frequency of left and right SC orienting responses to a six tone series (all 75 dB tones) and a ten tone series (including more intense 90 dB white noise stimuli and consonant-vowel stimuli), indicating that greater prefrontal area was associated with greater SC orienting. Correlations for the pons were also significant in all cases and ranged from .43 to .54. Correlations for left temporal area including the amygdala were significant (r = .47 to .53), but those for right temporal area were not. No significant correlations were observed for the control measures of posterior cortex and the cerebellum. No significant correlations were observed for medial prefrontal cortex (mid-sagittal cut), indicating that the significant prefrontal correlations from the coronal cut are likely to be attributable to dorsolateral or orbito-frontal area rather than medial prefrontal area. Correlations for the third ventricle were also non-significant.

## Interpretation of MRI Findings

The key findings from this study are that: (1) Larger areas of prefrontal, pons, and left temporal / amygdala regions are associated with greater SC orienting. (2) No such effects are observed for the third ventricle, and control measures of posterior cortex and the cerebellum. (3) These effects are obtained in normal, non-pathological humans, as opposed to clinical patients.

It should be noted that the significant correlations observed were not a function of outliers, as Spearman (rank order) correlations were employed to control for this possibility. Furthermore, significant relationships for frontal and pons area were not a function of greater brain size per se since correlations remained significant after expressing key areas as a ratio of overall brain size. However, the effects for left temporal area were no longer significant when expressed as a ratio to overall brain size, raising some doubt as to the significance of this brain area.

The conclusion that prefrontal area has an important excitatory influence on SC orienting is consistent with previous animal and human data. Of interest is the fact that some prefrontal-orienting correlations remained significant after partialling out the effects of both skin conductance level (SCL) and nonspecific fluctuations (NSFs) is consistent with the work of Kimble et al. (1965), who demonstrated a relationship between lateral prefrontal lesions and SC orienting deficits in monkeys which was independent from differences in NSFs. There are several studies which suggest that it is specifically the dorsolateral area of prefrontal cortex that is implicated in orienting. For example, lesions of this area in humans have been found to attenuate P300 event related potential orienting responses recorded over prefrontal cortex (Knight 1984), while lesions of dorsolateral prefrontal cortex in monkeys result in SC orienting deficits (Grueninger et al. 1965). Future MRI studies which can selectively assess this specific region of prefrontal cortex are required to test this hypothesis.

The mixed findings for temporal area including the amygdala from this MRI study are in accord with the mixed findings from the PET study. Three recent human neurological case studies have all failed to show any effect of bilateral amygdala damage on simple SC orienting (Tranel and Damasio, 1989; Tranel and Hyman, 1990, Lee et al. 1988). These findings warrant some re-evaluation of the role of the amygdala. It is interesting that dorsolateral prefrontal cortex was spared bilaterally in the patient tested by Tranel and Damasio (1989), and these authors speculate that prefrontal cortex may play an important role in mediating SC orienting. Certainly these human studies conflict with the early but limited monkey data implicating the amygdala as an excitatory center for SC activity (Bagshaw et al. 1965, Bagshaw and Benzies, 1968). Although recent human findings cast doubt on the role of the amygdala, it is quite possible that different regions of the amygdala have both excitatory and inhibitory influences on SC, just as they are differentially known to influence aggression, and this is an area where further animal research could be particularly informing.

More positive results were obtained from this MRI study compared with those obtained from CT studies. This is probably because MRI has much greater spatial resolution relative to CT, allowing for specific structures of relevance to SC orienting to be visualized and quantified. However, it is also possible that positive findings were a function of the use of normal subjects as opposed to pathological groups used in CT studies. We investigate this latter possibility next.

## Two Possible Neural Bases for SC Hyporesponsivity in Patients

The positive findings in Raine et al. (1991) were obtained using normal subjects who had been matched to schizophrenics on age, parental social class, and education level. However, no significant findings emerged from similar analyses conducted on groups of schizophrenic and affective disorder patients on whom the same variables had been collected. In this sense, the MRI findings are more consonant with the previous CT findings, which are generally non-significant.

One possible explanation for this discrepancy lies in the fact that a greater range is observed for SC orienting frequency in the normals relative to patient groups. In our MRI study, schizophrenic and affective disorder groups showed significantly reduced SC orienting relative to the normal control group, and did not differ from one another. Such hyporesponsivity in both affective and schizophrenic patients is consistent with previous research (Zahn, 1986; Iacono and Ficken, in this volume). However, this may have resulted in floor effects for schizophrenic and affective disorder groups: the mean number of responses for the schizophrenic and affective patient groups were 0.95 and 0.85 respectively, while the normal controls averaged 2.55 responses. Such restricted range in SC scores could suppress the size of brain structure - SC correlations in these two groups.

This restriction in range, combined with the view that schizophrenia is a disorder that may be heterogeneous in etiology, has led us to speculate that it may be of value to seek categorical relationships between brain structure and SC in pathological groups rather than the type of continuous, correlational patterns we observed in the normal control group. That is, individual differences in SC orienting may not relate in a linear fashion to individual differences in prefrontal area because schizophrenics may be characterized by multiple brain deficits that compromise SC orienting in different ways. For example, there could be a sub-group of schizophrenics whose reduced SC orienting could be explained by prefrontal deficits, while SC deficits in another schizophrenic sub-group could be explained by, for example, ventricular enlargement. We noted above that the study by Hazlett et al. (in press) found that two groups of patients with significant differences in brain functioning nevertheless had equal deficits in CPT performance. Similarly, it is likely that the orienting reflex depends for its integrity on a number of neural structures, rather than one discrete brain area being responsible for orienting.

Consequently, we have recently employed cluster analysis as a statistical technique to help identify discrete sub-groups of patients who may show similar deficits in SC orienting but differ in terms of the neural substrate of that deficit (Lencz et al. 1991). There were two steps to these analyses. The first consisted of ascertaining if and how subjects cluster with respect to SC orienting and brain anatomy. The second step consisted of determining whether these resulting clusters were related in any systematic way to psychiatric classification.

In the first analysis stage 45 subjects (15 schizophrenics, 15 affective disorder patients, and 15 normal controls) were entered into a cluster analysis. Three clustering variables were used: frequency of SC orienting responses, prefrontal area, and lateral VBR (measured from a transverse MRI cut taken at the mid-ventricular level). These latter two variables were selected because ventricular enlargement is one of the best replicated findings in schizophrenia, and it has also recently been observed in affective groups (Andreasen et al. 1990). As such, it could account for SC orienting deficits reliably observed in both of these groups. Prefrontal area was entered because both MRI and PET studies indicate that it plays a role in SC orienting, and because schizophrenics have been found to show reduced prefrontal area (Raine et al. in press; DeMeyer et al. 1988). The images used for this study did not have the resolution to allow for measurement of smaller structures, such as the hippocampus, amygdala, and thalamus. Other variables (e.g., temporal lobes) were not included in order to simplify this preliminary analysis; cluster analysis is susceptible to misleading results when too many variables are entered (Aldenderfer and Blashfield, 1984). Future cluster analytic studies might fruitfully examine some of these structures.

Variables were z-transformed and entered into an agglomerative hierarchical cluster analysis. Based on the dendrogram and a plot of the fusion coefficients, three clear clusters were identified. One-way ANOVAs were conducted on the clustering variables in order to determine the defining characteristics.

Results of this analysis are reported in Table 2. It can be seen that Cluster 1 consisted of subjects with reduced SC orienting, reduced prefrontal area, but normal ventricles. Cluster 2 also had reduced SC orienting, but had ventricular enlargement and normal prefrontal area. Cluster 3 showed normal values on all three measures. It should be noted that the terms "normal" and reduced" are used in a relative sense; that is, subjects in Clusters 1 and 2 had reduced SC responses relative to Cluster 3, as determined by the ANOVAs. Consequently, this cluster analysis indicates that there may be at least two neural bases to SC orienting deficits.

**Table 2.** Characteristics of three clusters with respect to skin conductance orienting activity (SC), prefrontal area, and lateral ventricle / brain ratio (Lencz et al. 1991).

|            | N  | SC               | PREFRONTAL    | VENTRICLES        |
|------------|----|------------------|---------------|-------------------|
| Cluster 1  | 12 | Hyporesponsivity | Reduced Area  | Normal            |
| Cluster 2  | 16 | Hyporesponsivity | Normal        | Ventriculomegaly  |
| Cluster 3  | 17 | Normal           | Normal        | Normal            |

A related but separate question concerns whether these three clusters bear any relationship to psychiatric grouping (diagnostic status was not a variable entered into the cluster analysis. The chi-square statistic ($X^2 = 11.18$, $p < .05$) indicated a significant relationship between psychiatric group classification and cluster membership. Results of this chi-square are shown in Table 3. It can be seen that Cluster 1 (reduced orienting, reduced prefrontal) was over-represented by schizophrenics. Interestingly, the 3 normals (20%) who fell into Cluster 1 (prefrontal and orienting deficits) were among the top four scorers on a measure of schizotypal personality (STA, Claridge and Broks, 1984) a finding consistent with the notion that subjects with tendencies towards schizotypal personality would share characteristics of schizophrenics. Cluster 2 (reduced orienting, enlarged ventricles) was over-represented by affective patients, while cluster 3 (normal SC, normal MRI) was over-represented by normal controls. Consequently, these analyses suggest an association between schizophrenia / schizotypy, reduced SC orienting, and prefrontal deficits on the one hand, and affective disorders, reduced SC orienting, and ventricular enlargement on the other. It should be noted that the three clusters did not significantly differ from each other with respect to brain area posterior to the prefrontal region, nor did they differ in age height, weight, education, or social class.

However, Table 3 also shows that schizophrenics were fairly evenly spread across the three clustering groups, illustrative of the heterogeneity of schizophrenia. Specifically, a third of the schizophrenics fell into cluster 2. Thus, while some schizophrenics may have SC orienting deficits produced by prefrontal deficits, others have orienting deficits which may be more explained by ventricular enlargement. Four of the schizophrenics (28%) were normal on all three measures. This is consistent with the notion that structural brain deficits and psychophysiological deficits have rarely if ever been found to characterize all schizophrenics. Interestingly, three out of the five female schizophrenics fell into this third cluster, while 9 of the 10 male schizophrenics fell into the more "pathological" clusters 1 and 2. Furthermore, cluster 3 schizophrenics had significantly higher scores on positive symptoms (delusions and hallucinations) than the other two clusters ($F=4.01$, $p<.05$). Consequently the schizophrenics falling into the "normal" cluster 3 are characterized by females and positive symptomatology, and as such may be more likely to have a good prognosis. Schizophrenics in the three clusters did not significantly differ on age, age at onset, duration of illness, or degree of negative symptomatology.

**Table 3.** Relationship between cluster membership and psychiatric group status (Lencz et al. 1991).

| | SC HYPORESPONDING | | NORMAL SC |
| --- | --- | --- | --- |
| | REDUCED PREFRONTAL | ENLARGED VENTRICLES | NORMAL MRI |
| | Cluster 1 | Cluster 2 | Cluster 3 |
| Schizophrenics | 6 | 5 | 4 |
| Affectives | 3 | 9 | 3 |
| Normals | 3 | 2 | 10 |
| Total | 12 | 16 | 17 |

**Comments on Findings from Cluster Analysis**

The findings of Lencz et al. (1991) may be best viewed as heuristic in value given the relatively small sample size employed. Nevertheless this analysis serves to illustrate a number of issues. First, the generally non-significant findings from CT studies may not only be a function of relatively weak imaging technology, but also from the attempt to seek out continuous relationships within pathological groups which are heterogenous with respect to neural deficits. Re-analyses of these data sets using cluster analytic techniques may result in clearer links between SC orienting measures and anatomical measures.

Second, these analyses illustrate the potential value of attempting to identify discrete sub-groups of schizophrenics who differ from each other in terms of underlying biological markers, with results indicating at least two possible neural bases to SC deficits in schizophrenics, one mediated by prefrontal deficits, and one by ventricular enlargement. Third, the analyses also suggest that the strategy of researching individual differences in schizotypal personality as an alternative "high risk" approach to schizophrenia may be justified; trends in Lencz et al. (1991) indicate that schizotypals, like a sub-group of schizophrenics, may be characterized by prefrontal deficits in association with SC orienting deficits. Finally, the fact that some schizophrenics fell into the second cluster which was otherwise characteristic of patients with affective disorder raises the possibility that some schizophrenics may belong to an etiological spectrum with the affective disorders, while others may not. As such, these data help to illustrate how research into the neuroanatomy of SC activity, while representing a "basic science" approach, can also help inform more clinical research into schizophrenia and affective disorders, and demonstrates the applied value of physiological research on EDA.

## CONCEPTUAL AND METHODOLOGICAL ISSUES: GUIDELINES FOR FUTURE RESEARCH

### Neuroanatomical Issues

MRI represents a significant advance over CT in the ability to differentiate structures within the cortex. Even so, our MRI studies have been neuroanatomically crude, in that these structures, such as the temporal lobe have been measured as a whole and related to SC. It is possible that some aspects of the thalamus or temporal cortex may have an excitatory role with respect to SC, while other parts of these same structures play an inhibitory role. Future MRI studies which can achieve greater resolution should attempt a more fine-grained division of structures such as the thalamus and the amygdala.

This suggestion is particularly salient with respect to assessment of the prefrontal cortex. Prefrontal cortex in man makes up 29% of all cortex, and we know little about the specific functions of localized areas of this complex structure. One realistic goal over the next few years would be to separately assess dorsolateral, orbito-frontal and medial areas of prefrontal cortex to more specifically assess the hypothesis that it is dorsolateral prefrontal cortex that most specifically relates to SC orienting. Currently it is difficult to identify clear neuroanatomical landmarks to make this division using MRI, but new three-dimensional volumetric scoring software developed recently should aid this process. PET studies measuring glucose metabolism from different prefrontal regions may conceivably make faster progress than MRI studies in this respect.

Similarly, previous imaging studies have been somewhat (perhaps necessarily) vague concerning the neuroanatomical significance of enlargement of the lateral ventricles, and there has been little discussion of this issue in the schizophrenia literature. However, there have been two factor analytic studies (Rossi et al. 1988; Cannon et al. 1989) which have demonstrated that enlargement of the lateral ventricles is independent of cortical atrophy in schizophrenics. It therefore seems reasonable to conclude that lateral ventriculomegaly reflects damage to the deep periventricular region. Inspection of the brain atlas of DeArmond et al. (1989) indicates that at the mid-ventricular level in the transverse plane the lateral ventricles are surrounded by white matter - largely from the splenium and genu of the corpus callosum. A cut 4mm superior to the body of the lateral ventricles again shows that radiations of the corpus callosum surround the superior portions of the lateral ventricles. However, a slice below the mid-ventricular level shows that thalamic nuclei surround the more inferior aspects of the body of the lateral ventricles. It could be argued therefore that enlargement of the lateral ventricles might reflect tissue loss to two main structures: (a) the thalamus and (b) the corpus callosum. While we did not have adequate resolution to delineate the thalamus in our MRI study, we did assess area of the corpus callosum (Raine et al. 1990). Correlations were computed between corpus callosum measures and SC orienting measures, but none were significant. By inference therefore, it is possible that enlargement of the lateral ventricles may be linked to reductions in SC orienting via tissue loss to the thalamus. However, this must remain a tentative hypothesis until tested by future MRI studies of SC orienting.

Imaging studies to date have largely identified brain areas which may play an excitatory role in SC orienting. An important question however concerns which brain areas may play an inhibitory role in SC orienting. Roy (in this volume) suggests that the medulla and periaqueductal gray areas may have important inhibitory influences on EDA, while Edelberg (1972) has implicated premotor cortex and ventromedial aspects of the bulbar reticular formation as inhibitory with respect to SC. Identification of such inhibitory areas in future imaging studies may give important clues as to mechanisms which may underlie SC nonresponding in schizophrenia, affective disorders, (Iacono and Ficken, in this volume), and schizotypal forms of antisocial behavior (Crider, in this volume).

CT, MRI, and PET studies have so far sought out brain mechanisms which may underlie orienting in isolation of one another. The challenge open to future researchers lies in moving away from such relatively simplistic notions and towards attempting to identify the neural network or networks activated during orienting. For example, PET studies could usefully intercorrelate glucose metabolism at prefrontal and thalamic sites to show that these areas function in unison during an orienting challenge task, in much the same way as coherence analysis in EEG helps identify integrated neural sites of activity.

## PET Methodology

The use of a CPT challenge task in PET may not be the best way of assessing SC orienting - brain function links. Isotopes with relative long half-lives require lengthy tasks such as a 32 minute CPT used in Hazlett et al. (in press). Ideally however, the brain mechanisms that underlie SC orienting might be most usefully explored by using the orienting paradigm itself as an uptake task, repeatedly presenting subjects with orienting stimuli over a short period of time. Such an experiment could be conducted using $^{15}$O which has a short half-life of only two minutes, and by testing subjects in both a baseline condition and an orienting condition. The former could be subtracted from the latter to more precisely assay which brain areas are specifically activated by the orienting paradigm. The simultaneous recording of PET and SC, using orienting as the challenge task, would clearly present a very potent strategy for understanding the brain mechanisms underlying SC orienting.

## SC Recording Methodology in Brain Imaging Studies

The imaging technology used in previous studies of SC orienting has so far been highlighted, with the clear indications being that more advanced imaging technologies (MRI and PET) have produced more positive findings than the seven studies which have used CT technology. In contrast, Table 4 summarizes the methodology used in the nine imaging studies to record SC orienting. It can be seen that almost all of the studies used silver/ silver chloride electrodes, with the one exception being Cannon et al. (1988) who used Zinc electrodes, explainable by the fact that recordings were taken in 1962. Most studies also used either sodium chloride or potassium chloride as electrolyte medium, in accordance with recommendations made by Fowles et al. (1981). Latency windows for scoring SCRs were appropriately conservative, with the modal window being 1-3 seconds. The criterion for minimal amplitude varied, but was most frequently .05 microsiemens. As would be expected, tone intensities varied from 54 - 85 dB, but all were within the orienting range.

The greatest degree of methodological discrepancy occurred for recording site. Four studies recorded from the medial phalange, three from the distal phalange, one from the thenar / hypothenar site, and one from the proximal site. Some studies recorded SC from the same dermatome (e.g. first and second fingers), while other studies crossed thedermatome (e.g. fingers one and three) and thus record from fingers which are differentially innervated. Examining the final column of Table 4, it can be seen that there was an association between outcome and SC recording site. That is, studies recording SC from distal sites tended to report significant relationships between SC orienting and neuroanatomical measures, whereas, studies recording from medial sites tended not to report significant findings. Specifically, all three studies recording from distal sites reported significant relationships, whereas only two of five studies recording SC from the medial site produced significant results.

This discrepancy may be because the distal site appears to be more active than the medial site. We have recently shown, for example, that SC amplitudes recorded from the

**Table 4.** Skin conductance recording methodology used in brain imaging studies. Scoring window is in seconds. Response criterion is in microsiemens. Intensity is in dB. Numbers after recording site refer to fingers used to record SC, e.g., Medial 12 = medial site using first and second fingers. The final column indicates whether significant relationships between neuroimaging variables and SC were reported.

| | ELECTRODE | ELECTROLYTE | SCORING WINDOW | RESPONSE CRITERION | INTENSITY | RECORDING SITE | SIGNIFICANT FINDINGS |
|---|---|---|---|---|---|---|---|
| Zahn et al. (1982) | Ag/AgCl | KCl | 1-4 | .002 | 72 | Distal 23 | Yes |
| Alm et al. (1984) | Ag/AgCl | --- | 1-4 | .05 | 80 | Medial 12 | No |
| Bartfai et al. (1987) | Ag/AgCl | NaCl | 1-5 | .0043 (log) | 85 | Thenar/Hypothenar | No |
| Cannon et al. (1988) | Zinc | $ZnSO_4$ | --- | --- | 54 | Distal 12 | Yes |
| Schnur et al. (1989) | Ag/AgCl | Beckman | 1-3 | .05 | 60 | Proximal 13 | Yes |
| Raine et al. (1991) | Ag/AgCl | KCl | 1-3 | .01 | 75 | Medial 12 | Yes |
| Lencz et al. (1991) | Ag/AgCl | KCl | 1-3 | .01 | 75 | Medial 12 | Yes |
| Katsanis et al. (1991) | Ag/AgCl | NaCl | 1-3 | .05 | 85 | Medial 13 | No |
| Katsanis & Iacono (1992) | Ag/AgCl | NaCl | 1-3 | .05 | 85 | Medial 13 | No |
| Hazlett et al. (1992) | Ag/AgCl | NaCl | 1-3 | .05 | 78 | Distal 12 | Yes |

distal site are 3.5 times higher than amplitudes recorded from the medial site in the same subjects (Scerbo et al. 1992). All 17 subjects who consistently produced SCRs showed this site effect. SC levels were twice as large at distal relative to medial sites. Furthermore, distal sites were more sensitive than medial sites to manipulations such as stimulus intensity.

One imaging study recorded from the thenar and hypothenar eminences of the hand, a site which is more responsive than medial sites (Edelberg, 1967), and interestingly produced a trend towards significance. The two analyses using medial sites (Raine et al., 1991; Lencz et al. 1991) which obtained significant effects employed more sensitive imaging technology, which might have compensated for the "weaker" SC recording methodology. It is interesting to note that the one study which used both strong imaging technology (PET) and recorded from the more sensitive distal site (Hazlett et al. in press) obtained the strongest effect sizes of all nine studies. Future psychophysiological studies might usefully record from the distal phalange in order to maximize the possibility of significant findings and minimize Type II errors.

**Methodological Directions for the Future**

In an ideal world, researchers would assess subjects on both PET and MRI in conjunction with SC orienting. In reality, it may be a long time before both structural and functional imaging studies of SC orienting are conducted on the same subjects. In the meantime, MRI studies could more easily assess brain function using appropriate neuropsychological tests. One interesting example of this approach may be found in the CT study of Katsanis and Iacono (1992) who found that neuropsychological measures of temporal lobe functioning (but not of frontal functioning) correlated positively with SC responding. Alternatively, EEG mapping techniques may also be a reasonable alternative to assessing function in structural imaging studies (Rippon, this volume). It must be remembered however that neuropsychological test performance is multiply determined by a variety of brain sites. For example, Hazlett et al. (in press) found that responding and nonresponding schizophrenics differed radically in terms of brain glucose metabolism, but not in terms of behavioral performance on the CPT.

In the long-term brain imaging will become cheaper, easier, and more available. For example, single photon emission computed tomography (SPECT) is a functional imaging technique that makes use of commercially available tracers, and as such does not require an expensive cyclotron, sophisticated associated facilities, and a team of specialists to operate. Several test conditions can be quickly run, and resolution for the latest SPECT is comparable with older PET (approximately 8 mm full width at half maximum). Indeed, SPECT is likely to be the imaging procedure most readily available to psychophysiologists in the future.

Perhaps the most promising technological development is fast MRI, a technique that uses magnetic resonance imaging for both structural and functional imaging simultaneously. Fast MRI has the potential to combine the structural detail of MRI with the ability to measure the functioning of the various brain regions by tracking the flow of blood in the brain. This technique, which is still in the earliest pilot stage, has a temporal resolution measured in seconds, as opposed to 30 minutes for standard PET. Thus, this method holds out the possibility of measuring changes in brain functioning in real time, while at the same time linking the function to structure. The main weakness of fast MRI is that it measures blood flow, which is a relatively crude measure of functioning compared to the direct measurement of glucose metabolism available in PET.

Brain imaging studies are only beginning to inform us on mechanisms underlying SC activity. Both animal and human neurological research is more advanced in having implicated many more structures than brain imaging research has to date. One good example from neurological studies to date can be found in the asymmetric role thought to be played by parietal cortex in mediating SC activity (Zoccolotti, this volume). Similarly, Sequeira and Roy (this volume) has highlighted the roles of parietal cortex and the pericruciate cortex in SC activity in the cat, while Roy (this volume) has outlined the inhibitory role of the medulla and periaqueductal gray. Such potentially important structures await quantification in brain imaging studies of SC activity.

Furedy (this volume) suggests that the psychophysiological utility of SC measures has been diminished by focussing on the physiological mechanisms which underlie SC, arguing that the focus should always be on psychological processes. It is hoped that the study of Lencz et al. (1991) goes some way to addressing this concern, in that this study illustrates how knowledge of the mechanisms underlying SC orienting can provide potentially valuable information on psychological and psychiatric problems such as the relationship between schizophrenia, schizotypal personality disorder, and affective disorder. In this context, we feel that an understanding of the brain mechanisms underlying SC orienting is non-trivial. Rather than focussing only on psychological aspects of psychophysiology, we can advance more by using research on the neuroanatomical bases of SC, combined with the psychological manifestations of SC, to better integrate physiological with psychological processes. We view psychophysiological research from an interactionist perspective, in which basic biological research can inform and direct psychological research, and vice versa. Psychological phenomena have sufficient complexity to be studied from both directions, and scientists working on any side of a problem are well served by remaining aware of "the big picture". As stated by Dawson (1990), psychophysiology lies at the interface of clinical science, cognitive science, and neuroscience, and as such is a tool that can and should be used for multiple purposes.

## SUMMARY

To date there have been 9 studies which have employed three different brain imaging techniques alongside SC recording. One study has employed positron emission tomography (PET). Seven of the nine studies have employed computerized tomography (CT), while one has used magnetic resonance imaging (MRI). It will be argued that, taken together, these studies implicate prefrontal cortex, the thalamus, pons, and hippocampus as having excitatory influences on skin conductance activity. Findings for the temporal lobes, the amygdala, and the third ventricle are more mixed. Studies which have recorded SC activity from the distal phalanges of the hand have tended to produce stronger findings than studies recording SC from the medial phalange, and it is suggested that this may be because SC activity is substantially greater in magnitude when recorded from the distal site. Results from a recent study using cluster analytic techniques suggest that there are at least two neural bases underlying SC hyporesponsivity in schizophrenics and patients with affective disorders, one mediated by the prefrontal area, and one by periventricular areas adjacent to the lateral ventricles.

## REFERENCES

Aldenderfer, M.S., and Blashfield, R.K., 1984, "Cluster Analysis," Sage Publications, Beverly Hills.
Alm,T., Lindstrom, L.H., Ost, L.G. and Ohman, A., 1984, Electrodermal nonresponding in schizophrenia: relationships to attentional, clinical, biochemical, computed tomographical and genetic factors, *Int. Journal of Psychophys.* 1:195-208.
Andreasen, N.C., Swayze, V.W., Flaum, M., Alliger, R., and Cohen, G., 1990, Ventricular abnormalities in affective disorder: clinical and demographic correlates. *Am. J. Psychiatry.* 147:893-900.
Bagshaw, M.H. and Benzies, S., 1968, Multiple measures of the orienting reaction and their dissociation after amygdalectomy in monkeys, *Exp. Neurol.* 20:175-187.

Bagshaw, M.H., Kimble, D.P. and Pribram, K.E., 1965, The GSR of monkeys during orienting and habituation and after ablation of the amygdala, hippocampus, and infero-temporal cortex, *Neuropsychologia.* 3:111-119.

Bartfai, A., Levander, S.E., Nyback, H. and Schalling, D., 1987, Skin conductance nonresponding and non-habituation in schizophrenic patients, *Acta Psychiatrica Scand.* 75:321-329.

Barr, M.L., 1979, "The Human Nervous System (3rd Edition)," Harper and Row, Hagerstown, MD.

Bloch, J.D. and Bonvallet, M., 1960, Le declenchement des responses electrodermales a partir du systeme reticulaire facilitateur, *Journal de Physiol.* 52:25-26.

Buchsbaum, M.S., 1987, Positron emission tomography in schizophrenia, *in:* "Psychopharmacology: The Third Generation of Progress," H.Y. Melzer, ed., Raven Press, New York.

Buchsbaum, M.S., Gillin, J.C., Wu, J., Hazlett, E., Sicotte, N., Dupont, R.M. and Bunney, W.E., 1989, Regional cerebral glucose metabolic rate in human sleep assessed by positron emission tomography, *Life Sci.* 45:1349-1356.

Buchsbaum, M.S., Nuechterlein, K.H., Haier, R.J., Wu, J., Sicotte, N., Hazlett, E., Asarnow, R., Potkin, S. and Guich, S., 1990, Glucose metabolic rate in normals and schizophrenics during the continuous performance test assessed by positron emission tomography, *Br. J. Psychiatry.* 156:216-227.

Cannon, T.D., Fuhrmann, M., Mednick, S.A., Machon, R.A., Parnas, J. and Schulsinger, F., 1988, Third ventricle enlargement and reduced electrodermal responsiveness, *Psychophys.* 25:153-156.

Cannon, T.D., Mednick, S.A., and Parnas, J., 1989, Genetic and perinatal determinants of structural brain deficits in schizophrenia, *Arch. Gen. Psychiatry.* 46:883-889.

Cannon, T.D., Raine, A., Herman, T.M., Mednick, S.A., Schulsinger, F. and Moore, M., 1992, Third ventricle enlargement and lower heart rate levels in a high risk sample, *Psychophys.* 29:294-301.

Claridge, G., and Broks, P., 1984, Schizotypy and hemisphere function-I: theoretical considerations and the measurement of schizotypy, *Person. Indiv. Diff.* 5:633-648.

Crider, A., 1993, Electrodermal response lability - stability: individual difference correlates, *In:* "Electrodermal Activity: From Physiology to Psychology," J.C. Roy, W. Boucsein, D.C. Fowles and J. Gruzelier, eds., Plenum, New York.

Dallakyan, I.G., Latash, L.P., and Popova, L.T., 1970, Certain regular relationships between the expressivity of the galvanic skin response and changes of the EEG in local lesions of the limbic (rhinencephalic) structures of the human brain, *Dokl. Akad. Nauk.* 190:991-999.

Damasio, A.R., Tranel, D. and Damasio, H., in press, Somatic markers and the guidance of behavior: theory and preliminary testing. *In:* "Frontal Lobe Function and Injury," H. Levin, H. Eisenberg and A. Benton, eds., Oxford University Press, New York.

Darrow, C.W., 1937, Neural mechanisms controlling the palmar galvanic skin reflex and palmar sweating, *Arch. Neurol. Psychiatry.* 37:641-663.

Dawson, M.E., 1990, Psychophysiology at the interface of clinical science, cognitive science, and neuroscience. *Psychophys.* 27:243-255.

DeArmond, S.J., Fusco, M.M., and Dewey, M.M., 1989, "Structure of the Human Brain: A Photographic Atlas (Third Edition)," Oxford University Press, New York.

DeMyer, M.K., Gilmor, R.L., Hendrie, H.C., DeMyer, W.E., Augustyn, G.T. and Jackson, R.K., 1988, Magnetic resonance brain images in schizophrenic and normal subjects : influences of diagnosis and education. *Schizophr. Bull.* 14:21-37.

Edelberg, R., 1972, Electrical activity of the skin: its measurement and uses in psychophysiology, *In:* "Handbook of Psychophysiology," N.S. Greenfield and R.A. Sternbach, eds., Holt, Rienhart and Winston, New York.

Fowles, D.C., Christie, M.J., Edelberg, R., Grings, W.W., Lykken, D.T. and Venables, P.H., 1981, Publication recommendations for electrodermal measurements, *Psychophys.* 18:232-239.

Furedy, J., 1993, Electrodermal activity as a tool for differentiating psychological processes in human experimental preparations: focus on the psyche of psychophysiology, *In:* "Electrodermal Activity: From Physiology to Psychology," J.C. Roy, W. Boucsein, D.C. Fowles and J. Gruzelier, eds., Plenum, New York.

Grueninger, W.E., Kimble, D.P., Grueninger, J. and Levine, S., 1965, GSR and corticosteroid response in monkeys with frontal ablations, *Neuropsychologia* 3:205-216.

Gruzelier, J.H. and Venables, P.H., 1972, Skin conductance orienting activity in a heterogenous sample of schizophrenics, *J. Nerv. Ment. Dis.* 155:277-287.

Hazlett, E., Dawson, M., Buchsbaum, M.S.. and Nuechterlein, K., in press, Reduced regional brain glucose metabolism assessed by PET in electrodermal nonresponder schizophrenics: A pilot study, *J. Abn. Psych.*

Iacono, W.G. and Ficken, J.W., 1993, Family studies of electrodermal habituation and psychopathology,

    *In*:"Electrodermal Activity: From Physiology to Psychology," J.C. Roy, W. Boucsein, D.C. Fowles and J. Gruzelier, eds., Plenum, New York.

Isamat, F., 1961, Galvanic skin responses from stimulation of limbic cortex, *J. Neurophysiol.* 4:176-181.

Katsanis, J., Iacono, W. and Beiser, M., 1991, Relationship of lateral ventricular size to psychophysiological measures and short-term outcome, *Psychiatry Res.* 37:115-129.

Katsanis, J. and Iacono, W.G., 1992, Temporal lobe dysfunction and electrodermal nonresponding in schizophrenia, *Biol. Psychiatry* 31:159-170.

Kimble, D.P., Bagshaw, M.W. and Pribram, K.H., 1965, The GSR of monkeys during orienting and habituation after selective partial ablations of the cingulate and frontal cortex. *Neuropsychologia* 3:121-128.

Knight, R.T., 1984, Decreased responses to novel stimuli after prefrontal lesions in man, *Electroenceph. Clin. Neurophys.* 59:9-20.

Lang, H., Tuovinen, T., and Valleala, P., 1964, Amygdaloid after-charge and galvanic skin response, *Electroenceph. Clin. Neurophys.* 16:366-374.

Lee, G.P., Arena, J.G., Meador, K.J., Smith, J.R., Loring, D.W. and Flanigan, H.F., 1988, Changes in autonomic responsiveness following bilateral amygdalectomy in humans. *Neuropsychiatry Neuropsychol. Behav. Neurol.* 1:119-130.

Lencz, T., Raine, A., 1991, Two possible neural bases of electrodermal hyporesponsivity, Presented at the annual convention of the Society for Psychophysiological Research, Chicago.

Luria, A.R. and Homskaya, E.D., 1970, Frontal lobe and the regulation of arousal processes.
    *In*:"Attention : Contemporary Theory and Research," D. Mostofsky, ed., Appleton Century Crofts: New York.

Raine, A., Harrison, G.H., Reynolds, G.P., Sheard, C., Cooper, J.E., Medley, I., 1990, Structural and functional characteristics of the corpus callosum in schizophrenics, psychiatric controls, and normal controls: a magnetic resonance imaging and neuropsychological evaluation, *Arch. Gen. Psychiatry.* 47:1060-1064.

Raine, A., Reynolds, G.P., and Sheard, C., 1991, Neuroanatomical correlates of skin conductance orienting in normal humans: a magnetic resonance imaging study. *Psychophys.* 28:548-558.

Raine, A., Lencz, T., Reynolds, G., Harrison, G., Sheard, C., Medley, I., Reynolds, L. and Cooper, J.C., in press, Evidence for both structural and functional prefrontal deficits in schizophrenia : Converging evidence from magnetic resonance imaging, neuropsychological, and psychophysiological measures, *Psychiatry Res.*

Rippon, G., Hemispheric differences and electrodermal asymmetry - task and subject effects,
    *In*:"Electrodermal Activity: From Physiology to Psychology," J.C. Roy, W. Boucsein, D.C. Fowles and J. Gruzelier, eds., Plenum, New York.

Rossi, A., Stratta, P., Gallucci, M., Pasariello, R., and Casacchias, M., 1988, Brain morphology in schizophrenia by magnetic resonance imaging (MRI), *Acta Psychiatrica Scand.* 77:741-745.

Roy, J.C., 1993, Subcortical control of electrodermal activity: excitatory and inhibitory mechanisms,
    *In*:"Electrodermal Activity: From Physiology to Psychology," J.C. Roy, W. Boucsein, D.C. Fowles and J. Gruzelier, eds., Plenum, New York.

Scerbo, A., Freedman, L., Raine, A., Dawson, M.E., and Venables, P.H., 1992, A major effect of recording site on electrodermal activity, *Psychophys.* 29:241-246.

Schnur, D.B., Bernstein, A.S., Mukherjee, S., Loh, J., Degreef, G. and Reidel, J., 1989, The autonomic orienting response and CT scan findings in schizophrenia, *Schizophr. Res.* 2:449-455.

Schwartzbaum, J., Wilson, W. and Morrissette, J.R., 1961, The effects of amygdalectomy on locomotor activity in monkeys. *J. Comp. Physiol. Psychology* 54:334-336.

Sequeira, H., Roy, J.C., 1993, Cortical and hypothalamo-limbic control of electrodermal responses.
    *In*:"Electrodermal Activity: From Physiology to Psychology," J.C. Roy, W. Boucsein, D.C. Fowles and J. Gruzelier, eds., Plenum, New York.

Thompson, R.F., 1967, "Foundations of Physiological Psychology," Harper and Row, New York.

Tranel, D. and Damasio, H., 1989, Intact electrodermal skin conductance responses after bilateral amygdala damage, *Neuropsychologia* 27:381-390.

Tranel, D. and Hyman, B.T., 1990, Neuropsychological correlates of bilateral amygdala damage, *Arch. Neurol.* 47:349-355.

Venables, P.H. and Christie, M.J., 1973, Mechanisms, instrumentation, recording techniques, and quantification of responses, *In*:"Electrodermal Activity in Psychological Research," W.F. Prokasy and D.C. Raskin, eds., Academic Press, New York.

Wang, G.W., 1964, "The Neural Control of Sweating," University of Wisconsin Press, Madison.

Yokata, T., Sato, A., and Fujimori, B., 1963, Inhibition of sympathetic activity by stimulation of the limbic system, *Japanese J Physiol* 13:137-143.

Zahn, T.P., vanKammen, D.P., Schooler, C. and Mann, L.S., 1982, Autonomic activity in schizophrenia: relationships to cortical atrophy and symptomatology, *Psychophys.* 19:593.

Zahn, T.P., 1986, Psychophysiological approaches to psychopathology, *In*:"Psychophysiology: Systems, Processes, and Applications," M.G.H. Coles, E. Donchin, and S.W. Porges, eds., Guilford, New York.

Zoccolotti, P., 1993, Electrodermal activity in patients with unilateral brain damage, *In*:"Electrodermal Activity: From Physiology to Psychology," J.C. Roy, W. Boucsein, D.C. Fowles and J. Gruzelier, eds., Plenum, New York.

# GATEWAYS TO CONSCIOUSNESS:

# EMOTION, ATTENTION, AND ELECTRODERMAL ACTIVITY

Arne Öhman, Francisco Esteves, Anders Flykt, and Joaquim J. F. Soares

Department of Clinical Psychology
University of Uppsala, P.O. Box 1225
S-751 42 Uppsala, Sweden

## INTRODUCTION

### The Role of Autonomic Activity in Emotion

Hardly anyone would dispute that activation of the autonomic nervous system provides an important ingredient of emotion. The heart races in rage, or sinks in disgust and fear of a mutilated body. Butterflies seem to invade the stomach in anxious anticipation, and perfuse perspiration may occur in fear. Everyday observations of this type have led some investigators (e.g., James, 1884) radically to equate the emotion with the bodily response. Others have postulated that autonomic activation is necessary but not sufficient for genuine emotion (e.g., Mandler, 1984), whereas still others have claimed only that it contributes to emotional experience (e.g., Schachter & Singer, 1962). Thus, laymen and academics concur in giving autonomic arousal a central place in the psychology of emotion.

This emphasis on autonomic nervous system activity in emotion puts the topic squarely within the domain of psychophysiology (see e.g., Öhman, 1987). As psychophysiology primarily is a field organized around techniques to measure bodily responses, it provides the investigator with a set of techniques for monitoring autonomic changes as a function of experimentally induced emotion (e.g., Ax, 1953). Electrodermal activity has been one of the favorite tools in this context. Partly, this can be attributed to the ease of its measurement. Only simple electronic circuitry is required to record electrodermal activity, and the recorded changes typically are so obviously related to, e.g., environmental events, that no advanced computational algorithms are necessary to transform them into numbers. Thus, there are scores of papers reporting the use of electrodermal activity as markers of autonomic arousal in emotion or other related contexts.

The aim of this chapter is not to provide a comprehensive coverage of this extensive literature. Rather, we will develop a theoretical framework for viewing electrodermal activity within an emotional context, and then we will proceed to review a series of studies illustrating the usefulness of this measure in illuminating aspects of emotion.

## Aspects of Emotion

**Defining Emotion.** Emotion, of course, is one of the psychological concepts that is hardest to define. Indeed, one could argue that it is, at the present time, wasted effort to quibble about the specific meaning of this term. Unequivocal definition is a result of research, not a prerequisite for it (Frijda, 1986; Öhman, 1987). Thus, rather than providing an explicit definition of the term emotion, the aim may be lowered to capture aspects of the underlying concept by referring to *emotional phenomena* (Frijda, 1986). Such phenomena are related to stimuli that for one reason or the other may be understood as significant to the person; further, they are manifested in enhanced physiological activity, behavioral responses such as approach or avoidance, and in verbal reports, typically suggesting affective evaluation of the stimulus (e.g., like-dislike) (Öhman & Birbaumer, 1993). This way of delineating emotional phenomena has several important implications.

**Emotion and Stimulus Significance.** The proposed definition requires that emotional phenomena concern events that are significant to the person. Such events include those that are important because of survival contingencies. Thus, one could say that they are "objectively" significant in the sense that they are important for all individuals of a given species. They involve, for example, stimuli related to basic motivational states such as hunger, thirst, sex or social attachment, but also stimuli related to past predatory pressures and social dominance conflicts, e.g., reptiles and faces expressing threat (Öhman, Dimberg, & Öst, 1985). However, most significant stimuli are unique to the individual. They reflect his or her particular learning history, and they imply quite advanced information processing on part of the person. This, in turn, implies that what is emotionally provocative for one person goes unnoticed by another.

The significance of a stimulus, however, is not sufficient for inducing an emotional state. A stimulus can be significant purely in an informational, nonemotional sense, e.g., by providing critical information for task execution. However, even though it is insufficient for emotion, there are strong claims that stimulus significance is sufficient for eliciting electrodermal orienting responses (e.g., Bernstein, 1981). Emotional stimuli, therefore, provide an important subset of stimuli that are effective in eliciting the orienting reflex.

**Emotion and Physiological Arousal.** We have stipulated that for something to qualify as an emotional phenomenon, it must be associated with enhanced physiological activity. Physiological arousal is a central component of emotion. Indeed, for some theorists, the arousal or activation theorists (e.g., Malmo, 1959; Lindsley, 1951), it was *the* central component. They postulated a unidimensional continuum of activation ranging from deep sleep, over relaxed wakefulness and alertness, to panic or terror, which was supposed to reflect activity in the brain stem ascending reticular formation and to be operationalizable in indices of central, skeletal, and autonomic activity. This activation dimension was then used as a powerful explanatory construct to organize several data domains, including emotion, psychophysiology, learning, and performance. However, in an influential critique of this position, Lacey (1967) adduced evidence to suggest that the various physiological domains presumed to be closely interrelated indices of activation only showed poor covariation with each other. Similarly, the neurophysiological underpinning of the arousal continuum turned out to be much more complex than its original location in the reticular formation suggested (e.g., Thompson, 1967). Nevertheless, although important aspects of the original activation theory were shattered by data, a concept of arousal has proved useful in many contexts, where it is given a more specific meaning (see e.g., Hockey, Gaillard, & Coles, 1986). For example, Kahneman (1973) fruitfully related various physiological arousal indices to the availability of cognitive capacity (see below).

Like significance, however, physiological arousal is insufficient to capture the meaning of emotional phenomena. For example, in some instances, such as during concentrated work, we may be quite activated, but not in an emotional sense. Indeed, a distinction between cognitive and emotional activation may be justified on the basis of electrodermal data. Bohlin (1976) showed that skin conductance level rose when a cognitive task was introduced, but was not further increased in a condition where threat of electric shock was added. Spontaneous skin conductance responses, on the other hand, rose both with the task and the shock threat. Thus, in contrast to skin conductance level, they were sensitive both to the cognitive and the emotional demands of the situation.

Factor analyses of emotional stimuli typically bring out a pervasive arousal factor, along with factors reflecting stimulus evaluation, i.e., valence, and dominance (e.g., Russell, 1980). Greenwald, Cook and Lang (1989) examined physiological responses to pictorial stimuli that were selected to vary in rated arousal and valence (i.e., liking). They reported that skin conductance responses to these pictures very sensitively and specifically tracked their arousal value, but were unrelated to their valence. Thus, again, it appears that electrodermal activity is closely and specifically associated with emotional arousal processes.

**Approach, Avoidance and Affect.** It is a natural presumption that we approach what we like and avoid what we dislike. Thus, approach or avoidance at the behavioral level appears easily tied to the experienced valence of a situation, i.e., whether it is liked or disliked. It is often taken as a necessary defining feature of emotional phenomena that they, one way or the other, can be related to underlying positive or negative appraisals (Ortony, Clore, & Collins, 1988). From this broad perspective, psychological events may be seen as unfolding in a space where approach/avoidance provides a pervasive dimension (Schneirla, 1959). This notion was used by Lang, Bradley, and Cuthbert (1990) in a novel theory of emotion. They viewed emotion as action sets organized along appetitive-aversive and arousal dimensions. The former dimension defines the general direction of behavior (approach or avoidance; positive or negative affect), whereas the latter defines the effort or energy exerted in the behavior. These dimensions were understood in *strategical* terms, that is to say, they were viewed in terms of the unitary underlying organization in the pursuit of broad end goals. As strategies, they were distinguished from the diverse, specific, and context-bound *tactical* action patterns governing organismic activity at any given moment. Although the tactics are subordinated to the strategies, their relationship is a flexible one. Thus, a tactical withdrawal may be part of an overall attack strategy. According to Lang and coworkers (1990), it is this tactical flexibility and variability in the moment-to-moment action and its associated physiology that has muddled the attempts to relate physiology to positive and negative affects. However, they suggested that the strategic orientation was uniquely associated with differential reflex facilitation and inhibition. Specifically, an approach orientation was associated with facilitation of appetitive reflexes and inhibition of defensive ones, whereas the opposite was held to be true for an avoidance disposition. From this premise, they went on to demonstrate empirically that blink responses to background startle probes were facilitated by an aversive context (e.g., a picture of a mutilated body) but were inhibited by an emotionally positive context (e.g., picture of a smiling baby). Thus, they argued that the startle probe technique allows diagnosis of the overall strategical disposition of the organisms in terms of its overall likelihood to approach or avoid the environment. The data presented by Greenwald et al. (1989), reviewed earlier, suggested that skin conductance responses were equally diagnostic with regard to the arousal dimension, but were unrelated to the appetitive-defensive dimension. Thus, electrodermal activity may taken as related to one of the two cardinal dimensions defining emotion (Lang et al., 1990). However, electrodermal activity may not reflect solely the strategic arousal disposition, but is clearly also sensitive to tactical behavioral processes, which, e.g., denotes some specific stimuli as currently significant.

## ELECTRODERMAL ACTIVITY AND EMOTION: THEORETICAL THEMES

### "Gateways to consciousness"

There are several interrelated theoretical themes that run through our analysis of electrodermal activity in emotion. The central theme derives from the fact that emotions are represented in consciousness. This is essentially what we mean when we say that an emotion is experienced. What is consciously represented, be it a tiger out there or a racing heart in the chest cage, is, by definition, at the center of voluntarily controlled attention. Electrodermal activity has, indeed, been specifically tied to conscious experience (Johnson & Lubin, 1972). For example, Ojeman and van Buren (1967) examined psychophysiological responses to electrical stimulation of the human diencephalon during brain surgery. In contrast to cardiovascular and respiratory changes, electrodermal responses were clearly associated with points of stimulation prompting reports of perceptual experience from the patient. However, this finding appears hard to reconcile with more recent neuropsychological data from prosopagnosic patients. These patients suffer from brain lesions in the visual association cortices, as a result of which they have grave difficulties in recognizing persons from their faces. Both Bauer (1984) and Tranel and Damasio (1985) reported electrodermal evidence of facial recognition in such patients, in spite of complete failures on the part of the patients in correctly naming the faces. To reconcile these findings, one could argue that electrodermal responses primarily reflect processes bringing perceptual input into the focus of consciousness (Öhman, 1988). Thus, although normally closely associated, the processes related to electrodermal activity may be dissociable from verbalized output from consciousness. Following this lead, our focus will be on the psychological events that precede conscious representations rather than on the conscious representations *per se*. Accordingly, we shall discuss processes that allow (or deny?) emotionally associated perceptual input to become consciously represented. The primary theoretical reason for this emphasis is the notion that electrodermal responses, as components of the orienting reflex, are intimately related to such processes (see Öhman, 1979). Hence, the title "Gateways to consciousness".

### Preattentive Processes

Somewhat more formally stated, the aim of the chapter is to examine the role of preattentive processes in attention and emotion. These processes differ from conscious, voluntary attention in that they cannot be suppressed intentionally once initiated. That is to say, they are automatic rather than controlled. Further, they work in parallel rather than sequentially on stimulus input, they do not interfere with focal attention, they are not easily distracted by attended activities, and they are not represented in consciousness. Thus, they require special experimental techniques for their elucidation.

As observers of ourselves, we are exposed only to the results of the preattentive processes. They determine what in the enormous amount of currently available sensory information will be selected for further controlled and conscious analysis. Thus, one notices only what is let through, but remains unaware of the gatekeeping activity itself. Put in this way, it is easy to imagine the replacement of "gatekeeping activity" by a "gatekeeper", a Freudian censor who decides what material is let through, and who may provide pacifying distortions of input in order to save consciousness from anxiety. Such a censor, however, is alien to the approach taken here. The aim is to uncover some of the rules governing the preattentive processes rather than to introduce yet another homunculus with a privileged causal status (see Öhman, in press). Yet, in the end, this analysis should be capable of explaining some of the observations that prompted Freud (e.g., 1900/1959) to postulate the Unconscious (Power & Brewin, 1991; Öhman, in press).

The emphasis on preattentive processing in the present analysis in some respects runs counter to the commonly held notion that emotion results from elaborate cognitive activity (e.g. Lazarus, Kanner, & Folkman, 1980; Mandler, 1984). What is suggested here is that emotions may be relatively automatically elicited and thus in effect precede later more conscious cognitive interpretation and elaboration. In this respect, our analysis conforms to Zajonc's (1980) influential slogan that "affect precedes inference." However, the perceptual/cognitive analysis of an emotional stimulus is by no means completed by the preattentive processing. Rather their effects, e.g., on physiological arousal, should be understood as setting the stage for further analysis in subsequent interacting information processing stages (see Öhman, in press).

## Cognitive resource theory

Cognitive capacity or cognitive resources (see Kramer & Spinks, 1991) provides a central theoretical notion for the analysis. This notion implies an economical perspective on cognitive function, where different types of cognitive activities have to compete for cognitive capacity. It is, of course, an old notion that consciousness, or, if you prefer, focal attention, is selective in the sense that it can deal with only one thing at a time. To quote James' (1890) famous definition of attention: "It is the taking possession by the mind, in clear and vivid form, of one out of what seems several simultaneously possible objects or trains of thought...It implies withdrawal from some things in order to deal effectively with others" (p. 403-404). A capacity view of this selectivity implies that the limitations are strategic rather than structural, that the resources can be flexibly allocated over activities depending on overall current plans and motivation. Furthermore, of special interest in the present context is that their overall availability may be dependent on physiological arousal processes (Kahneman, 1973).

From this perspective, the important point with the preattentive processes is that they do not compete for cognitive resources. Rather they should be viewed as automatic routines set up to relieve consciousness and focal attention from having to deal with the standard events of the situation. The automatic preattentive information processing routines may derive their origin from biological evolution, or, perhaps more commonly, they reflect overlearned activities. Thus, you can leave the routine parts of driving a car to the preattentive processes, while you devote your cognitive capacity to day dreaming, listening to the radio, or playing peek-a-boo with the infant facing you from the other front seat.

This arrangement is very convenient, but it is also risky. If something unforeseen should happen, the preattentive processes may be ill prepared to deal with the contingencies, because by nature they can handle only standard, routine matters. Thus, there must be effective means of switching control from the preattentive to the conscious, controlled level of processing. When the preattentive mechanisms no longer can manage the situation, e.g., because a novel event interferes, or a threatening stimulus appears, there must be a quick call for cognitive capacity as the control over information processing is transferred to the conscious channel. This call is associated with the orienting reflex (Öhman, 1979), and its most direct effect is a reallocation of capacity to deal with the situation. Often it also results in an overall increase in the available capacity, as a correlate of the arousal increase associated with the orienting reflex. Because the electrodermal response provides the most accessible and reliable index of orienting, such responses are held to be closely associated with the entering of a stimulus into the controlled processing mode (Öhman, 1979). Thus, from this perspective, electrodermal activity becomes intimately related to the selection of material for conscious processing. Furthermore, combining Lang et al. (1990) and Kahneman (1973), the larger the electrodermal response, the more aroused the conscious-controlled processing system (Lang et al., 1990), and the more cognitive resources are mobilized to deal with the situation (Kahneman, 1973).

## The Role of the Orienting Reflex

The theoretical notions advanced here (see Öhman, 1987, 1992, in press, for more complete accounts) suggest that preattentive processes have a key role to play in emotion. Almost by definition, emotional stimuli are significant to the person. Thus, the preattentive stimulus analysis mechanisms may be primed to locate emotionally relevant stimuli wherever an attribute suggesting such a stimulus is found in the perceptual field. As a result, there is a reflexive shift of attention toward this stimulus, with an associated reallocation of cognitive resources for its further analyses. As enumerated by Öhman (1987, pp. 104-106) there is considerable overlap between emotion and orienting. First, both emotion and orienting are related to stimulus significance. For example, Hamburg, Hamburg, and Barchas (1975, p. 239) suggested that emotions have a "signal function which warns the organism and other individuals significant to him that something is wrong, attention must be paid, learning capacities utilized, resources mobilized to correct the situation." Second, both orienting (e.g., Graham, 1979) and emotion theorists (e.g., Izard, 1979) emphasise the role of the respective processes in sensitizing the organism to environmental input. Third, both orienting (e.g., Lynn, 1966) and emotion (e.g., Folkman, Schaeffer, & Lazarus, 1979) are said to result in the interruption of ongoing behavior, presumably as control is withdrawn from the preattentive mechanisms in charge of routinized behavior. Fourth, stimuli eliciting orienting and emotion distract ongoing cognitive activity by turning attention away from it (e.g., Waters, McDonald and Koresko, 1977; Folkman et al., 1979). Finally, the conditions for evoking the autonomic components of orienting shows considerable overlap with those mobilizing autonomic arousal in emotion, with major roles given to discrepancy, conflict, and interruptions of integrated sequences of thought or behavior (e.g., Mandler, 1984). From this analysis it follows that the orienting reflex as manifested, e.g., in electrodermal responses, is intimately engaged in the initiation of emotion. Such initiation of emotion always involves that the eliciting stimulus captures focal attention, and such capturing, furthermore, is associated with orienting. Thus, emotion, attention and orienting are overlapping processes with regard to bringing events into the focus of consciousness. Hence, they may all be referred to as "gateways to consciousness."

## Preparedness

Although not a focal theme for the chapter, the concept of preparedness (Seligman, 1970) still is behind most of the empirical work that will be reviewed. The preparedness concept implies that the associative apparatus of organisms is constrained by evolution. Thus, animals (and humans as well) are assumed to learn more easily to associate some events rather than others, as a result of selection pressures in the long past. In the present case, it is assumed that common phobic stimuli, such as small animals or human facial expression suggesting condescension or threat, easily become associated with fear and anxiety (Öhman, 1993; Öhman et al., 1985). Once such selective, prepared associations have been formed, the resulting fear is assumed to be very persistent and to resist information suggesting that the stimulus in effect is innocuous (Seligman, 1971). In the perspective of the theoretical notions outlined previously, it may be assumed that some attributes of common fear stimuli have privileged access to the arousal system (Öhman, in press) via the orienting reflex (Öhman, 1992) so that a fear response may be initiated even before the eliciting stimulus reaches a full conscious analysis. Thus, most of the empirical work reviewed below will deal with electrodermal responses to fear-relevant stimuli, such as pictures of snakes, spiders or angry human faces.

## Summary

The view of emotion adopted here suggests that emotional processes are related to the transaction between organism and environment. Specifically, the emotional state of an organism may be located in a two-dimensional space defined by overall strategical dispositions of approach/avoidance and arousal. Electrodermal activity, it is held, reflects specifically the arousal aspects of emotion but is unrelated to the approach/avoidance, or valence, dimension.

While an emotion invariably ends up in consciousness, at the center of attention, the focus of the present analysis is on the preceding preattentive processing stages. Emotional stimuli are, by definition, significant to the organism, and as such they can be located by preattentive perceptual mechanisms, working in parallel on sensory input independently of the current focus of voluntarily controlled attention. As a significant stimulus is located, there is an automatic switch of attention to this stimulus, which involves a reallocation of cognitive capacity to deal with the situation. At the same time there is an arousal increase that may result in a general increase of the available cognitive resources. This arousal increase is marked by the elicitation of an orienting reflex, which is most reliably indicated by an electrodermal response. Some stimuli, for which an evolutionarily determined emotional potency is likely (e.g., snakes or angry human faces), may be particularly effective in this preattentive catching of attention.

In the remaining part of the chapter, a research program starting from the theoretical premises outlined here will be described. Thus, after a brief outline of some central methodological aspects, we shall proceed to examine a series of electrodermal experiments performed in the Uppsala laboratory.

# BACKWARD MASKING AS A TOOL TO ISOLATE PREATTENTIVE PROCESSING

## Theoretical Foundation

Human electrodermal responding is a final product of the complete information processing system. Thus, there is no way to dissect the response to determine what part of it can be attributed to the preattentive mechanisms that are at the focus of our analysis. The instruments of dissection must be sought in another direction, the one concerned with experimental design. What is needed is a methodological tool to guarantee that the stimulus of interest is subjected to a preattentive perceptual analysis, yet is denied access to conscious, controlled processing. There are several techniques available for nonconscious presentation of stimuli, each more or less dependent on below-threshold stimulus exposure. For example, stimuli may be presented below the threshold of conscious perception either because of low applied energy or short duration, visual stimuli may be presented extra-foveally, or the stimuli may be hidden in a nonattended channel, e.g., in a dichotic listening task (see Holender, 1986, for a critical review).

We have chosen to use backward masking to dissociate preattentive from conscious processing. In this technique, the stimulus of interest, the *target* stimulus, is presented briefly, and then followed by another stimulus, the *mask*, either immediately or after a short empty interval. By varying the *stimulus-onset asynchrony* (SOA) between target and mask, recognition of the target may be manipulated from random performance to confident, correct recognitions.

The backward masking technique is theoretically appealing, because, given that information processing is something that unfolds over time, it implies that processing of the target is disrupted by the mask. Thus, introducing the mask provides an active control of the amount of processing allowed. This situation is clearly better than the one resulting from non-masked short stimulus durations, because the mask disrupts the sensory icon that may persist several hundred milliseconds after the physical termination of a stimulus (e.g., Massaro, 1975).

Adding to the theoretical appeal of backward masking, Marcel (1983) introduced a theory of unconscious and conscious perception, which provides a viable rationale for using the technique precisely for the purpose of allowing preattentive, but denying conscious, processing of a stimulus. According to this theory, there are unconscious perceptual mechanisms that redescribe sensory data "into every other representational form that the organism is capable of representing, whether by nature or by acquisition" (Marcel, 1983, p. 244). These redescribed codes provide input to further processing mechanisms, and output from these units can also unconsciously support behavior such as, for example, orientation in space and postural adjustments. Thus, these sensory codes are derived from sensory data in a data-driven, bottom-up type of processing. A conscious percept is formed when these codes meet a conceptually driven, top-down derived hypothesis in a perceptual recovery process, which selects one of the very many potential percepts among the unconscious sensory codes. It is this act of recovery which specifically is assumed to be disrupted by backward masking. Thus the masking technique leaves heaps of perceptual data unconsciously lingering in the system, where they, for example, already may connect to response mobilization processes initiating emotional processes.

**Empirical Data**

From this account of backward masking, it is clear that this technique is promising for use in the analysis of preattentive processing of emotional stimuli. The emotional stimuli used in the studies are pictures of biologically fear-relevant stimuli such as snakes, spiders, and angry faces. Emotionally neutral control stimuli are pictures of flowers, mushrooms, and happy faces. These stimulus classes have been used in an extensive series of conditioning studies performed in our laboratory over a 20-year period. These studies document that the fear-relevant stimuli readily become associated with aversive unconditioned stimuli, and in particular electric shock. The skin conductance responses that result from such conditioned association have proven unusually resistant to extinction (see Öhman, 1993, for a recent review of this work). In the work to be described here, stimuli of these types were presented masked by other stimuli, in order to allow electrodermal assessment of the preattentive effects. However, before reviewing the electrodermal studies, it is necessary with a short digression to describe perceptual and memorial effects of masked stimuli in order to delineate the stimulus parameters to be used.

Esteves and Öhman (1992) examined recognition of masked facial stimuli in an extensive series of experiments. Typically, a forced-choice procedure was used, where the subjects were required to guess the emotional expression of a target face preceding the mask portraying an emotionally neutral expression. They were also asked to rate their confidence in the sensory decisions. Target-mask face pairs with SOAs varying from 20 to over 300 ms were presented in random order. The data showed that a SOA of about 100 ms was needed in order to give confident correct recognitions. A 30 ms SOA did not result in above chance performance, and according to the confidence ratings, the subjects felt that they merely were guessing. Furthermore, according to subjects asked to indicate whether they perceived one or two stimuli, a 30 ms SOA was perceived as one stimulus in about 90% of the trials. These general relations were quite robust over experimental conditions, e.g., with regard to mask duration, unfilled or filled target-mask interval, and intensity relations between the stimuli.

Parra, Esteves, and Öhman (submitted) reported very similar results from a series of recognition memory experiments. Subjects were first exposed to pairs of target and mask faces with SOAs varying between 30 and 330 ms, and were then asked to recognize unmasked presentations of target faces. Again, above chance performance appeared to require a 100-200 ms SOA in the study phase, whereas no evidence of recognition was obtained with a 30 ms SOA.

Öhman and Soares (1993) reported a series of similar experiments using animal and control stimuli. Their subjects were required to identify target stimuli that were pictures of snakes, spiders, flowers or mushrooms. The masks were similar pictures which had been randomly cut to pieces and then randomly reassembled so that any recognizable central object in the picture was lost. Again, a SOA of about 100 ms was needed for consistent, confident recognitions, whereas a SOA of 30 ms resulted in random performance. In one of the experiments, the subjects were exposed to random electric shock stimuli (subjectively defined as uncomfortable but not painful) interspersed among the pictures to examine whether the identification function would be altered when the subjects were activated. However, the shocks had no effects whatsoever. A similar shock experiment using facial stimuli was reported by Esteves, Dimberg, Parra and Öhman (submitted), again with no effects of the shocks.

Taken together these data demonstrate that a SOA of 30 ms definitely is below the threshold of perceptual identification for all of our studied subjects. As the SOA is lengthened to 50 or 60 ms there is reliable above chance performance, albeit with low confidence in the decisions. Only when the SOA is increased to about 100 ms is there consistent confident recognition of the target stimuli. Thus, if one wants to study preattentive processing uncontaminated by conscious, controlled processes it appears safe to use a SOA of 30 ms.

## PREATTENTIVE ELICITATION OF ELECTRODERMAL RESPONSES: EMPIRICAL DATA

### Responses to phobic stimuli presented outside of awareness

The most basic assertion of the present theoretical framework is that emotional responses may be initiated by preattentive processing mechanisms of which the subjects remain unaware. Backward masking appears to provide a convenient method by which access to conscious perception can be blocked, so that the pure effect of preattentive processing can be examined. Thus, by this technique, it should be possible to evoke emotional responses without the subjects being aware of the stimulus to which they are responding. This basic hypothesis was tested in the first experiment to be reported here (Öhman & Soares, in press).

In order to be able to induce genuine emotions, it was decided to expose phobic subjects to pictorial representations of their feared object. It is well documented that such stimuli result in strong autonomic responses, including electrodermal ones, when presented to phobic subjects (e.g., Fredrikson, 1981; see Sartory, 1983, for review). Consequently, questionnaires measuring snake and spider fears were distributed to a large pool of university students. From 800 answered questionnaires, subjects were selected so that they were either highly snake fearful or highly spider fearful. That is to say, they had to be above the 95th percentile in one of the distributions (e.g., snake fears) and below the 50th percentile in the other (e.g., spider fear). Non-fearful control subjects had to score below the 50th percentile on both questionnaires. Thus, we ended up with three groups of 16 subjects each: Snake fearful, spider fearful, and nonfearful controls.

All subjects were exposed to the same stimulus sequence. It consisted of pictures of snakes, spiders, flowers, and mushrooms, with 8 exemplars in each of the categories. This randomly ordered series of pictures was presented twice. In the first presentations, the pictures were masked with a 30 ms SOA, thus preventing their conscious recognition. That is to say, a 30 ms exposure of the target stimulus was immediately followed by a 100 ms mask (randomly cut and reassembled pictures). The second series consisted of unmasked stimulus presentations with 130 ms exposure time. After each of the stimulus series, examples of each stimulus type, as well as new stimuli of the same type, were rated in terms of valence, arousal, and dominance, and the subject was asked to identify the masked or nonmasked pictures and whether each had been part of the original set.

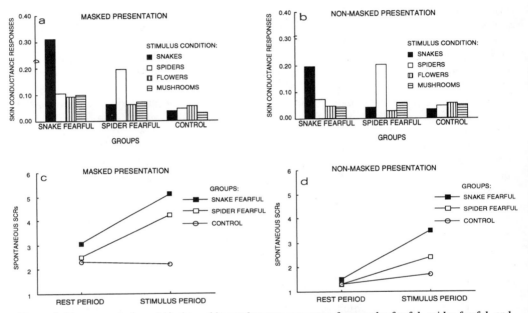

*Figure 1.* Upper panels (a and b) show skin conductance responses from snake fearful, spider fearful, and nonfearful controls to effectively masked (a) and nonmasked (b) presentations of pictures of snakes, spiders, flowers and mushrooms. Fearful subjects showed elevated responding to their feared stimulus even if it was prevented from entering conscious perception by backward masking (panel a). Lower panels show spontaneous skin conductance responses (SCRs) in the intervals between stimulation. Whereas controls did not change from rest during stimulation, the fearful subjects showed enhanced spontaneous responding suggesting that they became anxious after both masked (c) and nonmasked (d) presentations of feared stimuli.

The psychophysiological dependent variables were skin conductance responses to the pictures and spontaneous fluctuations in skin conductance in the interstimulus intervals.

The results were quite dramatic and are presented in Figure 1. Regardless of masking conditions, the snake fearful subjects showed elevated skin conductance responding to snake stimuli, and the spider fearful subjects showed elevated responding to spider pictures, whereas the control subjects did not differentiate the four stimulus types. These results were confirmed by a highly significant interaction between groups and stimuli, with associated Tukey follow-up tests to support the elevated responding to fear stimuli in fearful subjects (see Öhman & Soares, in press, for details). The only difference between the masked and nonmasked stimulus series pertained to overall larger responses in the former series. Because of the fixed order of presentation of the series, this effect most probably reflected overall habituation from the first to the second series. Thus it was clear that the subjects differentiated as well between the feared and nonfeared stimuli when they were not able to recognize them (i.e., the masked series) as when they were clearly recognizable (i.e., the nonmasked stimulus series). As shown in the two lower panels of Fig. 1, effects of the fear stimuli were discernible also in spontaneous skin conductance responses. Thus, the rate of spontaneous fluctuation became elevated if the stimulus series contained a relevant fear stimulus (e.g., a snake for a snake fearful subject), regardless of whether the fear stimulus was masked or not. The effect was somewhat clearer during the masked stimulus series, which, again, probably can be attributed to the fact that this series came first.

The skin conductance data were exactly paralleled in the emotional ratings. Thus, snake and spider fearful subjects rated themselves as more disliking, more aroused and less in control when they were exposed to their feared stimulus, even if the presentation was masked. However, the overall emotional intensity was rated as higher during nonmasked stimulus presentation.

These results give full support to the contention that emotional responses are initiated at a preattentive level of information processing. Indeed, some surprise may be voiced regarding the general lack of difference between the two masking conditions. From these data it appears that most of the emotional effect has its basis at the preattentive level.

## The Origin of Phobic Responses: Pavlovian Conditioning

According to the preparedness theory of phobias (Öhman et al., 1985; Seligman, 1971) phobias are acquired through biologically prepared Pavlovian conditioning. Because most phobias involve potentially dangerous situations such as snakes, dogs, heights, or enclosed spaces, Seligman (1971) argued that evolution has put a survival premium on genes promoting rapid fear learning and subsequent avoidance of such stimuli. This theory has received a fair amount of experimental support (McNally, 1987; Öhman, 1993). If this theory is correct, it should be possible to produce effects similar to those observed in fearful subjects in normals conditioned to potentially phobic stimuli. Thus, one would expect that skin conductance responses conditioned to pictures of snakes or spiders should be elicited even when the conditioned stimuli (CSs) are presented during masking conditions preventing their recognition. This hypothesis was tested by Öhman and Soares (1993) and Öhman, Dimberg and Esteves (1989).

Öhman and Soares (1993) used a differential conditioning paradigm to condition different groups of subjects to either fear-relevant (snakes or spiders) or fear-irrelevant (flowers or mushrooms) stimuli. Subjects in the fear-relevant groups were shown two pictures portraying snakes and spiders, respectively. Subjects in the fear-irrelevant groups were shown pictures of flowers and mushrooms. After a few habituation trials, there was an acquisition phase where one of the stimuli was followed by an electric shock unconditioned stimulus (US), with a .5 s interstimulus interval. This picture was designated the CS+. The other picture (e.g., a spider if the CS+ was a snake) was designated the CS-. With this paradigm the difference in skin conductance response to the CS+ and the CS- reflects pure conditioning effects uncontaminated by sensitization, initial responding, etc. (see Öhman, 1983). In the extinction phase that terminated the experiment, the CS+ and the CS- were presented without any USs. Half of the subjects conditioned to fear-relevant and fear-irrelevant stimuli, respectively, were extinguished with masked stimuli and the other half without any masks. Thus, subjects in the masked groups had both the CS+ and the CS-masked by a randomly cut and reassembled picture with a 30 ms SOA, exactly as in the experiment on fearful subjects reported by Öhman and Soares (in press).

The results were clear-cut. Both the groups extinguished without masks showed reliable differential skin conductance responding to the CS+ and the CS-, suggesting continuing conditioning effects in both groups. In fact, these groups did not differ from each other. This failure to obtain the standard preparedness effect may perhaps be attributed to the short interstimulus interval used during training. For the groups extinguished with masked CSs, however, fear relevance made a dramatic difference. Whereas masking completely abolished differential responding in the group conditioned to fear-irrelevant stimuli, differential responding to the CS+ and the CS+ remained in the group conditioned to snakes or spiders. The result for this group therefore paralleled those obtained with fearful subjects in the previous experiment (see Fig. 1). Exactly parallel conditioning and extinction data were reported by Öhman et al. (1989) using angry and happy faces as CS+ and CS-, respectively. Thus, in support of the preparedness theory, it appears that masking takes away differential responding to neutral stimuli but leaves differential responding to fear-relevant CSs+ and CSs- virtually intact.

Soares and Öhman (in press) took this analysis one step further. On the basis of a development of preparedness theory by Öhman et al. (1985), they argued that subjects fearful of, e.g., snakes, should have an enhanced readiness to associate fear to any animal stimuli, such as, e.g., spiders. This hypothesis derives from the proposition that all animal fear goes back to a common predatory defense system, which has evolved to help animals survive predation pressure (Öhman et al., 1985). To test this hypothesis, Soares and Öhman recruited fearful and nonfearful subjects by criteria similar to those used by Öhman and Soares (in press). Then half of the subjects fearing snakes were conditioned to pictures of spiders, with pictures of rats as control stimuli, whereas half of the spider fearful subjects were conditioned to snakes. Thus the fearful subjects were conditioned to a non-feared but still fear-relevant animal stimulus. The remaining halves of the fearful groups were conditioned to fear-irrelevant stimuli (flowers and mushrooms). Half of the normal controls were conditioned to fear-relevant stimuli (snakes or spiders) and half to fear-irrelevant stimuli. Then all subjects were extinguished with masked CSs. The results were straightforward but devastating to the specific hypothesis: The fear-relevance of the CS turned out to be the only important factor in promoting differential response to masked stimuli. Both fearful and nonfearful subjects showed remaining differential response to the CS+ and the CS- during masked extinction if the CSs were fear-relevant, but no differential response if they were fear-irrelevant, with no effect whatsoever of fearfulness. Thus, fearing one animal was not associated with any increased readiness to acquire fear of other animals. In other words, preparedness appeared to be specific to the type of animal.

In a final experiment of this series, Soares and Öhman (1993) examined the interaction between fear-relevance, masking, and instructed extinction (i.e., the effects of instructions explicitly informing subject that no more shock would be presented). Lack of voluntary control is considered a hallmark of phobias (Marks, 1969). Accordingly, information about the actual innocuousness of the phobic situation has little effect in alleviating phobic fear. In agreement with this notion, Hugdahl and Öhman (1977) reported that instructed extinction had no effect on skin conductance responses conditioned to fear-relevant stimuli (snakes or spiders), but removed differential response completely to fear-irrelevant stimuli (flowers or mushrooms). In the present experiment, half of the subjects were conditioned to fear-relevant and the other half to fear-irrelevant stimuli in a differential conditioning paradigm with shock US presented at a .5 s interstimulus interval during acquisition. These main groups were subdivided into halves and extinguished with or without masks. Finally, these four groups were further subdivided according to whether they were informed about shock omission during extinction or not, leaving 8 groups with 16 subjects each. For the informed subjects, the experimenter entered the cubicle where the subject was seated before extinction started, told the subject that no more shocks would be presented, and removed the shock electrodes. For noninformed subjects, he entered the cubicle allegedly to check the skin conductance electrodes, but did not mention anything about the shocks. The results showed that instructions and masking, independently and additively, removed differential response to fear-irrelevant stimuli, but left reliable differential response to fear-relevant stimuli. Thus, even the fear-relevant group exposed to both masking and instruction showed reliable differential response during extinction.

This series of studies shows quite convincingly that skin conductance responses conditioned to fear-relevant stimuli (snakes/spiders or angry faces) reliably survives backward masking, whereas a differential response to fear-irrelevant stimuli is abolished by this procedure. This surviving response is automatic in the sense that it is not affected by instruction, and the effect appears specific to a particular stimulus category, such as snakes *or* spiders.

## Competition for Cognitive Resources

The data reviewed so far demonstrate that electrodermal responses related to emotional processes indeed require only a preattentive analysis of the stimulus for their elicitation. According to the notion of preattentive mechanisms adopted earlier, this implies that elicitation of these responses do not compete for cognitive resources. Rather they are assumed to result in the reallocation of cognitive resources in the form of an attentional switch, without drawing on the resources themselves. However, reason to question this simple notion has started to accumulate (see Öhman, 1992; Spinks & Kramer, 1991). Rather than to digress into an extensive treatment of these problems here, we will proceed to describe an experiment that seems to imply that the preattentively derived call for a reallocation of cognitive resources may indeed itself provide a source of competition for these resources.

One way to examine this issue would be to introduce attentional demands into the experimental situation. In the experiments reviewed so far, the subjects have been left to deploy their attention in any way they wish. Because the preattentive processing was assumed to be independent of the direction of voluntary attention, there was no need to actively control attention. However, if the preattentive effect of emotionally relevant stimuli actually is dependent on resources, it should be sensitive to the attentional context. In particular, one would expect competition between the target and the mask in the capture of attention. Indeed, Parra et al. (submitted) demonstrated that attention to the mask was a very powerful determinant of the effect of masking on recognition memory. Thus, in the experiment to be reported here, attention to the mask was experimentally manipulated. Following the theoretical outline developed earlier, with a short SOA allowing only preattentive processing, attention to the mask should have no effect on the elicited skin conductance responses. With a long SOA, however, giving room for conscious, controlled processing, attention to the mask should interfere with further controlled processing of the target.

To test these predictions, two levels of attention to the masks were orthogonally crossed with a short and a long masking interval during a series of extinction trials following conditioning training with facial stimuli as CSs (Esteves, Dimberg, & Öhman, submitted). The acquisition phase involved conditioning with an angry face serving as CS+ and a happy face as the CS-. The US was an electric shock and the interstimulus interval was .5 s. In the extinction phase, all subjects had the CSs masked by male and female neutral faces. Half of the subjects had a 30 ms SOA precluding recognition of the target CS, whereas the other half had a 180 ms SOA allowing at least some recognition of the target CSs (see Esteves & Öhman, in press). Within each of the SOA groups, half of the subjects were instructed to count the number of female faces they detected in the mask position, whereas the other half were not given any instructions about the masks. For the no instruction groups, there were, as expected, reliably larger responses to the masked CS+ than to the masked CS-, both for the 30 ms and 180 ms SOA groups. However, contrary to the hypothesis, attention to the mask wiped out the differential response regardless of SOA. Thus, attention to the mask provided competition with the elicitation of a skin conductance response to the target stimulus even at the short, effective, SOA, which suggests that some cognitive resources were needed by the preattentive mechanisms (see Öhman, 1992, for a more complete discussion of these issues).

## Direct assessment of Cognitive Resources

**Probe RT as a Secondary Task**. The secondary task technique allows a direct assessment of cognitive resource utilization. The assumption is that the amount of resources, as well as the changes in resources, invested in the primary task can be tracked by impeded performance in the secondary task (see Kramer & Spinks, 1991). One of the most frequently used secondary tasks is the probe RT. With this technique, the subjects are instructed to concentrate their effort on the primary task, but they are also required to press a response key whenever a probe stimulus is presented. Thus, slowing of RT during performance of the primary task as compared to a control condition not involving this task is then taken to reflect the investment of resources in performing the primary task.

In an innovative study, Dawson, Schell, Beers and Kelly (1982) applied the secondary probe RT technique to human Pavlovian conditioning. They presented RT probes in the intertrial intervals as well as during defined points in the CS-US interval during a differential conditioning paradigm of the type previously discussed. The CS+ and the CS- were different coloured lights, the US was an electric shock and the RT probes were tones. The probe position 300 ms after onset of the CS+ showed marked RT slowing compared to similarly placed probes during the CS-, which suggested that more resources were allocated to analyse the CS+ than the CS-. After this time point the RT returned to control level for the remaining CS-US interval, but it remained slower during the CS+ than the CS-, which actually suggests some facilitation of the RT during the latter stimulus. Of considerable interest from our perspective was the finding that subjects showing larger skin conductance orienting responses to the CSs showed more RT slowing, suggesting a relation between the orienting reflex and resources allocation, as postulated by Öhman (1979). The fruitfulness of this technique has been documented in further work by Dawson and colleagues (e.g., Dawson, Filion, & Schell, 1989) and Siddle and colleagues (e.g., Siddle & Spinks, 1992).

Given the central role of resource allocation in the present theoretical framework, it appears an important step to incorporate direct measurement of this process by means of the probe RT technique. From the background results presented in this chapter and reviewed elsewhere (Öhman, 1993), one would expect that fear-relevant stimuli draw more resources than fear-irrelevant ones. Furthermore, from the experimental results of attentional competition between target and mask, one would expect that this resource demand by fear-relevant stimuli should be obvious already at the preattentive level of information processing. We have recently initiated a research program to examine these hypotheses.

**Ratings of US Expectancy**. As a first step, we wanted to examine resource allocation during conditioning and extinction to fear-relevant and fear-irrelevant stimuli. Furthermore, we wanted to assess simultaneously shock expectancy during conditioning to these stimuli. Starting from the demonstration by Tomarken, Mineka and Cook, (1989) that subjects show a bias to overestimate the relation between fear-relevant stimuli (snakes and spiders) and aversive events, Davey (1992) argued that the preparedness effect is completely attributable to such expectancy biases. Assessment of expectancy is appealing also because it gives a purer measure of controlled conscious processing during conditioning, since it is obviously based on the subjects' awareness of the relations between CSs and USs. Continuous assessment of expectancy, e.g., by requiring the subjects to manipulate a lever or knob, has proven quite useful in electrodermal conditioning research (e.g., Booth, Siddle, & Bond, 1989; Davey, 1992; Schiffman & Furedy, 1972). However, requiring the subject to continuously indicate his or her shock expectancy introduces an additional primary task into the situation, which may be expected to compete for cognitive resources. If, in addition, the probe RT task were to be used, the task that is presumed to be the primary one, Pavlovian conditioning to the CSs, may, in fact, be relegated to the background, because it makes less direct claims for the subject's involvement than the more active rating and RT tasks. Thus, we wanted to design the study so that we could assess the effect of these additional tasks.

**Design of the Study**. In order to be able to accomplish this goal, performing the RT probe task or not was orthogonally combined with providing ratings of US expectancy or not in subjects conditioned either to an angry face or a happy face CS+, with the other facial expression serving as CS-. The US was an electric shock and the CS-US interval was 3.5 s, in order to allow ratings in the interval. After 6 habituation trials, there was an acquisition phase of 20 reinforced CSs+ and 20 nonreinforced CSs-, and then followed an extinction phase involving 20 presentations of each CS. To sum up, first, two groups of subjects, one conditioned to an angry and the other to a happy face, were exposed only to the differential conditioning contingency. Second, two other groups (one with an angry and the other with a happy CS+) were, in addition, required to operate a voice key to produce RTs to an occasionally occurring tone stimulus. Third, two groups (one angry and one happy) were required to indicate continuously their US expectancy by rotating a knob. Fourth, the remaining two groups performed both tasks, i.e., they both produced RTs to the probes and indicated their shock expectancy.

RT probes were presented in the intertrial intervals and at 300 or 3000 ms SOAs after CS onset. Four (out of 20) CSs+ and 4 CSs- were probed with each of the CS-probe intervals both during acquisition and extinction. Sixteen probes were presented at random points in the intertrial intervals.

**Probe RT Results**. The RT data collapsed for the two groups that performed this task are presented in Figure 2. During acquisition (left panels) the RT was overall more slowed to the CS+ than to the CS-, suggesting that more resources were allocated to the analysis of the former stimulus. The slowing was more apparent immediately after the CS onset than immediately before the US, and this effect was more obvious in the group conditioned to angry faces. There is a hint in the acquisition data to suggest that there was an earlier differentiation in RT slowing between the CS+ and the CS- for this group, but this effect was not confirmed by the statistical analysis. During extinction (right panels) there was larger overall slowing in the group conditioned to angry than in the groups conditioned to happy faces (compare upper and lower right panels), and more slowing at 300 than at 3000 ms after CS onset. As shown by a reliable interaction between CS and groups, only the group conditioned to the fear-relevant angry faces showed more slowing to the CS+ than to the CS-. Furthermore, as shown by the reliable interaction between CS, group, and SOA, this differential effect of the CS+ and the CS- pertained specifically to the 300 ms post-CS onset probe position. Thus, the only RT evidence of lasting conditioning effects during extinction pertained to the early probe position for the fear relevant stimuli.

**Expectancy ratings**. During acquisition, the subjects quickly picked up the correct CS-US contingency so that it took only a few trials to judge shock as virtually certain after the CS+ and as very unlikely after the CS-. These effects yielded very high F-ratios for the CS and CS x Trials factors. The data for the ratings during extinction are shown in the two middle panels of Figure 3. The subjects rated the shock as less likely after the CS- than the CS+ and this effect was more obvious for those conditioned to a fear-relevant angry CS+, as shown by the reliable interaction between CS and group. In addition, extinction was demonstrated in the sense that shock was rated as progressively more unlikely over trials and that this trend was more obvious for the CS+ than the CS-.

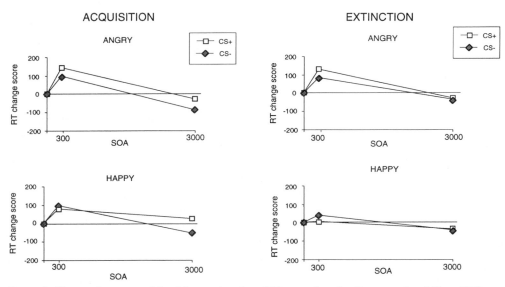

*Figure 2*. Changes from control level in reaction time (RT) to probe stimuli presented at 300 or 3000 ms stimulus-onset asynchrony from onset of the reinforced (CS+) and nonreinforced (CS-) conditioned stimuli. Control probes were presented in the intertrial intervals. The left panels show acquisition data for groups conditioned with an angry (upper panel) or happy (lower panel) face as the CS+. The right panels show extinction data.

**Skin conductance responses**. Interpretation of the skin conductance data was complicated by before-conditioning differences in responding between subjects conditioned to angry and happy CSs+. Data from the extinction series are shown in the left-most column of panels in Figure 3. A reliable four-way interaction between group (angry vs. happy CS+), CS, RT task and rating prompted evaluation with separate t-test to examine differential response in each of the eight groups. For subjects only exposed to the conditioning contingency (upper left panel), reliable differential response to the CS+ and the CS- was obtained only for those conditioned to the angry fear-relevant stimulus. Thus, these groups replicated the standard preparedness effect with these stimuli (Öhman & Dimberg, 1978). When the rating task was added (second panel from top in the left column), only subjects conditioned to happy CSs+ showed reliable differential response. None of the groups doing only the RT task (third panel from top) showed differential response, and in the subjects performing both tasks (lowest left panel) only those conditioned to an angry CS+ showed differential response. Further examinations of the left four panels in Figure 3 reveals that the rating task resulted in reliably increased skin conductance responding, whereas the RT task tended (nonsignificantly) to depress responding. However, according to the reliable interaction between RT and CS, performing the RT task resulted in overall less differential response to the CS+ and the CS-.

**Discussion**. There are several interesting aspects of these results. First, preparedness effects, defined as larger resistance to extinction to fear-relevant stimuli, were demonstrated in all measures. For skin conductance responses this was true only for the groups that had no other task than the differential conditioning contingency (see upper left panel of Figure 3). For expectancy ratings, the resistance to extinction was larger to the fear-relevant (angry) CS+, regardless of whether the subjects performed an additional RT task or not. For probe RT slowing, finally, there was a clear preparedness effect for the probe position close to CS

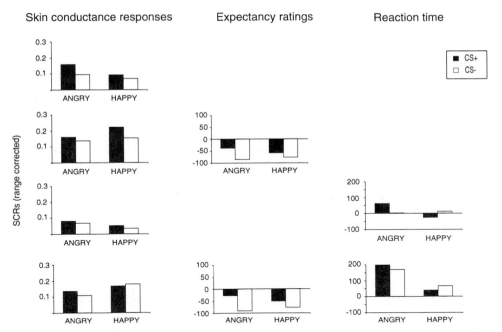

Skin conductance responses     Expectancy ratings     Reaction time

*Figure 3.* Range-corrected skin conductance responses (SCRs), expectancy ratings ("-100"=sure of no shock; "0"=shock and no shock equally likely; "100"=sure of shock), and change in reaction time (RT) from control level to probe presented 300 ms after onset of the reinforced and nonreinforced conditioned stimuli (CS+ and CS-, respectively) during extinction. Two groups of subjects (N=10 in each) were conditioned to angry and happy CSs+, with no rating or RT task (first row), two groups were required to continuously rate their shock expectancy (second row), two groups performed the RT task (third row) and two groups both did the ratings and performed the RT task (fourth row). The data in the left and middle panels are taken from trials with no probe stimuli.

onset (see Figure 3). However, as shown by the two RT panels of Figure 3, this effect was most clear-cut for subjects doing only the RT task. If they in addition were required to do the ratings, the increased task demands resulted in more overall RT slowing but less differential response to the CS+ and the CS-.

The effect of the rating task on RTs is merely one example of task interactions in the present data. Perhaps most interestingly, skin conductance responses were very sensitive to the task demands imposed by ratings and probe RTs. First, adding the ratings to the conditioning contingency had two important effects. Overall responding was increased, probably because the rating task gave additional signal value both to the CS+ and the CS-. More importantly, the preparedness effect that was obvious in the no task group (upper left panel of Fig. 3) was lost, and even replaced by an effect in the opposite direction with larger remaining differential response to fear-irrelevant stimuli. These data effectively call into question Davey's (1992) attempt to account for the preparedness effect in terms of expectancy biases. By introducing the expectancy rating task, the situation is significantly changed as compared to a condition without this task. Thus, this is a case where the assessment procedure changes the phenomenon one wants to assess. No doubt there is an expectancy bias to fear-relevant stimuli of the type that Davey (1992) described, but it distorts rather than explains the skin conductance preparedness data.

Second, the probe RT task, too, interfered with the skin conductance data. Probably because it directed attention to another stimulus modality, it resulted in (nonsignificantly) smaller responses overall, and in reliably less differential response to the CS+ and the CS-. Moreover, the skin conductance preparedness effect was lost.

The results from this experiment show quite clearly that at least part of the preparedness effect can be attributed to more effective demands on cognitive resources by fear-relevant stimuli. Whether this demand for resources begins to be manifested already at the preattentive level of information processing remains to be empirically determined. To answer this question, the experiment must be repeated, using backward masking as a way to allow only preattentive processing. Thus, the interesting question pertains to whether we will obtain similar results with masked stimuli.

The results also demonstrate the exquisite sensitivity of skin conductance responses to the cognitive resource demands of the experimental situation. Thus, great care must be taken in the design of electrodermal experiments not to let this sensitivity confound the phenomena in which the investigator is primarily interested.


## SUMMARY AND CONCLUSIONS

To recapitulate, we started out by arguing that an important part of the information processing action with regard to emotion occurs at a preattentive level, outside of the person's awareness. The preattentive processes may be understood as a monitoring system, automatically keeping track of important aspects of what is going on in the environment. When this system locates emotionally significant stimuli, there is an automatic switch of attention to bring the stimulus into the focus of voluntary, conscious attention. The monitoring system is assumed to be especially sensitive to biologically fear-relevant stimuli that have been associated with survival threats during the evolution of mankind. The shift of attention occasioned by relevant stimuli is associated with the orienting reflex, and, hence, with electrodermal responding. Electrodermal responses, therefore, are closely tied to overlapping processes of orienting, attention and emotion, that collectively may be denoted as "gateways to consciousness."

These theoretical notions were empirically examined using backward masking as a procedure to separate preattentive from conscious information processing. With this technique it was demonstrated that the elevated skin conductance responses shown by fearful subjects exposed to their feared stimuli did not depend on conscious information processing. In fact, full-blown emotional responses, including ratings of disliking, arousal and lack of control were obtained to masked stimuli, where the subjects remained unaware of the emotionally relevant target. Similar results were also obtained from normals who had been conditioned to fear-relevant stimuli (snakes, spiders, angry faces).

The concept of cognitive capacity or cognitive resources was given a central position in the theoretical analysis. It was argued that the preattentively originated shift of attention to emotional stimuli resulted in a reallocation of cognitive resources to deal effectively with the situation. Such resource allocation should limit the resources available for other tasks. Using a secondary RT probe task to assess resource utilization, it was demonstrated that more resources were recruited by fear-relevant than by fear-irrelevant stimuli. Furthermore, it was demonstrated that manipulating attention to the mask affected skin conductance responding to the masked stimuli, which suggests that competition for resources may occur already at the preattentive level of information processing.

Taken together the theoretical formulation advanced here and the associated empirical data provide a few steps toward the understanding of how emotions are activated. The empirical part attests to the sensitivity and utility of electrodermal activity in pursuing this important task. Thus, there is no question that the electrodermal system provides an important tool for the investigation of emotion.

## REFERENCES

Ax, A. (1953). The physiological differentiation between anger and fear in humans. *Psychosomatic Medicine*, **15**, 433-442.

Bauer, R. M. (1984). Autonomic recognition of names and faces in prosopagnosia: A neuropsychological application of the Guilty Knowledge Test. *Neuropsychologia*, **22**, 457-469.

Bernstein, A. S. (1981). The orienting response and stimulus significance: Further comments. *Biological Psychology*, **12**, 171-185.

Bohlin, G. (1976). Delayed habituation of the electrodermal orienting response as a function of increased level of arousal. *Psychophysiology*, **13**, 345-351.

Booth, M. L., Siddle, D. A. T., & Bond, N. W. (1989). Effects of conditioned stimulus fear-relevance and preexposure on expectancy and electrodermal measures of human Pavlovian conditioning. *Psychophysiology*, **26**, 281-291.

Davey, G. C. L. (1992). An expectancy model of laboratory preparedness effects. *Journal of Experimental Psychology: General*, **121**, 24-40.

Dawson, M. E., Filion, D. L., & Schell, A. M. (1989). Is elicitation of the autonomic orienting response associated with allocation of processing resources? *Psychophysiology*, **26**, 560-572.

Dawson, M. E., & Schell, A. M., Beers, J. R., & Kelly, A. (1982). Allocation of cognitive processing capacity during human autonomic classical conditioning. *Journal of Experimental Psychology: General*, **111**, 273-295.

Esteves, F., Dimberg, U., & Öhman, A. (submitted). Automatically elicited fear: Conditioned skin conductance responses to masked facial expressions.

Esteves, F., Dimberg, U., Parra, C., & Öhman, A. (submitted). Implicit emotional learning: Pavlovian conditioning of skin conductance responses to masked fear-relevant facial stimuli.

Esteves, F., & Öhman, A. (in press). Masking the face: Recognition of emotional facial expressions as a function of the parameters of backward masking. *Scandinavian Journal of Psychology*.

Folkman, S., Schaeffer, C., & Lazarus, R. S. (1979). Cognitive processes as mediators of stress and coping. In V. Hamilton & D. M. Warburton (Eds.). *Human stress and cognition: An information processing approach*. Chichester: Wiley.

Fredrikson, M. (1981). Orienting and defensive responses to phobic and conditioned stimuli in phobics and normals. *Psychophysiology*, **18**, 456-465.

Freud, S. (1900/1959). The interpretation of dreams. In J. Strachey (Ed.) *The standard edition of the complete psychological works of Sigmund Freud*. (Vol. 4). London: The Hogarth Press.

Frijda, N. H. (1986). *The emotions*. Cambridge: Cambridge University Press.

Graham, F. K. (1979). Distinguishing among orienting, defense, and startle reflexes. In H. D. Kimmel, E. H. van Olst, & J. F. Orlebeke (Eds.) *The orienting reflex in humans*. Hillsdale, N. J.: Erlbaum.

Greenwald, M. K., Cook, E. W., III, & Lang, P. J. (1989). Affective judgement and psychophysiological response: Dimensional covariation in the evaluation of pictorial stimuli. *Journal of Psychophysiology*, **3**, 51-64.

Hamburg, D. A., Hamburg, B. A., & Barchas, J. D. (1975). Anger and depression in perspective of behavioral biology. In L. Levi (Ed.) *Emotions: Their parameters and measurement*. New York: Raven.

Hockey, G. R. J., Gaillard, A. W. K., & Coles, M. G. H. (Eds.). (1986). *Energetics and human information processing*. Dordrecht, The Netherlands: Nijhoff.

Holender, D. (1986). Semantic activation without conscious identification in dichotic listening, parafoveal vision, and visual masking: A survey and appraisal. *Behavioral & Brain Sciences*, **9**, 1-66.

Hugdahl, K., & Öhman, A. (1977). Effects of instruction on acquisition and extinction of electrodermal responses to fear-relevant stimuli. *Journal of Experimental Psycholog: Human Learning and Memory*, **3**, 608-618.

Izard, C. E. (1979). Emotions as motivations: An evolutionary-developmental perspective. In H. E. Howe, Jr. & R. A. Dienstbier (Eds.) *Nebraska symposium on motivation 1978*. Lincoln: University of Nebraska Press.

James. W. (1884). What is an emotion? *Mind*, 9, 188-205.

James, W. (1890/1950). *The principles of psychology*. Vol. 1. New York: Dover.

Johnson, L. C., & Lubin, A. (1972) On planning psychophysiological experiments. Design, measurement, and analysis. In N. S. Greenfield & R. A. Sternbach (Eds.) *Handbook of psychophysiology* (pp. 125-158). New York: Holt, Rinehart, and Winston,

Kahneman, D. *Attention and effort*. Englewood Cliffs, NJ: Prentice-Hall.

Kramer, A., & Spinks, J. (1991). Capacity views of human information processing. In J. R. Jennings, & M. G. H. Coles (Eds.) *Handbook of cognitive psychophysiology. Central and autonomic nervous system approaches* (pp. 179-250). Chichester: Wiley.

Lacey, J. I. (1967). Somatic response patterning and stress: Some revisions of activation theory. In M. H. Appley & R. Trumbull (Eds.) *Psychological stress: Issues in research* (pp. 14-38). New York: Appleton-Century-Crofts

Lang, P. J., Bradley, M. M., & Cuthbert, B. N. (1990). Emotion, attention, and the startle reflex. *Psychological Review*, 97, 377-395.

Lazarus, R. S., Kanner, A. D., & Folkman, S. (1980). Emotions: A cognitive-phenomenological analysis. In R. Plutchik & H. Kellerman (Eds.) *Emotion: Theory, research, and experience. Vol. 1: Theories of emotion*. New York: Academic Press.

Lindsley, D. B. (1951). Emotions. In S. S. Stevens (Ed.) *Handbook of experimental psychology*. New York: Wiley.

Lynn, R. (1966). *Attention, arousal, and the orientation reaction*. Oxford: Pergamon Press.

McNally, R. J. (1987). Preparedness and phobias: A review. *Psychological Bulletin*, 101, 283-303.

Malmo, R. B. (1959) Activation: A neuropsychological dimension. *Psychological Review*, 66, 367-386.

Mandler, G. (1984). *Mind and body: Psychology of emotion and stress*. New York: Norton.

Marcel, A. (1983). Conscious and unconscious perception: An approach to the relations between phenomenal experience and perceptual processes. *Cognitive Psychology*, 15, 238-300.

Marks, I. M. (1969). *Fears and phobias*. London: Heineman Medical Books.

Massaro, D. W. (1975). *Experimental psychology and information processing*. Chicago: Rand McNally.

Öhman, A. (1979). The orienting response, attention, and learning: An information processing perspective. In H. D. Kimmel, E. H. van Olst, & J. F. Orlebeke (Eds.), *The orienting reflex in humans* (pp. 443-472). Hillsdale, N. J.: Erlbaum.

Öhman, A. (1983). The orienting response during Pavlovian conditioning. In D. A. T. Siddle (Ed.), *Orienting and habituation: Perspectives in human research* (pp. 315-369). Chichester: Wiley.

Öhman, A. (1987). The psychophysiology of emotion: An evolutionary-cognitive perspective. *Advances in psychophysiology*, 2, 79-127.

Öhman, A. (1988). Nonconscious control of autonomic responses: A role for Pavlovian conditioning? *Biological Psychology*, 27, 113-135.

Öhman, A. (1992). Orienting and attention: Preferred preattentive processing of potentially phobic stimuli. In B. A. Campbell, H. Haynes, & R. Richardson (Eds.) *Attention and information processing in infants and adults. Perspectives from human and animal research*. Hillsdale, N. J.: Erlbaum.

Öhman, A. (1993). Stimulus prepotency and fear: Data and theory. In N. Birbaumer & A. Öhman (Eds.) *The organization of emotion: Cognitive, clinical and psychophysiological perspectives*. Toronto: Hogrefe.

Öhman, A. (in press). Fear and anxiety as emotional phenomena: Clinical phenomenology, evolutionary perspectives, and information processing mechanisms. In M. Lewis & J. M. Haviland (Eds.) *Handbook of emotions*. New York: Guiford.

Öhman, A., & Birbaumer, N. (1993). Psychophysiological and cognitive-clinical perspectives on emotion: Introduction and overview. In N. Birbaumer & A. Öhman (Eds.). *The organization of emotion: Cognitive, clinical, and psychophysiolgoical aspects*. Toronto: Hogrefe and Huber.

Öhman, A., & Dimberg, U. (1978). Facial expressions as conditioned stimuli for electrodermal responses: A case of "preparedness"? *Journal of Personality and Social Psychology*, 36, 1251-1258.

Öhman, A., Dimberg, U., & Esteves, F. (1989). Preattentive activation of aversive emotions. In T. Archer and L.G. Nilsson (Eds.) *Aversion, Avoidance, and Anxiety*, Hillsdale, New Jersey: Erlbaum.

Öhman, A., Dimberg, U., & Öst, L.G. (1985). Animal and social phobias: Biological constraints on learned fear responses. In S. Reiss & R. R. Bootzin (Eds.), *Theoretical issues in behavior therapy* (pp. 123-178). New York: Academic Press.

Öhman, A., & Soares, J. J. F. (1993). On the automaticity of phobic fear: Conditioned skin conductance responses to masked phobic stimuli. *Journal of Abnormal Psychology*, 102, in press.

Öhman, A., & Soares, J. J. F. (in press). Unconscious anxiety: Phobic responses to masked stimuli. *Journal of Abnormal Psychology*

Ojeman, G. A., & van Buren, J. M. (1967). Respiratory, heart rate, and GSR responses from human diencephalon. *Archives of Neurology*, 16, 74-88.

Ortony, A., Clore, G. L., & Collins, A. (1988). *The cognitive structure of emotions*. New York: Cambridge University Press.

Parra, C., Esteves, F., & Öhman, A. (submitted). Recognition memory for masked facial stimuli.

Power, M., & Brewin, C. R. (1991). From Freud to cognitive science: A contemporary account of the unconscious. *British Journal of Clinical Psychology*, 30, 289-310.

Russell, J. A. (1980). A circumplex model of affect. *Journal of Personality and Social Psychology*, 39, 1161-1178.

Sartory, G. (1983). The orienting response and psychopathology: Anxiety and phobias. In D. Siddle (Ed.) *Orienting and habituation: Perspectives in human research* (pp. 449-474). Chichester: Wiley.

Schachter, S., & Singer, J. (1962). Cognitive, social, and physiological determinants of emotional state. *Psychological Review*, 69, 379-399.

Schiffman, K., & Furedy, J. J. (1972). Failures of contingency and cognitive factors to affect long interval differential Pavlovian autonomic conditioning. *Journal of Experimental Psychology*, 96, 215-218.

Schneirla, T. C. (1959). An evolutionary and developmental theory of biphasic processes underlying approach and withdrawal. *Nebraska Symposium of Motivation: 1959* (pp. 1-42). Lincoln: University of Nebraska Press.

Seligman, M. E. P. (1970). On the generality of the laws of learning. *Psychological Review*, 77, 406-418.

Seligman, M. E. P. (1971). Phobias and preparedness. *Behavior Therapy*, 2, 307-320.

Siddle, D. A. T., Spinks, J. A. (1992). Orienting, habituation, and the allocation of processing resources. In B. A. Campbell, H. Haynes, & R. Richardson (Eds.) *Attention and information processing in infants and adults. Perspectives from human and animal research.* (pp. 227-262). Hillsdale, N. J.: Erlbaum.

Soares, J. J. F., & Öhman, A. (1993). Preattentive processing, preparedness, and phobias: Effects of instruction on conditioned electrodermal responses to masked an non-masked fear-relevant stimuli. *Behaviour Research and Therapy*, 31, 81-95.

Soares, J. J. F., & Öhman, A. (in press). Backward masking and skin conductance responses after conditioning to non-feared but fear-relevant stimuli in fearful subjects. *Psychophysiology*.

Spinks, J., & Kramer, A. (1991). Capacity views of human information processing: Autonomic measures. In J. R. Jennings & M. G. H. Coles (Eds.) *Handbook of cognitive psychophysiology. Central and autonomic nervous system approaches*. Chichester: Wiley.

Thompson, R., F. (1967). *Foundations of physiological psychology*. New York: Harper & Row.

Tomarken, A. J., Mineka, S., & Cook, M. (1989). Fear-relevant selective associations and covariation bias. *Journal of Abnormal Psychology*, 98, 381-394.

Tranel, D., & Damasio, A. R. (1985). Knowledge without awareness: An autonomic index of facial recognition by prosopagnosics. *Science*, 228, 1453-1454.

Waters, W. F., McDonald, D. G., & Koresko, R. L. (1977). Habituation of the orienting response: A gating mechanism subserving selective attention: *Psychophysiology*, 14, 228-237.

Zajonc, R. B. (1980). Feeling and thinking: Preferences need no inferences. *American Psychologist*, 35, 151-175.

# ELECTRODERMAL HABITUATION PATTERNS: EFFECT OF

# RELATIVE REFRACTORINESS, EXTRAPOLATION OF

# STIMULUS CONDITIONS, OR GESTALT PERCEPTION?

Rüdiger Baltissen

Physiological Psychology
University of Wuppertal
5600 Wuppertal 1  Germany

## INTRODUCTION

The electrodermal response (EDR) is the most extensively used dependent variable in the study of orienting and habituation. As a consequence tests of the appropriate theoretical account of the phenomena of orienting and habituation are based mainly on results from electrodermal recordings (Siddle, 1991).

Theories of habituation can be divided broadly into comparator or two-stage theories and noncomparator or one-stage theories (Lynn, 1966). One of the essential features of the comparator theories is that they emphasize the extrapolatory properties of the information processing system. The comparison is said to be between anticipated and actual stimulation (Siddle, Bond & Packer, 1988). Noncomparator theories, on the other hand, hold that the decline in response magnitudes is due to a change in elements which intervene between stimulus and response.

Experiments that are considered as suitable to distinguish between comparator and noncomparator theories are those in which the temporal structure of the stimuli is varied. "The most interesting are the experiments where the "nerve model of the stimulus" reflects the temporary sequence of signals equal in strength and quality... It may be said that by observing the pecularities of the incoming signal for a long time the nervous system extrapolates its future value. The orienting reaction arises if the prediction...does not coincide with the value of the incoming signal" (Sokolov, 1966; pp. 347-348). The "missing stimulus effect", the occurrence of a previously habituated response to the absence of a regularly presented event, has been identified as a crucial manipulation to confirm Sokolov's assumption. The empirical evidence, however, is far from convincing. At best, only a fraction of subjects exhibit a response to the omission of a regularly presented stimulus (Siddle, 1991).

Another way to test the extrapolatory properties of the information processing system and to induce regularity or redundancy in the stimulus sequence may be achieved by presenting subjects with a pattern of interstimulus intervals (ISIs). A sequence with alternating intervals, for example, is as redundant as a sequence with one constant interval (Attneave, 1965). In the experiments reported here alternating intervals were used in a habituation paradigm and the EDR was recorded as an indicator of the information processing of stimulus sequences. The aim of these studies is to show the effect of patterned stimulation on the EDR and to answer the question whether the resulting electrodermal changes have to be considered simply as an effect of the relative refractoriness of the electrodermal system, as an effect of the extrapolatory properties of the nervous system, or may be due to the perception of the temporal pattern as a Gestalt.

## PATTERNING OF EDRS WITH PATTERNED STIMULATION: EFFECT OF RELATIVE REFRACTORINESS?

In an experiment by Baltissen, Schaefer and Kimmel (1989), 1sec 1000 Hz tones of 90dB(A) intensity were presented with alternating ISIs of 30-50sec and with another of 10-70sec as well as a constant ISI of 40sec. Thus all series had the same average ISI and took the same time. In this experiment a striking pattern of trial-by-trial alternation in EDR magnitude (skin conductance response) occurred in the 10-70sec groups.

As can be seen in Figure 1, large responses tended to occur following the 70sec interval while small responses followed the 10sec interval. For the 70-10sec group, even trials followed a 70sec ISI; conversely for the 10-70sec group. The magnitude curves of

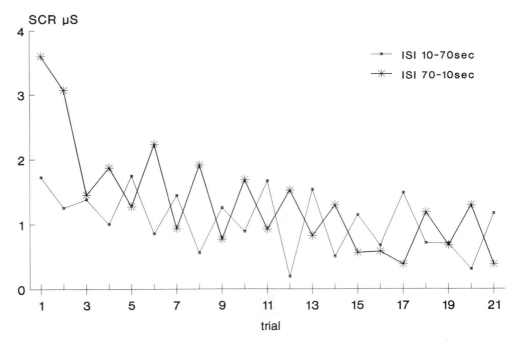

**Figure 1.** Mean magnitude of EDR to a 1sec 1000Hz tone of 90dB(A) intensity presented with alternating intervals of 10-70sec and 70-10sec across 21 trials .

160

the two subgroup's responses are one trial out of phase, since one group started with 70sec and the other with 10sec intervals. Given that large responses followed the 70sec intervals and small responses followed the 10sec intervals, at first glance, the oscillating pattern of responding seemed to be attributable to a relatively trivial mechanistic process.

It is well-established by Furedy and Scull (1971) as well as by Grings and Schell (1973) that the response to the second of two successive stimuli is directly proportional to the time between stimuli. Results of this type are easily to explain on the basis of a relative refractory period of the electrodermal system following an elicited EDR. The longer the time the greater the recovery from refractoriness, and thus the larger the response. This possible interpretation of the data was tested by subjecting the individual response curves to multiple regression analyses, with log of trial number and time since last stimulus as predictors. It was expected that time since last stimulus would account for a significant percentage of variance of the individual response curves. Log of trial number accounted for 25.1% of the variance in the EDR magnitude and time since last stimulus accounted for an additional 25%, appearently confirming a refractoriness interpretation.

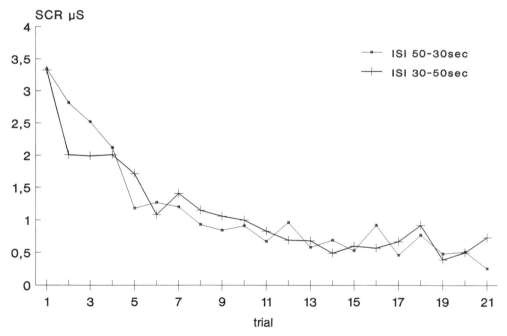

**Figure 2.** Mean magnitude of EDR to a 1sec 1000 Hz tone of 90 dB(A) intensity presented with alternating intervals of 50-30 sec and 30-50 sec across 21 trials.

The EDR magnitude data of the 30-50sec and 50-30sec subgroups are shown in Figure 2. Here it can be seen that the trial-by-trial oscillation in the EDR magnitude was minimal. It was assumed that these findings reflect the fact that the time difference between 30 and 50sec was so much smaller than the one between 10 and 70 s that the effect of relative refractoriness was considerably reduced; indeed, the 30sec interval was long enough so that very little refractoriness was to be expected. Multiple regression analyses of the EDR magnitudes showed that 42.7% of the variance was accounted for by log trial number and only 5% additional variance by the time since last stimulus (n.s.).

To further test the relative refractoriness hypothesis two additional control groups were run. These groups received two different random sequences of all intervals that had been used in the other three groups, i.e. 10, 30, 40, 50 and 70sec.

As the trial-by-trial changes in Figure 3 show, rate of habituation in the control groups did not differ from those of the other groups. However, the multiple regression analyses of the two groups were of singular significance. Log trial number accounted for 38.7% of the variance in trial-by-trial responding. But the time since last stimulus accounted for only 7% of the variance. It must be emphasized that subjects in this condition received intervals ranging from as small as 10sec to as large as 70sec. The regression analyses of the random groups' responses provided strong evidence that the effect of time since last stimulus, as was seen in the 10-70sec and 70-10sec subgroups, cannot be explained as a mechanical refractoriness effect, since this kind of influence should have also occurred in the random groups. Therefore, it was not the time since last stimulus, in the trivial sense, that was accounting for 25% of the variance in EDR magnitudes. Instead, it may have been the fact that an alternating sequence of intervals was employed, a sequence that could very easily be registered by the subject.

## PATTERNED ELECTRODERMAL RESPONDING:
## EFFECT OF SEQUENCE DETECTION AND ANTICIPATION?

Assuming that time since last stimulus is not itself the critical factor determining the patterning effect in the 10-70sec and 70-10sec conditions, but that the alternating

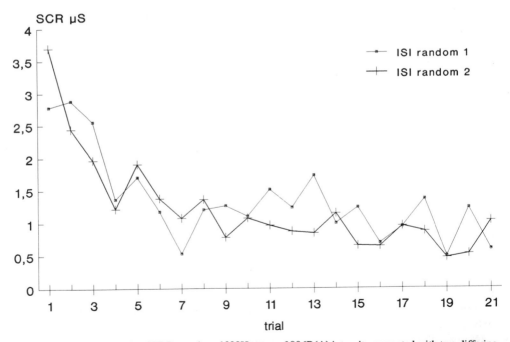

**Figure 3.** Mean magnitude of EDR to a 1sec 1000Hz tone of 90dB(A) intensity presented with two differing random orders across 21 trials.

sequence of short and long intervals is also critical, one wonders why only minimal patterning was observed in the 30-50sec and 50-30sec condition (i.e. why the percentage of variance attributable to the time since last stimulus did not differ significantly from zero in these alternating conditions). The answer could be that the time difference between 30sec and 50sec was not large enough to be reliably registered by the subjects. Therefore, the pattern of alternation of ISIs was inadequately registered and only weakly mirrored in the subject's responses.

An even more relevant question that must be raised is why the time since last stimulus influenced the magnitude of responding significantly when an alternating temporal pattern was administered and registered but not when the intervals varied randomly. It seems reasonable to assume that subjects receiving patterned stimulation will be able to anticipate each forthcoming stimulus, and that it is easier to anticipate the next stimulus when the interval is 10sec than when it is 70sec. On the further assumption that responses to anticipated stimuli are likely to be smaller than to unanticipated stimuli, the patterned responding could be explained.

To further substantiate this interpretation, one should consider the experimental procedure from the subject's viewpoint. The subject heard the same tone over at different intervals. The development of "knowledge" regarding these events requires that there be some basis for organizing the tones by means of relating them to one another. Fortunately, some of the subjects in the 10-70sec and 70-10sec conditions spontaneously reported how they did this. In an informal, unstructured interview conducted at the end of the experimental session, the subjects were asked to describe their experience during the experiment in their own words. Some of them reported having heard two tones followed by a long interval, afterwards two tones followed by a long interval etc. In other words, they grouped the two stimuli that were 10sec apart, and thus reported only one interval. From this perspective, only the first one of the grouped stimuli is really important, therefore evoking the larger response.

These post-experimental descriptions of what the subject experienced are consistent with expectations based on the Gestalt law of proximity. The temporal patterning phenomenon could be a manifestation of this law. Perhaps, the subject's perceptual field organizes its input to produce the "best" auditory figure, so that the two adjacent tones tend to join experientially. This would be a kind of auditory phi-phenomenon. Alternatively, the patterning could be interpreted in terms of the information processing theories of habituation which focus on the encoding of the stimulus pattern in the neuronal model (Sokolov, 1963). This is considered to account for the extrapolatory mechanism of the nervous system, i.e. its tendency to predict what will come next after the first stimulus of the stimulus pair has been presented.

When trying to explain the phenomenon within the context of current information processing theories of habituation, one finds Sokolov (1969) being quite explicit in describing the subject's responses to a sequence of stimuli. When the subject detects a sequence in the order of stimuli he/she will exhibit an orienting reaction to each first stimulus of the sequence signalling the occurrence of all other stimuli of that sequence. As a consequence, the response to the first stimulus of the sequence will be largest, because it has signal value and predicts the occurrence of all other stimuli which are part of the sequence. It seems reasonable to assume that a simple sequence consisting of only two stimuli can easily be detected, learned and encoded in the neuronal model.

If one further assumes that the stimuli are encoded in the neuronal model as stimulus pairs, any disruption of the sequence either by presentation of an unexpected additional stimulus out of sequence or by omission of an expected one should lead to a reinstatement of the OR as a result of the mismatch between expected and actual stimulation.

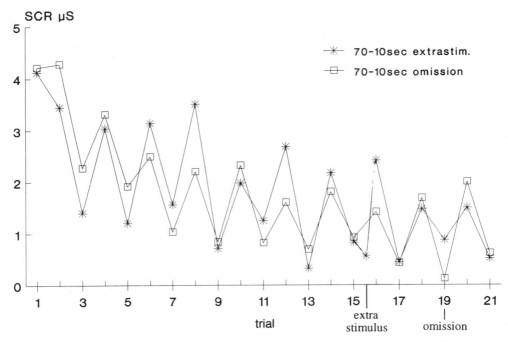

**Figure 4**. Mean magnitude of EDR to a 1sec 1000Hz tone of 90dB(A) intensity presented with alternating intervals of 70-10sec across 21 trials for a condition in which an extra stimulus was presented between trial 15 and trial 16 and a condition in which the stimulus was omitted in trial 19.

As can be seen in Figure 4, neither the presentation of an additional stimulus between trial 16 and 17 in a sequence of 70-10-10sec intervals nor the omission of a second stimulus of a pair in trial 19 led to a reinstatement of the OR. However patterned responding was found throughout all trials, and regression analyses of the responses showed an average variance of 24% accounted for by the time since last stimulus. Interpretation of the results is straight-forward suggesting that the stimuli are not encoded in the neuronal model as stimulus pairs.

However, the manipulations to test Sokolov's hypothesis might have been relatively weak for two reasons. Firstly, the stimulus omission effect appears to be especially fragile in terms of the low number of subjects who display the phenomenon, and there has been little success in delineating the conditions under which the effect occurs most strongly (Siddle, 1991). Secondly, the change in a sequence of intervals is an infrequently used method to induce OR reinstatement. Thus, there are no data available to estimate the effectiveness of this procedure (cf. Siddle, Stephenson & Spinks, 1983). Furthermore, the change may have been too small to be detected by the subjects and may have been dependent upon the subject's attention which was not especially directed to the interval duration.

Therefore, a more direct procedure was introduced to influence the development of the neuronal model in order to test the memory representation hypothesis of stimulus pairs. A direct method to vary the formation of the neuronal model has been provided in an experiment by Iacono and Lykken (1983), in which the effects of instructions and a distraction story on electrodermal habituation were examined.

A secondary task like listening to a distracting story while hearing tones is expected to delay or even prevent the establishment of a neuronal model of the tone stimuli in the same manner as instructions to ignore the tones. On the other hand, attend-instructions to count the stimuli or to make judgements with regard to their quality gives signal value to the stimuli and therefore should result in a faster and more precise encoding of the stimuli in the neuronal model.

In applying the procedure used by Iacono and Lykken (1983), 6 groups in a 3 by 2 factorial design with instruction varied in 3 levels (attend, ignore and neutral) and distraction in 2 levels (radio crime play vs none) were run. Subjects in the attend groups were instructed to count the stimuli, while subjects in the ignore groups were instructed to tune out the stimuli. Subjects in the neutral groups were only informed that a series of tones would be presented. Half of the subjects in each group heard the radio story. Again, tones were presented with alternating intervals of 10 and 70sec. Less patterned responding was expected in the conditions with distractor and in the ignore instruction groups, while a stronger patterning should occur in the conditions without distractor and in the attend instruction groups.

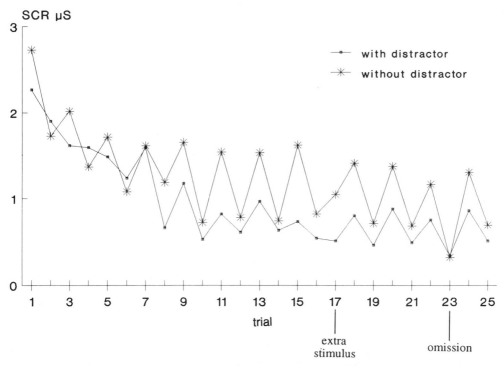

**Figure 5**. Mean magnitude of EDR to a 1sec 1000Hz tone of 90dB(A) intensity presented with alternating intervals of 10-70 sec across 25 trials for a condition with distractor (story) and without distractor(no story).

As can be seen in the Figure 5, the presentation of the distracting story reduced the patterning of the EDRs. Regression analyses revealed that time since last stimulus accounted for 20% of the variance in the groups without a distractor, compared with only 8.7% in the groups with a distractor. Although patterned responding appeared to be more reliable in the attend as compared to the other groups, regression analyses showed only a marginal effect of instruction, thus increasing the variance accounted for by the time since last stimulus in the attend groups to 19% as compared to 11 % and 12.3 % in the ignore and neutral instruction groups.

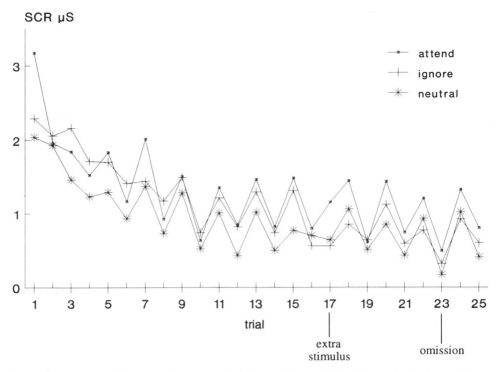

**Figure 6**. Mean magnitude of EDR to a 1sec 1000Hz tone of 90dB(A) intensity presented with alternating intervals of 10-70sec and different instructions. In trial 17 an extra stimulus was presented after a short interval of 10sec where a 70sec interval was expected and in trial 19 the tone after a short interval of 10sec was omitted

However, as Figure 6 shows, the attend instruction to count the stimuli led to a significantly increased responding to the presentation of an additional stimulus after a short interval in trial 17, where a long interval was expected (see "extrastimulus"), while in the neutral and ignore groups a slight decrease or no change at all occurred. Again, responses to the omission of an expected stimulus were not increased, either in the attend or in the neutral and ignore groups.

So far, results show that the presentation of a distracting story reduces the patterned responding. It does so presumably because attention is drawn away from the alternation of the intervals, thereby preventing subjects from clearly registering the difference between long and short intervals. Thus the development of the neuronal model of stimulus pairs is somewhat delayed and less pronounced although not totally abolished. The OR reinstatement to the disruption of the sequence - although occurring only selectively in the attend groups - seems to provide some indirect evidence for the assumption that generally the stimuli are encoded as stimulus pairs in the neuronal model. The question remains as to why was there no OR reinstatement in the neutral and ignore instruction groups. One could argue that the disruption must have some meaning to the subject in order evoke a response. The disruption became meaningful to the subjects in the attend groups because they had to count the stimuli and tried not to dismiss one. This interpretation could also explain why no OR reinstatement could be observed in the previous experiment.

The interpretation of the patterned responding in terms of the development of a neuronal model of the stimulus sequence and the interpretation of the decreased response magnitude to the second stimulus in terms of the predictability of its occurrence was subjected to further testing.

166

When the patterned responding is attributed to the registration of a sequence and the response decrement to the predictability of the stimuli within the sequence, no patterning should occur in a random sequence of 10sec and 70sec intervals. This is because a random sequence does not allow the subject to predict the time of the occurrence of the next stimulus.

However, as can be seen in Figure 7, patterning was present in the random condition even in the first sequence of 10 and 70sec intervals, and it was also present in a 10-70sec control condition. Regression analyses showed 22% of the variance accounted for by the time since last stimulus in the random condition and 18.7% in the control condition. This result is in serious conflict with an interpretation of patterning in terms of predictability or anticipation of the second stimulus of a stimulus pair. Instead, the results suggest that the intervals themselves and especially the relation of intervals is of major importance for the occurrence of the patterned responding.

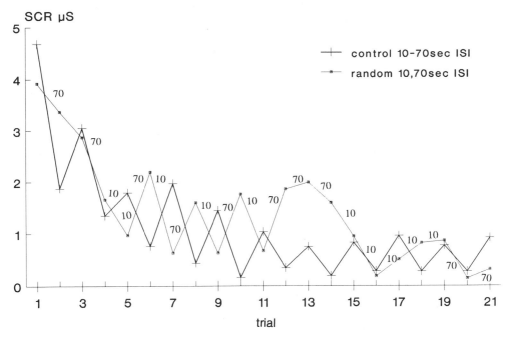

**Figure 7**. Mean magnitude of EDR to a 1sec 1000Hz tone of 90dB(A) intensity for a control condition with alternating intervals of 10-70sec and a condition with a random order of 10sec and 70sec intervals.

## PATTERNED ELECTRODERMAL RESPONDING: EFFECT OF GESTALT PERCEPTION ACCORDING TO THE LAW OF PROXIMITY?

Focussing on relations between elements of stimuli is characteristic for Gestalt psychology. Since Gestalt perception is always a relational perception, stimuli, which are spatially or temporally related are typically perceived as going together. However, in determinations of perceptual grouping, it is not the absolute distances among elements - as in contiguity theory - but rather the relative distances in the array which are of importance. The likelihood that two events will be perceptually grouped depends not only on their distance from each other but also on the distance of each one from other elements in the display. However, most of the Gestalt work on the phenomenon of grouping by proximity has dealt with visual stimuli, in which all of the potentially groupable elements are simultaneously present. The organization of temporally separate elements, such as the stimuli in the experiments reported here, present a somewhat different situation. Köhler (1947), however, has argued that experienced time has certain characteristics in common with experienced space. He further stated that the factors on which temporal grouping depends may be the same as those on which spatial grouping depends. "Suppose that I knock three times at short intervals on my table, and that after waiting for a second I repeat the performance, and so forth. People who hear this sequence of sounds experience groups in time." He continues: "Physically, all these sounds are, of course, independent events. ...there is no grouping in the physical sequence." (Köhler, 1947; p.89).

This example demonstrates that a Gestalt does not develop, but is forced (Köhler, 1947). Assuming that a Gestalt is forced and that the response pattern mirrors the subject's Gestalt perception, then the immediate occurrence of the patterned responding at the beginning of the series can be explained on that basis. Furthermore it can explain why patterning occurs in a random sequence of 10-70sec intervals, whenever that particular sequence of 10-70sec is presented. This concept constitutes an alternative interpretation of the data in Figure 7 which otherwise may imply a refractory effect.

If it is the relation of intervals which is the most important for the occurrence of the patterned responding, then the gestalt qualities as described by Ehrenfels (1890) should apply to the above series of stimuli. The qualities are "Übersummativität" (oversummativity, i.e. the whole is more than its parts) and "Transponierbarkeit" (transposability). The best illustration for "Transponierbarkeit" is found in music. A melody may be transposed to another key and still retains its structure or Gestalt. When transposing the relation of 1:7 between the intervals to other absolute durations by doubling or halfing the original 10-70sec arrangement, using 20-140sec and 5-35sec, the pattern should still be present. From a contiguity or predictability point of view one would

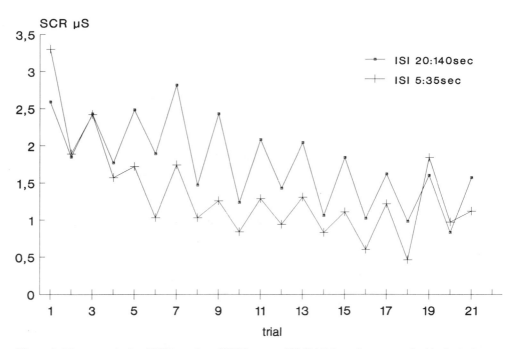

**Figure 8**. Mean magnitude of EDR to a 1sec 1000Hz tone of 90dB(A) intensity presented with alternating intervals of 5-35sec and 20-140sec across 21 trials.

expect stronger evidence of patterning with the 5-35sec than with the 20-140sec sequence, while from a Gestalt point of view there should be no differences in strength of patterning. The trial-by-trial magnitudes of the EDRs for these conditions are shown in Figure 8.

At first glance, patterning appears to be greater in the 20-140sec condition than in the 5-35sec condition. However, regression analyses showed, that the time since last stimulus accounted for 19.5% of the variance in the 20-140sec group and 17.8% of the variance in the 5-35sec group. Therefore, it has to be concluded that patterning was significantly present in both groups, but not differentially. This result is not in accordance with a contiguity or predictability interpretation. Rather it is consistent with a Gestalt interpretation.

To examine the temporal limits of the patterning, an experiment of a large scale of interval ratios ranging from 5-75, 15-65, 20-60, 25-55 to 35-45sec was conducted. 10-70sec and 30-50sec conditions were not included, since the outcome of these arrangements was already known. Patterned responding was expected to occur with intervals from 5-75sec up to 20-60sec i.e. to a minimum of 1:3.

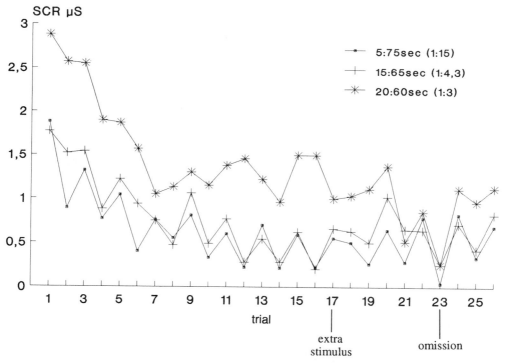

**Figure 9.** Mean magnitude of EDR to a 1 sec 1000Hz tone of 90dB(A) intensity presented with alternating intervals of 5-75sec, 15-65sec and 20-60sec across 26 trials.

As can be seen in Figure 9, patterned responding was present in the 5-75sec and 15-65sec condition but not in the 20-60sec condition. Regression analyses revealed that the time since last stimulus accounted for 14.8% of the variance in the 5-75sec, and for 10.8% of the variance in the 15-65sec group, but only for 2.6% of the variance in the 20-60sec condition.

Figure 10 shows the trial-by-trial changes for the 25-55sec and 35-45sec conditions. Responses were not dependent on the interval, and the regression analyses showed that the time since last stimulus accounted for only 3.3% of the variance in the 25-55sec condition and for 1.7% of the variance in the 35-45sec condition. On the basis of these results we can conclude that patterned responding occurs when the relation between intervals exceeds a value of 1:4.

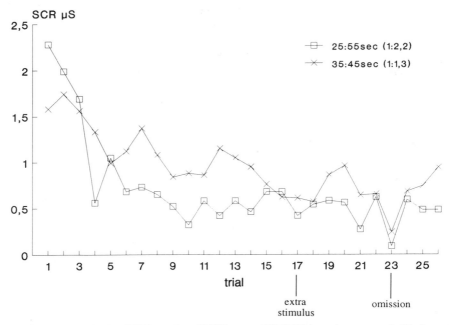

**Figure 10**. Mean magnitude of EDR to a 1sec 1000Hz tone of 90dB(A) intensity presented with alternating intervals of 25-55sec and 35-45sec across 26 trials.

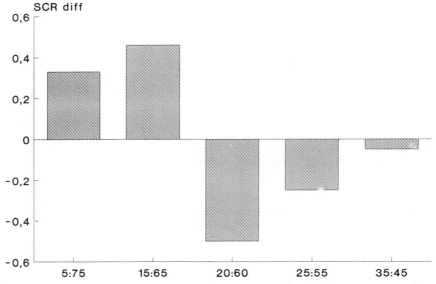

**Figure 11**. Mean difference in the magnitude of the EDR between the response to the extra stimulus (trial 17) and the preceding trial (trial 16) for the different interval conditions.

The same manipulations to induce reinstatement of the OR were applied as in previous experiments by presenting an additional stimulus after a short interval where a long one was expected and by omitting the second stimulus of a stimulus pair in trial 23. Figure 11 shows the difference in response magnitude between the response to an additional stimulus on trial 17 and the previous trial for each interval condition.

There were decreases from the 16th to the 17th trial in the three groups which did not show patterned responding and increases in the two which did. The reason for the substantial decrease in the 20-60sec group remains to be explained. These results again strongly suggest that the pattern of stimulation is encoded in the neuronal model and that the OR reinstatement to the disruption of the sequence results from mismatch between expected and actual stimulation.

What then about the Gestalt interpretation of the patterned responding? One could argue that during presentation of the first 3 or 4 stimulus pairs the law of proximity operates on the stimuli and the tones are grouped by the subject. After presentation of the first 3 or 4 pairs subjects have learned that there are two stimuli followed by a long interval, two stimuli followed by a long interval etc. Therefore, in later trials an association may have developed between the two stimuli. However this association is - as Koehler (1947, p.163) stated - only an aftereffect of the perceptual organization of the two stimuli.

## CONCLUSION

It is obvious that we do not know enough about the phenomenon to arrive at a definite conclusion regarding its theoretical explanation. We are left with the problem of differentiating more clearly between an associatively based explanation of the phenomenon in terms of learning of stimulus contingencies on the one hand and Gestalt interpretation or relational pattern perception hypothesis on the other hand. Furthermore this ambiguity may be resolved in future experiments by using more complex sequences which have a periodicity over more than two trials. With such paradigms, one may put to the test the question weather a response pattern develops more slowly or occurs immediately in the sense of a preorganized Gestalt.

## REFERENCES

Attneave, F. 1965, "Informationstheorie in der Psychologie", Huber, Bern.

Baltissen, R., Schaefer, F., and Kimmel, H.D., 1989, Der Einfluß von zeitlicher Verteilung bei konstanter Häufigkeit der Reize auf die Habituation der Orientierungsreaktion, *Zeitschrift für experimentelle und angewandte Psychologie, 36*, 181-198.

Grings, W. W. and Schell, A. M., 1969, Magnitude of electrodermal response to a standard stimulus as a function of intensity and proximity of a prior stimulus, *Journal of Comparative and Physiological Psychology, 67*, 77-82.

Furedy, J. J., and Scull, J., 1971, Orienting-reaction theory and an increase in the human GSR following stimulus change which is unpredictable but not contrary to prediction, *Journal of Experimental Psychology, 88*, 292-294.

Iacono, W. G., and Lykken, D. T., 1983, The effects of instructions on electrodermal habituation, *Psychophysiology, 20*, 71-80.

Koehler, W., 1947, "Gestalt Psychology, An Introduction to New Concepts in Modern Psychology", Liveright, New York.

Lynn, R., 1966, "Attention, Arousal and the Orientation Reaction", Pergamon Press, Oxford.

Siddle, D. A. T., Bond, N. W., and Packer, S., 1988, Comparator theories of habituation: A comment on Mackintosh's analysis, *Biological Psychology, 27,* 59-63.

Siddle, D. A. T., Stephenson, D., and Spinks, J. A., 1983, Elicitation and habituation of the orienting response, *in*: "Orienting and habituation: Perspectives in Human Research", D. Siddle, ed., Wiley, Chichester.

Siddle, D. A. T., 1991, Orienting, habituation, and resource allocation: An associative analysis, *Psychophysiology, 28,* 245-259.

Sokolov, E. N., 1963, "Perception and the conditioned reflex", Pergamon Press, Oxford.

Sokolov, E. N., 1966, Orienting reflex as information regulator. *in*: "Psychological research in the USSR (Vol. 1)", A. N. Leontiev, A. R. Luria, E. N. Sokolov, and O. S. Vinogradova, ed., Progress Publishers, Moscow.

Sokolov, E. N., 1969, The modeling properties of the nervous system, *in*: "A Handbook of Contemporary Soviet Psychology", M. Cole, and I.Maltzman, ed., Basic Books, New York .

# ELECTRODERMAL RESPONSE LABILITY-STABILITY:
# INDIVIDUAL DIFFERENCE CORRELATES

Andrew Crider

Department of Psychology
Williams College
Williamstown, MA 01267 USA

## INTRODUCTION

The aim of this chapter is to review a sizable literature on electrodermal response (EDR) lability considered as an individual difference phenomenon. The exposition is divided into three parts. The first deals with questions of definition and measurement the second presents a first-order and an extended hypothesis regarding likely personality correlates, and the third reviews evidence for interpreting EDR lability as a concomitant of individual differences in characteristic levels of arousal along a sleep-wakefulness continuum.

## DEFINITION AND PSYCHOMETRIC PROPERTIES

The concept of EDR lability is rooted in a 1953 paper by Mundy-Castle & McKiever, who found that subjects who emitted a high frequency of nonspecific (spontaneous) electrodermal responses also responded with a high frequency of specific (elicited) responses to an iterated stimulus, whereas subjects who emitted few nonspecific responses showed few specific responses. This robust phenomenon is illustrated in Figure 1 (Dawson & Nuechterlein, 1984). The figure depicts skin conductance tracings from two hypothetical subjects during a brief rest period followed by three presentations of a nonsignal stimulus. The top tracing is that of a labile subject, who shows frequent nonspecific responses both before and during the stimulus presentations, as well as vigorous specific responses to each of the stimuli. The bottom tracing illustrates a stabile subject, who shows only one nonspecific and two specific responses.

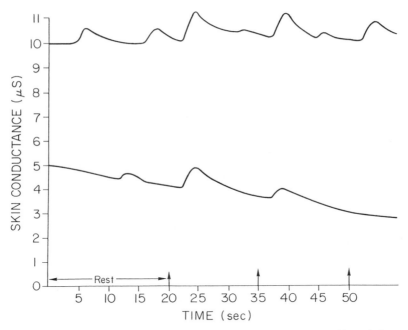

**Figure 1.** Idealized skin conductance tracings from labile (top) and stabile (bottom) subjects during a rest period followed by three nonsignal stimulus presentations. Reprinted with permission from Dawson & Nuechterlein (1984).

Since the original Mundy-Castle and McKiever (1953) observation, a number of studies have measured the covariation of specific and nonspecific EDR lability in iterated stimulus paradigms (e.g., Bohlin, 1973b; Bull & Gale, 1973; Carr et al., 1985; Crider & Lunn, 1971; Schell et al., 1988; Siddle & Herron, 1976; Vossel & Zimmer, 1988). In the typical procedure, subjects are presented with a discrete nonsignal stimulus that is repeated at varying intervals on the order of tens of seconds. Nonspecific responding is usually measured as the frequency of phasic EDRs reaching some minimal amplitude during an initial rest period. Specific responding is usually measured as the trial number at which the stimulus no longer elicits phasic EDRs of minimal amplitude. The correlations between these two measures reported in the seven studies cited above range from .50 to .75, with a median value in the mid .60's. With the exception of the Carr et al. (1985) study, which employed chronic pain patients, these findings were derived from normal samples. However, covariations of similar magnitude also characterize psychiatric samples (e.g., Edman et al., 1986; Rubens and Lapidus, 1978).

Schell et al. (1988) provided a categorical analysis of the covariation of specific and nonspecific EDRs. Fifty-seven subjects were tested in an iterated stimulus procedure on two occasions approximately one month apart. Subjects falling above median nonspecific EDR frequency in both sessions were classified as nonspecific labiles, and those falling below the median in both sessions were classified as nonspecific stabiles. Similarly, subjects falling above or below median specific EDR frequency in both sessions were classified into specific EDR labile and stabile groups. Of the subjects classified as nonspecific EDR labiles, 80% were also classified as specific EDR labiles; of those classified as nonspecific EDR stabiles, 82% were also classified as specific EDR stabiles.

The relationship of nonspecific to specific responding is often interpreted as showing that nonspecific EDR lability predicts electrodermal orienting response habituation. Indeed, specific EDR lability is often defined as an habituation parameter known as "trials to habituation" in studies informed by orienting response theory. Unfortunately, the distinction between specific EDR lability and EDR habituation is clouded by a lack of consensus on the conceptual and operational definition of habituation (Siddle et al., 1983). In particular, specific EDR lability (trials to habituation) is uncorrelated with regression measures of EDR amplitude decrement over trials, the latter measure being operationally closer to the concept of habituation than the former (Martin and Rust, 1976; Siddle et al., 1983). There is therefore reason to question the alignment of specific EDR lability with the concept of habituation.

The covariation between specific and nonspecific EDR lability can be interpreted without recourse to the concept of orienting response habituation: The data indicate that the two forms of lability share common variance and may therefore be controlled by a common mechanism. Or, to put the matter somewhat differently, the term EDR lability can be used to describe both the common variance between frequency measures of specific and nonspecific EDR activity and, by inference, their common psychophysiological mechanism (Carr et al., 1985; Crider and Lunn, 1971).

The observed correlation between specific and nonspecific EDR lability appears to be limited by the marginally adequate reliabilities of the individual measures. A number of studies have explicitly examined the test-retest stability of nonspecific EDR frequency for periods ranging from one week to several months (Baugher, 1975; Bohlin, 1973a; Corah & Stern, 1963; Crider & Lunn, 1971; Dykman et al., 1963; Hustmeyer & Burdick, 1965; Johnson, 1963; Schell et al., 1988; Siddle & Herron, 1976; Vossel & Zimmer, 1988). The eleven reported reliabilities in these ten studies ranged from .42 to .82, with a median of .61. Several studies have also assessed the test-retest stability of specific EDR frequency to iterated stimuli for a similar range of retest intervals (Bernstein, 1967; Crider & Augenbraun, 1975; Crider & Lunn, 1971; Iacono et al., 1984; Rachman, 1960; Schell et al., 1988; Siddle & Herron, 1976; Vossel & Zimmer, 1988). These eight studies reported nine reliability coefficients varying from .47 to .75, with a median of .58. Very similar findings were reported by Frexia i Baqué (1982) in an earlier review.

The temporal stability of specific and nonspecific EDR lability within the context of iterated stimulus procedures is somewhat lower than usually demanded of individual difference measures. This attenuated reliability may be in part due to substantial measurement error. One likely source of error is the restricted sampling of EDR lability in iterated stimulus procedures, which typically allow for only brief observations of both specific and nonspecific lability. Repeated assessments (e.g., Bull & Gale, 1973; Crider & Lunn, 1971) or the selection of extreme groups (O'Gorman, 1977) may be useful strategies for reducing measurement error. A procedure described by Wilson and Graham (1989) that combines both specific and nonspecific EDR frequency counts to identify labiles and stabiles also warrants further investigation.

It may also be possible to develop qualitatively different assessment procedures. Subjects tend to maintain their EDR lability rankings from resting conditions to conditions of task engagement (Bohlin, 1973a; Lacey & Lacey, 1958; O'Gorman & Horneman, 1979). This cross-situational consistency suggests the possibility of identifying assessment settings and procedures correlated with, yet more reliable than, measures derived from the iterated stimulus paradigm.

To summarize, EDR lability can be conceptualized as a psychophysiological trait indexed by frequency counts of either specific or nonspecific phasic activity. Increased attention to the requirements of measurement reliability would ostensibly increase the measured covariation of these two indices, as well as increase the validity of EDR lability with other individual difference measures.

## PERSONALITY CORRELATES

A relationship between EDR lability and personality dispositions would seem implausible. As O'Gorman (1983) pointed out, positive results require finding an association between widely disparate observational domains. EDR lability reflects the output of palmar sweat gland effectors in a laboratory setting, while personality dispositions summarize a range of behaviors, beliefs, and attitudes across disparate settings. The implausibility of such a relationship is supported by largely unsuccessful attempts to find correlations between lability indices and the personality factors of neuroticism on the one hand and extraversion on the other. The relevant literature has been thoroughly reviewed by O'Gorman (1977, 1983) in the context of research on individual differences in EDR habituation.

The search for a neuroticism-lability covariation can be justified under the hypothesis that EDR lability reflects individual differences in trait anxiety. O'Gorman (1977) cited a dozen studies that correlated a measure of neuroticism with specific EDR lability to an iterated stimulus. The studies were approximately evenly divided between those reporting significant and those reporting null findings. Of those studies reporting significant findings, some found a positive relationship and others a negative relationship between lability and neuroticism. Rappaport and Katkin (1972) produced evidence to support a lability-neuroticism relationship under threatening conditions, but this finding has not been confirmed (Kilpatrick, 1972; Kimmel and Bevill, 1985). In brief, a relationship between EDR lability and neuroticism is highly unlikely.

The search for an EDR lability-extraversion relationship is justified by an argument linking lability to the concept of arousal and thence to Eysenck's (1967) hypothesis of a negative relationship between extraversion and characteristic levels of arousal. O'Gorman's (1977) review included a dozen studies employing a measure of specific EDR lability and a measure of extraversion. The studies were fairly evenly divided between those finding and those failing to find a significant negative relationship between the two measures, although no study reported a positive relationship. This state of affairs continued to hold when several more studies were subsequently reviewed (O'Gorman, 1983). Both O'Gorman (1977) and Stelmack (1981) offered a variety of criticisms of those studies reporting null findings, most notably the use of low intensity stimuli in the assessment of specific lability. Nevertheless, the accumulated findings suggest a weak inverse relationship between EDR lability and extraversion. Unfortunately, it is not clear from the studies reported to date whether this relationship can be attributed either to the impulsivity or to the sociability component of broadly defined extraversion (Crider, 1979).

The rather meagre yield from studies attempting to relate EDR lability to neuroticism or extraversion has undoubtedly led to skepticism regarding the existence of any lability-personality correlates. Yet negative findings also operate to direct attention to alternative formulations. As a first-order approximation to such a reformulation, we will examine several studies that suggest a relationship between EDR lability and the personality factor of agreeableness-antagonism.

## Agreeableness-Antagonism and EDR Lability

Agreeableness-antagonism forms part of the emerging five-factor model of personality that also includes neuroticism, extraversion, conscientiousness, and openness to experience (Digman, 1990; McCrae & Costa, 1987; Norman, 1963). McCrae and Costa (1987) described antagonistic individuals as having a defective sense of attachment to others, shown by mistrustful and skeptical attitudes, callous and unsympathetic sentiments, and uncooperative, stubborn, and rude behavior. The agreeable pole of this dimension includes trusting, cooperative, and affiliative behavior. Agreeableness-antagonism is conceptually similar to Eysenck's psychoticism factor (Eysenck & Eysenck, 1975), although the latter appears to be a higher order factor that combines both agreeableness-antagonism and conscientiousness (Digman, 1990; McCrae & Costa, 1985).

Early indications of a relationship between EDR lability and agreeableness-antagonism appeared in studies by Jones (1950; 1960) and Block (1957). Both of these studies antedate contemporary conceptions of EDR lability and the convention of employing iterated stimulus paradigms for assessment purposes. Nevertheless, their results are not inconsistent with findings derived from iterated stimulus paradigms, as reported by Crider & Lunn (1971) and Raine and Venables (1984).

Jones' (1950; 1960) results are remarkable for having been derived from multiple observations of behavior and electrodermal activity over several years. As part of a longitudinal study of adolescents, Jones assessed electrodermal reactivity to a word association test in 100 mixed gender school children. Each child was tested eleven times during the six-year longitudinal period. Jones' reports do not detail his methods or measurement procedures. However, Jones appears to have identified extreme groups of 20 "high reactive" and 20 "low reactive" subjects in terms of the average amplitude of specific EDRs accompanying the word associations over the eleven assessments. In iterated stimulus procedures, average EDR amplitude is known to be correlated with the frequency of specific EDRs (Martin & Rust, 1976; Schell et al., 1988). Jones may therefore have employed an electrodermal measure correlated with EDR lability. The two groups were then compared on behavior ratings made by trained observers over the same six year period. The high reactive subjects were described as cooperative, deliberative, good-natured, and calm, while the low reactive subjects were described as irresponsible, impulsive, irritable, and excitable. In addition, Jones found the low reactive children to be more attention-seeking, talkative, animated, and assertive than the high reactives. The foregoing descriptors are very similar to items defining the antagonism-agreeableness factor reported by McCrae & Costa (1987).

Block (1957) undertook a conceptual replication of the Jones study, using 70 male medical school applicants as subjects. The subjects were tested in a pseudo lie-detection situation in which the examiner attempted to determine the subject's choice of specific digits, months, and colors. The subjects were instructed to respond with a simple "no" to all questions posed. Block identified extreme groups of 20 "reactors" and 20 "nonreactors" primarily on the basis of the number of EDRs emitted during the test without regard to specific or nonspecific form. The two groups were then examined for trait differences arising from an independently conducted California Q-Sort evaluation. The nonreactors were evaluated as relatively more hostile, autonomous, critical, and rebellious. The reactors were seen as more affiliative, submissive, ethical, and easily threatened. The characteristics of the nonreactors provide a good fit with antagonism items identified in a factor analysis of the California Q-Sort by

McCrae et al. (1986), although the traits of the reactors are less obviously related to Q-Sort items defining the agreeable pole.

More recent studies by Crider & Lunn (1971) and Raine & Venables (1984) assessed EDR lability in iterated stimulus paradigms and reported psychometric evidence consistent with the Jones and Block findings. In the Crider and Lunn (1971) study, specific and nonspecific EDR lability were assessed over two sessions of iterated auditory stimulation in a sample of 22 male undergraduates. The two lability measures were correlated with MMPI and CPI scales selected to reflect the traits described by Jones and Block. Both lability measures were positively correlated with the CPI responsibility and self-control scales and inversely correlated with the MMPI psychopathic deviate and hypomania scales. Elevations on these two MMPI scales is generally taken to indicate a poorly socialized, impulsive disposition indicative of psychopathy.

The subjects of the Raine and Venables (1984) study were 101 15-year-old males randomly selected from three schools. The subjects were assessed on specific EDR lability to iterated tones and on both a self-report measure and a teacher rating of antisocial behavior. The self report measure was specially constructed from a factor analysis of tests of antisociality, while the teacher rating employed the unsocialized-psychopathic scale of Quay and Parsons (1970). The principal finding was that both the self report measure and the teacher rating were negatively correlated with specific EDR lability. In an interesting follow-up study (Raine, Venables, & Williams, 1990), the original subjects were assessed ten years later for criminal status. A search of criminal records showed that 17 of the original sample had committed an average of 7.3 serious offenses. In the original testing, the mean nonspecific lability score of the 17 criminals-to-be was significantly lower than that of their noncriminal peers.

The hypothesis suggested by the foregoing studies is that individual differences in EDR lability are correlated with the broad personality factor of agreeableness-antagonism. In these studies labile subjects tend to be described as friendly, socialized, responsible, and controlled, whereas stabile subjects tend to be described as hostile, unsocialized, irresponsible, and impulsive.

The antagonistic pole of agreeableness-antagonism would appear to define conventional descriptions of psychopathy (McCrae & Costa, 1987). Curiously, the relationship between psychopathic status and EDR lability is at best tenuous. For example, Lippert & Senter (1966) found lower nonspecific lability in adolescent psychopaths than in controls during a recovery period following threat of punishment but not during the threat period or the preceding rest period. Schalling et al. (1973) found lower nonspecific lability during auditory stimulation and recovery in a group of antisocial male offenders relative to more socialized offenders but no differences during the preceding rest period. Siddle et al. (1973) were unable to distinguish socialized from unsocialized institutionalized adolescents in terms of either specific or nonspecific lability. These data suggest that high antagonism individuals are not necessarily EDR stabiles and that further differentiation of the agreeableness-antagonism factor is required for a more precise prediction of EDR lability differences.

## Schizoid Antagonism and EDR Lability

In their 1984 paper, Raine and Venables showed that although antisociality was negatively related to EDR lability, only a portion of their antisocial subjects were extreme EDR stabiles.  Raine and Venables adduced evidence suggesting that a "schizoid" subgroup of their antisocial subjects was particularly likely to be electrodermally unresponsive.  Somewhat earlier, Schalling (1978) made a similar distinction between "impulsive" and "detached" subtypes of antisocial personalities.  The impulsive subtype was described as thrill-seeking, aimless, indifferent to the future, and unable to profit from experience.  The second group, also referred to as "schizoid" by Schalling, was described as showing defective attachments, low empathy, lack of concern for others, poverty of affect, and suspiciousness.

The foregoing considerations suggest that EDR stability characterizes a schizoid subgroup of antagonistic individuals.  This extended hypothesis of the personality correlates of EDR lability is compatible with the presence of EDR anomalies in schizophrenia.  It is generally agreed that a large proportion of schizophrenic patients are EDR stabiles in that they are unresponsive to orienting stimuli. (e.g., Bernstein et al., 1982; Dawson et al., 1992).  Öhman et al. (1989) have further observed that EDR stability in the form of nonresponding is particularly characteristic of schizophrenic patients with a history of poor premorbid functioning.  Poor premorbid functioning is in turn characterized by antagonistic behavior patterns.  That is to say, developmental studies of schizophrenia have shown that behaviors such as hostility, mistrust, and alienation are markers of poor premorbidity (Parnas et al., 1982; Ricks & Berry, 1970; Watt & Lubensky, 1976).  In sum, schizophrenic patients who can also be described as antagonistic are particularly prone to EDR stability.

The schizoid trait or traits postulated by this extended hypothesis may be equivalent to or correlated with anhedonia as measured by the Chapman et al. (1976; 1982) physical anhedonia scale.  Designed as a measure of proneness to schizophrenia, the scale assesses impaired ability to experience pleasure in everyday experiences.  An inverse relationship between anhedonia and EDR lability was first demonstrated by Simons (1981), who found that a mixed gender sample of undergraduate students with elevated physical anhedonia scores showed less specific and nonspecific EDR lability than control subjects in an iterated stimulus procedure.  This finding was substantiated for specific EDR lability by Bernstein and Riedel (1987) in a similar sample of male and female students.  Similar results were reported by Raine (1987) for a sample of incarcerated criminals, although the measure of anhedonia was not strictly comparable.

A study by Blackburn (1979) provides some support for the hypothesis of EDR stability among schizoid antagonists.  Blackburn assessed both specific and nonspecific EDR lability in "primary" and "secondary" male psychopaths drawn from a population of incarcerated criminals.  Both groups showed the expected elevations on the MMPI psychopathic deviate and hypomania scales.  The group of so-called secondary psychopaths also showed elevations on the MMPI schizophrenia and depression scales.  The elevated depression is of special interest in light of the affinity of depression with anhedonia.  This group therefore resembled schizoid antagonists.  In an iterated stimulus procedure, the secondary psychopaths showed lower levels of both specific and nonspecific lability than the comparison group of primary psychopaths.

To recapitulate, the work of Schalling (1978) suggests that the personality factor of antagonism can be differentiated into impulsive and schizoid components.  Research and theory further suggest that the subgroup of schizoid antagonists is particularly prone to EDR stability.  This schizoid factor may be tentatively aligned with individual differences measured by the Chapman et al. (1976; 1982) physical anhedonia scale.  The extended hypothesis of EDR lability therefore holds that individuals who are both antagonistic and anhedonic are likely to be EDR stabiles and that agreeable, hedonic individuals are likely to be EDR labiles.

## EDR LABILITY AND AROUSAL

If EDR lability is in fact related to specific personality dispositions, a proper interpretation of this covariation requires a specification of the psychological process or processes underlying individual differences in lability. At least three types of evidence suggest that EDR lability reflects individual differences in characteristic levels of arousal along a sleep-wakefulness continuum.

One type of evidence is based on a consideration of task performance differences between EDR labiles and stabiles. Figure 2 presents an idealized but heuristically useful summary of labile-stabile performance differences. It follows Humphreys & Revelle (1984) in distinguishing between sustained information transfer (SIT) tasks and short-term memory (STM) tasks. SIT tasks require the subject to process a stimulus, associate an arbitrary response to it, and rapidly execute the response. Effective performance requires the ability to sustain attention to the stimulus field for lengthy periods. Examples of SIT tasks include reaction time, vigilance, and letter cancellation. In contrast, STM tasks require the subject to maintain information in a readily available state or to retrieve information that has not been attended to for a short period of time. Effective performance on such tasks requires good selective attention and ability to resist distraction. According to the Humphreys & Revelle (1984) formulation, high arousal facilitates performance on SIT tasks but impairs performance on STM tasks. That is, arousal energizes simple responses to discrete stimuli but interferes with information in short-term store.

| Performance Requirement | EDR Lability Group: Labile | EDR Lability Group: Stabile |
|---|---|---|
| Sustained Information Transfer (SIT) | Good | Poor |
| Short Term Memory (STM) | Poor | Good |

**Figure 2.** Heuristic illustration of the interaction of EDR lability with performance on SIT versus STM tasks.

There is good evidence that EDR labiles are superior to EDR stabiles on SIT tasks. For example, labiles are superior to stabiles on vigilance tasks that require the detection of infrequent signals over an extended monitoring period. Of seven studies reporting correct detection (hit) data, four found labiles to be superior to stabiles over the entire monitoring period (Coles & Gale, 1971; Crider & Augenbraun, 1975; Parasuraman, 1975; Vossel & Rossmann, 1984), and three found the labile superiority to emerge in the latter stages of the vigil (Hastrup, 1979; Siddle, 1972; Sostek, 1978). The relatively poor detection performance of stabiles may be due either to lessened perceptual sensitivity, greater reporting caution, or both (Munro et al., 1987). Those of the foregoing studies that have addressed these alternatives are not in agreement, and the matter remains unresolved. It is likely that the processes responsible for the labile-stabile detection difference will vary with the particular demands of different monitoring tasks (Parasuraman, 1979).

In addition, labiles show faster reaction time than stabiles over an extended trial series. This finding was originally reported by Lacey and Lacey (1958) using a rather complex apparatus to assess "motor impulsivity", and subsequent attempts to replicate were not uniformly successful (Doctor et al., 1964; Williams et al., 1965). However, more recent studies using either simple or choice reaction time procedures with signalled foreperiods report a labile superiority over varying foreperiod lengths (Kopp et al., 1987; Wilson, 1987; Wilson & Graham, 1989; Vossel, 1988).

The findings are less certain with regard to STM tasks, but some evidence supports superior EDR stabile performance in such situations. Thus Hustmyer & Karnes (1964) found that stabiles were better able than labiles to extract a simple figure from a more complex design in Witkin's Embedded Figures test, which presumably requires an STM component. Block (1957) found the same effect with the Rod and Frame test, which shares variance with the Embedded Figures test. An important study by O'Gorman and Lloyd (1988) found a stabile superiority in a dichotic listening procedure with an STM component. On each of 40 trials, three word pairs were presented to subjects through earphones. One word in each pair was presented to the right ear and the second was presented simultaneously to the left ear. At the end of each trial, subjects were asked to recall as many as possible of the six words. Stabiles recalled approximately 50 percent more of the words than did labiles. Finally, Zimmer et al. (1990) found stabiles to be superior to labiles in recognizing whether a complex visual probe was similar or not to one of two memory items presented ten seconds previously.

In sum, there appear to be arousal-dependent performance differences between labiles and stabiles. Labiles are clearly superior in situations calling for sustained attention to the external field and rapid response execution, but they may be relatively impaired on tasks requiring a short-term memory component and freedom from distraction.

A second type of evidence for the EDR lability-arousal hypothesis includes the lability enhancing effects of stimulant drugs and the lability damping effects of sedatives. For example, Lader (1969) reported a dose-response curve relating amphetamine and caffeine ingestion to nonspecific EDR lability. Similar results for high but not low doses of amphetamine were reported by Zahn et al. (1981) for both specific and nonspecific EDR lability. In contrast, sedative drugs reduce lability. The early work of Lader (1964) with barbiturates is well known, and subsequent work with benzodiazepines has produced similar results (Frith et al., 1984). Marcy et al (1985) have developed an animal model of benzodiazepine effects on specific EDR lability in mice. They reported a correlation between the receptor binding potency of eight benzodiazepines and the dose required to reduce specific lability by 50 percent.

Finally, several studies of EEG correlates of EDR lability suggest that stabiles are less alert than labiles (Bohlin, 1973a; Kaiser & Roessler, 1968; McDonald et al., 1964; Siddle & Smith, 1974). The most persuasive are the Bohlin and the Siddle and Smith studies. In both studies subjects were asked to sit quietly with eyes closed for approximately 30 minutes while being exposed either to an iterated tone or to no stimulation. Bohlin divided her subjects into high, medium, and low nonspecific lability groups and measured time to sleep onset by the disappearance of alpha waves from the EEG record for 60 seconds. The extreme labile group maintained alertness longer than the extreme stabile group in both conditions; the middling group fell between the extremes. Siddle and Smith divided subjects into labile and stabile groups in terms of specific EDR lability to an iterated stimulus. In both conditions, labile subjects showed no change in alpha output during the vigil, but stabiles showed a relatively rapid alpha decline in the direction of sleep onset.

In brief, evidence from different domains converges on the conclusion that EDR lability differences are a concomitant of an underlying arousal or sleep-wakefulness continuum, which interacts with the attentional demands of different types of tasks to produce differential performance effects.

## SUMMARY

The concept of EDR lability rests on the robust covariation between frequency measures of specific and nonspecific electrodermal responding, as most often observed in iterated stimulus procedures. EDR lability can be taken to describe the common variance of these two measures or, by inference, their common psychophysiological mechanism. The reliability of specific and nonspecific EDR lability measures typically found in iterated stimulus procedures is only marginally adequate for individual difference studies. Greater attention to the requirements of measurement reliability should pay dividends in the form of replicable findings with external criteria.

The psychophysiological mechanism of individual differences in EDR lability is, most likely, characteristic differences in level of arousal conceived of as a sleep-wakefulness continuum. Although the concept of arousal is often criticized as lacking empirical specificity, it nevertheless provides a unified explanation for the performance and EEG correlates of individual differences in EDR lability, as well as for the differential effects of stimulant and sedative drugs on lability. In particular, differential arousal explains the apparent interaction of EDR lability with sustained information transfer versus short-term memory tasks, as specified by the Humphreys-Revelle (1984) formulation.

The search for personality correlates of EDR lability has not been conspicuously successful. Nevertheless, the emerging five-factor model of personality provides an opportunity for rethinking past failures. Evidence stretching over many years suggests that EDR lability is correlated with individual differences in agreeableness-antagonism. An extended hypothesis suggests that anhedonic, or schizoid, antagonists are particularly likely to be EDR stabiles, whereas agreeable, hedonic individuals are likely to be EDR labiles. An obvious implication is that these contrasting personality types will also manifest performance and psychophysiological evidence of differential arousal. We have arrived at a promising juncture for further exploration of the relationships among EDR lability, personality, and performance.

## REFERENCES

Baugher, D. M., 1975, An examination of the nonspecific skin resistance response, *Bulletin of the Psychonomic Society*, 6:254.

Bernstein, A. S., 1967, The orienting reflex as a research tool in the study of psychotic populations, *in:* "Mechanisms of Orienting Reaction in Man," I. Ruttkay-Nedecky, L. Ciganek, V. Zikmund, and E. Kellerova, eds., Slovak Academy of Sciences, Bratislava.

Bernstein, A. S., Frith, C. D., Gruzelier, J. H., Patterson, T., Straube, E., Venables, P. H., and Zahn, T. P., 1982, An analysis of the skin conductance orienting response in samples of Americans, British, and German schizophrenics, *Biological Psychology*, 14:155.

Bernstein, A. S., and Riedel, J. A., 1987, Psychophysiological response patterns in college students with high physical anhedonia: Scores appear to reflect schizotypy rather than depression, *Biological Psychiatry*, 22:829.

Blackburn, R., 1979, Coritcal and autonomic arousal in primary and secondary psychopaths, *Psychophysiology*, 16:143.

Block, J., 1957, A study of affective responsiveness in a lie-detection situation, *Journal of Abnormal Social Psychology*, 55:11.

Bohlin, G., 1973a, Interaction of arousal and habituation in the development of sleep during monotonous stimulation, *Biological Psychology*, 1:99.

Bohlin, G., 1973b, The relationship between arousal level and habituation of the orienting reaction, *Physiological Psychology*, 1:308.

Bull, R. H. C., and Gale, M. A., 1973, The reliability of and interrelationships between various measures of electrodermal activity, *Journal of Experimental Research in Personality*, 6:300.

Carr, V., Minniti, R. and Pilowsky, I., 1985, Electrodermal activity in patients with chronic pain: Implications for the specificity of physiological indices in relation to psychopathology, *Psychophysiology*, 22:208.

Chapman, L. J., Chapman, J. P., and Miller E. N., 1982, Reliabilities and intercorrelations of eight measure of proneness to psychosis, *Journal of Consulting and Clinical Psychology*, 50:187.

Chapman, L. J., Chapman, J. P. and Raulin, M. L., 1976, Scales for physical and social anhedonia, *Journal of Abnormal Psychology*, 85:374.

Coles, M. G. H. and Gale, A., 1971, Physiological reactivity as a predictor of performance in a vigilance task, *Psychophysiology*, 8:594.

Corah, N. L. and Stern, J. A., 1963, Stability and adaptation of some measures of electrodermal activity in children, *Journal of Experimental Psychology*, 65:80.

Crider, A., 1979, The electrodermal response: biofeedback and individual difference studies, *International Review of Applied Psychology*, 28:37.

Crider, A. and Augenbraun, C. B., 1975, Auditory vigilance correlates of electrodermal response habituation speed, *Psychophysiology*, 12:36.

Crider, A. and Lunn, R., 1971, Electrodermal lability as a personality dimension, *Journal of Experimental Research in Personality*, 5:145.

Dawson, M. E., and Nuechterlein, K. H., 1984, Psychophysiological dysfuntions in the developmental course of schizophrenic disorders, *Schizophrenia Bulletin*, 10:204.

Dawson, M. E., Nuechterlein, K. H., and Schell, A. M., 1992, Electrodermal anomalies in recent-onset schizophrenia: Relationships to symptoms and prognosis, *Schizophrenia Bulletin*, 18:295.

Digman, J. M., 1990, Personality structure: Emergence of the five-factor model, *Annual Review of Psychology*, 41:417.

Doctor, R. F., Kaswan, J. W., and Nakamura, C. Y., 1964, Spontaneous heart rate and GSR changes as related to motor performance, *Psychophysiology*, 1:73.

Dykman, R. A., Ackerman, P. T., Galbrecht, C. R., and Reese, W. G., 1963, Physiological reactivity to different stressors and methods of evaluation, *Psychosomatic Medicine*, 25:37.

Edman, G., Asberg, M., Levander, S. and Schalling, D., 1986, Skin conductance habituation and cerebrospinal fluid 5-hdroxyindoleacetic acid in suicidal patients, *Archives of General Psychiatry*, 43:586.

Eysenck, H. J., 1967, "The Biological Basis of Personality", C. C. Thomas, Springfield, Illinois.

Eysenck, H. J., and Eysenck, S. B. G., 1975, "Manual of the Eysenck Personality Questionnaire," EdITS, San Diego, CA.

Frexia i Baqué, E., 1982, Reliability of electrodermal measures: A compilation, *Biological Psychology*, 14:219.

Frith, C. D., Stevens, M., Johnstone, E. C., and Owens, D. G., 1984, The effects of chronic treatment with amitriptyline and diazepam on electrodermal activity in neurotic outpatients, *Physiological Psychology*, 12:247.

Hastrup, J. L., 1979, Effects of electrodermal lability and introversion on vigilance decrement, *Psychophysiology*, 16:302.

Humphreys, M. S., and Revelle, W., 1984, Personality, motivation and performance: A theory of the relationship between individual differences and information processing, *Psychological Review*, 91:153.

Hustmyer, F. E. and Burdick, J. A., 1965, Consistency and test-retest reliability of spontaneous autonomic nervous system activity and eye movements, *Perceptual and Motor Skills*, 20:1225.

Hustmyer, F. E. and Karnes, E., 1964, Background autonomic activity and "analytic perception", *Journal of Abnormal and Social Psychology*, 68:467.

Iacono, W. G., Lykken, D. T., Haroian, K. P., Peloquin, L. J., Valentine, R. H., and Tuason, V. B., 1984, Electrodermal activity in euthymic patients with affective disorders: One-year retest stability and the effects of stimulus intensity and significance, *Journal of Abnormal Psychology*, 93:304.

Johnson, L. C., 1963, Some attributes of spontaneous electrodermal activity, *Journal of Comparative and Physiological Psychology*, 56:415.

Jones, H. E., 1950, The study of patterns of emotional expression, *in:* "Feelings and Emotions," M. L. Reymert, ed., McGraw-Hill, New York.

Jones, H. E., 1960, The longitudinal method in the study of personality, *in:* "Personality Development in Children," R. Iscoe and H. Stevenson, eds., University of Chicago Press, Chicago.

Kaiser, C. and Roessler, R., 1968, Stability and habituation of nonspecific GSRs, *Perceptual and Motor Skills*, 27:495.

Kilpatrick, D. G., 1972, Differential responsiveness of two electrodermal indices to psychological stress and performance of a complex cognitive task, *Psychophysiology*, 9:218.

Kimmel, H. D., and Bevill, M., 1985, Habituation and dishabituation of the human orienting reflex under instruction-induced stress, *Physiological Psychology*, 13:92.

Kopp, M. S., Katalin, M., Emese, L., and Bitter I., 1987, Electrodermally differentiated subgroups of anxiety patients. I. Automatic and vigilance characteristics, *International Journal of Psychophysiology*, 5:43.

Lacey, J. I., and Lacey, B. C., 1958, The relationship of resting autonomic activity to motor impulsivity, *Research Publications of the Association for Research in Nervous and Mental Disease*, 36:144.

Lader, M. H., 1964, The effect of cyclobarbitone on the habituation of the psycho-galvanic reflex, *Brain*, 87:321.

Lader, M. H., 1969, Comparison of amphetamine sulphate and caffeine citrate in man, *Psychopharmacologia*, 14:83.

Lippert, W. W., and Senter, R. J., 1966, Electrodermal responses in the sociopath, *Psychonomic Science*, 4:25.

Marcy, R., Quermonne, M., Raoul, J., Nammathao, B., and Smida, A., 1985, Skin conductance reaction (SCR)-habituation test, a tool to detect anxiolytic activity. Its justification by the correlation between SCR-habituation test activities and specific binding potencies in benzodiazepines, *Progress in Neuro-Psychopharmacology and Biological Psychiatry*, 9:387.

Martin, I. and Rust, J., 1976, Habituation and the structure of the electrodermal system, *Psychophysiology*, 13:554.

McCrae, R. R. and Costa, P. T., 1985, Comparison of EPI and psychoticism scales with measures of the five-factor model of personality, *Personality and Individual Differences*, 6:587.

McCrae, R. R. and Costa, P. T., 1987, Validation of the five-factor model of personality across instruments and observers, *Journal of Personality and Social Psychology*, 52:81.

McCrae, R. R., Costa, P. T., and Busch, C. M., 1986, Evaluating comprehensiveness in personality systems: The California Q-set and the five factor model, *Journal of Personality*, 54:2.

McDonald, D. G., Johnson, L. C. and Hord, D. J., 1964, Habituation of the orienting response in alert and drowsy subjects, *Psychophysiology*, 1:163.

Mundy-Castle, A. C., and McKiever, B. L., 1953, The psychophysiological significance of the galvanic skin response, *Journal of Experimental Psychology*, 46:15.

Munro, L. L., Dawson, M. E., Schell, A. M., and Sakai, L. M., 1987, Electrodermal lability and rapid vigilance decrement in a degraded stimulus continuous performance task, *Journal of Psychophysiology*, 1:249.

Norman, W. T., 1963, Toward and adequate taxonomy of personality attributes: Replicated factor structure in peer nomination personality ratings, *Journal of Abnormal and Social Psychology*, 66:574.

O'Gorman, J. G., 1977, Individual differences in habituation of human physiological responses: A review of theory, method, and findings in the study of personality correlates in non-clinical populations, *Biological Psychology*, 5:257.

O'Gorman, J. G., 1983, Individual differences in the orienting response, *in*: "Orienting and Habituation: Perspectives in Human Research", D. Siddle, ed., John Wiley, Chichester.

O'Gorman, J. G. and Horneman, C., 1979, Consistency of individual differences in non-specific electrodermal activity, *Biological Psychology*, 9:13.

O'Gorman, J. G. and Lloyd, J. E. M., 1988, Electrodermal lability and dichotic listening, *Psychophysiology*, 25:538.

Öhman, A., Öhlund, L. S., Alm, T., Wieselgren, I-M., Ost, L-G., and Lindstrom, L. H., 1989, Electrodermal nonresponding, premorbid adjustment, and symptomatology as predictors of long-term social functioning in schizophrenics, *Journal of Abnormal Psychology*, 98:426.

Parasuraman, R., 1975, Response bias and physiological reactivity, *Journal of Psychology*, 91:309.

Parasuraman, R., 1979, Memory load and event rate control sensitivity decrements in sustained attention, *Science*, 205:924.

Parnas, J., Schulsinger, F., Schulsinger, H., Mednick, S. A., and Teasdale, T. W., 1982, Behavioral precursors of schizophrenia spectrum, *Archives of General Psychiatry*, 39:658.

Quay, H., & Parsons, L. B, 1970, "The Differential Classification of the Juvenile Offender," Bureau of Prisons, Washington.

Rachman, S., 1960, Reliability of galvanic skin response measures, *Psychological Reports*, 6:326.

Raine, A., 1987, Effect of early environment on electrodermal and cognitive correlates of schizotypy and psychopathy in criminals, *International Journal of Psychophysiology*, 4:277.

Raine, A. and Venables, P. H., 1984, Electrodermal nonresponding, antisocial behavior, and schizoid tendencies in adolescents, *Psychophysiology*, 21:424.

Raine, A., Venables, P. H., and Williams, M., 1990, Relationships between central and autonomic measures of arousal at age 15 years and criminality at age 24 years, *Archives of General Psychiatry*, 47:1003.

Rappaport, H., and Katkin, E. S., 1972, Relationships among manifest anxiety, response to stress, and the perception of autonomic activity, *Journal of Consulting and Clinical Psychology*, 38:219.

Ricks, D. F., and Berry, J. C., 1970, Family and symptom patterns that precede schizophrenia, *in*: "Life History Research in Psychopathology (Vol 1.)", M. Roff and D. F. Ricks, eds., University of Minnesota Press, Minneapolis.

Rubens, R., and Lapidus, L., 1978, Schizophrenic patterns of arousal and stimulus barrier functioning, *Journal of Abnormal Psychology*, 87:199.

Schalling, D., Lidberg, L., Levander, S. E., and Dahlin, Y., 1973, Spontaneous autonomic activity as related to psychopathy, *Biological Psychology*, 1:83.

Schalling, D., 1978, Psychopathy-related personality variables and the psychophysiology of socialization, *in*: "Psychopathic Behaviour: Approaches to Research," R.D. Hare and D. Schalling, eds., John Wiley & Sons, Chichester.

Schell, A. M., Dawson, M. E. and Filion D. L., 1988, Psychophysiological correlates of electrodermal lability, *Psychophysiology*, 25:619.

Siddle, D. A. T., 1972, Vigilance decrement and speed of habituation of the GSR component of the orienting response, *British Journal of Psychology*, 63:191.

Siddle, D. A. T. and Heron, P. A., 1976, Reliability of electrodermal habituation measures under two conditions of stimulus intensity, *Journal of Research in Personality*, 10:195.

Siddle, D. A. T., Nicol, A. R., and Foggitt, R. H., 1973, Habituation and over-extinction of the GSR component of the orienting response in anti-social adolescents, *British Journal of Social and Clinical Psychology*, 12:303.

Siddle, D. A. T. and Smith, D. G., 1974, Effects of monotonous stimulation on cortical alertness in fast and slow habituation groups, *Journal of Research in Personality*, 8:324.

Siddle, D. A. T., Stephenson, D., and Spinks, J. A., 1983, Elicitation and habituation of the orienting response, *in:* "Orienting and Habituation: Perspectives in Human Research," D. Siddle, ed., John Wiley, Chichester.

Simons, R. F., 1981, Electrodermal and cardiac orienting in psychometrically defined high-risk subjects, *Psychiatry Research*, 4:347.

Sostek, A. J., 1978, Effect of electrodermal lability and payoff instructions on vigilance performance, *Psychophysiology*, 15:561.

Stelmack, R. M., 1981, The psychophysiology of extraversion and neuroticism, *in:* "A Model for Personality," H. J. Eysenck, ed., Springer-Verlag, Berlin.

Vossel G., 1988, Electrodermal lability, errors, and reaction times: an examination of the motor impulsivity hypothesis, *International Journal of Psychophysiology*, 6:15.

Vossel, G. and Rossman, R., 1984, Electrodermal habituation speed and visual monitoring performance, *Psychophysiology*, 21:97.

Vossel, G. and Zimmer, H., 1988, Scoring criteria for electrodermal habituation: Further research, *Psychophysiology*, 25:712.

Watt, N. F. and Lubensky, A. W., 1976, Childhood roots of schizophrenia, *Journal of Consulting and Clinical Psychology*, 44:363.

Williams, T. A., Schacter, J., and Rowe, R., 1965, Spontaneous autonomic activity, anxiety, and "hyperkinetic impulsivity": A psychophysiologic study of 46 college males, *Psychosomatic Medicine*, 27:9.

Wilson, K. G., 1987, Electrodermal lability and simple reaction time, *Biological Psychology*, 24:275.

Wilson, K. G. and Graham, R. S., 1989, Electrodermal lability and visual information processing, *Psychophysiology*, 26:321.

Zahn, T. P., Rapoport, J. L., and Thompson, C. L., 1981, Autonomic effects of dextroamphetamine in normal men: Implications for hyperactivity and schizophrenia, *Psychiatry Research*, 4:39.

Zimmer H., Vossel, G., and Frölich, D., 1990, Individual differences in resting heart rate and spontaneous electrodermal activity as predictors of attentional processes: effects on anticipatory heart rate deceleration and task performance, *International Journal of Psychophysiology*, 8:249.

# ELECTRODERMAL INDICES AS MARKERS FOR THE DEVELOPMENT OF SCHIZOPHRENIA

Peter H. Venables

Department of Psychology
University of York
Heslington, York, YO1 5DD, UK

## INTRODUCTION

Work on the psychophysiology of schizophrenia has extended from the stage at which studies were mainly carried out on schizophrenic patients so that it now encompasses a more widely ranging approach. Research now takes place in five areas: (1) on adult patients in the morbid state, (2) on adult patients in remission or recovery, (3) on children at risk for psychiatric breakdown, where in most studies risk has been defined as due to familial factors, (4) on normal relatives of schizophrenic patients, (5) on normal subjects with schizotypic characteristics, who for that reason may be considered to be at greater than normal risk for schizophrenia. This chapter will be particularly concerned with areas (3) and (5).

The use of the term marker in the title of this chapter deserves some discussion. It is convenient here to use the system outlined by Iacono (1985), which defines three types of marker: (1) Episode or state markers which are present only in patients in a state of exacerbation of their symptoms, (2) Vulnerability markers which identify those **prone** to psychosis and (3) Genetic markers, which are vulnerability markers for which there is evidence that the marker is a heritable trait. In this chapter, the concern is clearly with the second and third categories.

Electrodermal measurement in the investigation of schizophrenia may have a practical, clinical aim. It may be concerned with the identification of those who are likely to develop schizophrenia in the same way as one might use any behavioural test or clinical assessment. Valuable as this may be, it does not, in the main, lead to an understanding of the processes which are involved in the development of the disorder, an understanding which may lead eventually to a more fully rational clinical approach.

It must be acknowledged, of course, that the use of electrodermal measurement is only one, relatively small, part of the armamentarium which is available to the investigator of the mechanisms of schizophrenia. A general case is made for the use of relatively simple measures such as those of electrodermal and cardiovascular activity in Venables (Venables, 1991) in contrast to the more currently fashionable methods such as CT, MRI

*Progress in Electrodermal Research,* Edited by
J.-C. Roy *et al.* Plenum Press, New York, 1993

and PET scans on the grounds of non-invasiveness, low cost and ability to deal readily with the effects of single stimuli. However, a *prima facie* case may also be made to suggest that the use of electrodermal measurement may be more than just the use of a conveniently measured index. For illustrative purposes, this case may be approached in two ways, the first would be that it is acknowledged that some functions of the limbic system and frontal lobes may be reflected in electrodermal activity (EDA), (see, for example with the work of Pribram and his colleagues (Bagshaw, Kimble, & Pribram, (1965) Kimble, Bagshaw, & Pribram, (1965) and also the chapters by Raine, Roy and Sequeira-Martinho in this volume) and that disturbances of the function of the limbic system and the frontal lobes are probably involved in schizophrenia; e.g. (Seidman, 1983). Secondly, work on EDA in schizophrenia, has somewhat uniquely provided evidence of a heterogeneity among schizophrenic patients that is not immediately evident by other methods (Bernstein, Frith, Gruzelier, Patterson, Straube, Venables, et al., 1982; Gruzelier & Venables, 1972; Öhman, 1981). The evidence suggests that there are two classes of schizophrenic patients, one which does not show electrodermal responses to stimuli of intensity which would invoke an orienting response in normal subjects and the other which some evidence would suggest show electrodermal hyperactivity while other evidence would indicate at least normal orienting. These two cases for the value of EDA measurement in research on schizophrenia are not, by any means the only ones that may be cited, nor are they independent. They do, however, provide material which gives some indication of the important position which work in this field has held in the study of schizophrenia.

## EPIDEMIOLOGICAL CONCERNS IN "HIGH RISK FOR SCHIZOPHRENIA" STUDIES

This chapter is not primarily concerned with work on schizophrenic **patients** but rather with work on the **development** of schizophrenia. The start of work in this area where electrodermal activity was measured, can be traced very directly to the Copenhagen High-Risk study initiated by Mednick and Schulsinger in 1962 (Mednick, 1967; Mednick & Schulsinger, 1968). In Mednick and Schulsinger's study risk was defined on a familial basis. The theoretical origin of this sort of study is probably the paper by Pearson and Kley (1957), where it was advocated that investigators should pay attention to the expectation of breakdown with disorder among the population they were studying which was dependent on the base rate for that disorder in the population. Thus the low base rate of 1% lifetime risk for schizophrenia in the general population would mean that a very large population would have to be studied in a longitudinal project to achieve a workable sample of patients by the end of the study. In the Copenhagen study this base rate problem was tackled by the selection of an experimental group of children, mean age 15 years, selected on the basis that they had mothers who were schizophrenic, thus having an estimated 15% chance of developing schizophrenia, as against the 1% chance in the general population. A control group did not have any psychiatric disorder amongst their families. However, it should be noted, that the selection of the control group in such studies is not free of problems. In this instance, because the groups were matched on a number of variables including intactness of family, some of the control group came from broken homes, the reason for which later turned out to be that they contained a larger than normal number of parents who were criminal. Studies such as that by Loeb and Mednick (1977), showed that electrodermal indices, measured at age 15, particularly **long** SCR recovery, distinguished those who later became delinquent from a control group who did not. (Whereas, see below, it was reported that children of schizophrenic parents and those later to become schizophrenic exhibited **short** SCR recoveries) Thus, the control group, because of the inclusion of a subgroup that had particular electrodermal characteristics, might not provide the unbiased comparison group for the experimental group that was hoped for. When the Copenhagen study was started in 1962, the question of the existence of a spectrum of schizophrenic characteristics extending into the general population had not obtained general currency. However, in the same year, Meehl (1962), had put forward a theory, which has spawned a great deal of subsequent work, that schizophrenia could be considered to be the pathological end of a continuum which extended to normality through various degrees of "schizotypy". The underlying pathology, "schizotaxia", interacting with benign or malign social or environmental circumstances would result in, respectively, schizotypy or schizophrenia. This view, now more readily accepted than in 1962, advocating a dimensional rather than a categorical view of schizophrenia, leads to the idea that any normal control group will contain a number of subjects with schizotypic characteristics and if these have some of the same electrodermal characteristics as the "experimental" group, group differences will be attenuated. Given the acceptance of a dimensional account, it is logically not possible to draw a hard and fast line between pathology and abnormality, however accepting the view that what makes a patient a patient, is behaviour unacceptable to the person him/herself and those around him, it is possible to still identify those who may be called schizophrenic, on the basis of standard criteria (e.g. DSM-III) while another group, while not exhibiting the full schizophrenic disorder may be called borderline (a term which later became the paradigm for the DSM-III term "Schizotypal Personality Disorder", (SPD)). Using data from the 1962 Copenhagen study, it may be possible to estimate what is the base rate for those in the population who while not being amongst the 1% who manifest the full schizophrenic syndrome, nevertheless exhibit sufficient abnormality of behaviour for them to be thought of as "different" from normal. In a 10 year follow up of the subjects of the 1962 Copenhagen study, Schulsinger (1976), reported that while 55 of 173 (32%) children of schizophrenic mothers had a diagnosis of "borderline state", 4 out of 91 children of "normal" mothers were so diagnosed, a rate of 6%. This 6% rate is higher than the general expectation for schizophrenia and furthermore is based on a population that had not run the full risk period for the disorder. Another study by Baron and Risch (1987), indicates that DSM-III, SPD is on a genetic-environmental etiological continuum with schizophrenia and that the rate for SPD is 5.75 times greater than broadly defined schizophrenia, a figure very close to that estimated from Schulsinger's (1976) figures.

If the idea of markers for vulnerability to schizophrenia is to be extended so that includes the category of **genetic** markers then it is important that evidence is available on the heritability of EDA measures. Zahn, (1977) reviews the data available at that time and also provides some results from a twin study from his laboratory. Those components of SC in an orienting stimulation paradigm showing a significant genetic contribution were SCL, numbers of spontaneous SCRs, numbers of orienting responses and half recovery **rate**. There was no genetic contribution to SCR latency, rise time or amplitude. Bell, Mednick, Gottesman, and Sergeant (1977) report results from a twin study using orienting and conditioning paradigms. A significant genetic contribution is found for half recovery time in the orienting an part of the conditioning phase in data from the left but not the right hand. In the case of SCR amplitude in the orienting session, the genetic contribution approaches significance. These data are to be compared to those from a twin study by Kotchoubei (1987), examining responses to 80 and 105 dB tones which shows an important role for genetic factors in the determination of latency and amplitude of responses to both tone intensities, and also a significant contribution to habituation of responses. In summary, although the data are not entirely consistent there is sufficient evidence to suggest some genetic contribution to those measures which are to be of importance in the studies which are reviewed in later sections. (See also the chapter by Iacono and Ficken in this volume for more extensive data on this point)

# ELECTRODERMAL MEASUREMENT IN "HIGH-RISK" STUDIES

Five studies are reviewed in this section. The first, the Copenhagen study, has been used as a model for all those which follow it, with the possible exception of the Israeli study, and even this seeks to try to replicate the Copenhagen findings. It is probably a consequence of the time at which the studies were started that none take the point of view that schizophrenia itself may be a heterogeneous diagnosis, and none initially sought to relate the measurement of electrodermal activity to the central mechanisms which, related to electrodermal activity, might be shown to be dysfunctional in schizophrenia. To that extent, the studies which follow up the Copenhagen study may be thought to be disappointing. Work on the Copenhagen study has subsequently, however, made use of other developments in work on schizophrenia to extend the usefulness of the electrodermal measurements made at the start of the study.

## Copenhagen High-Risk Study

The use of electrodermal measurement in the Copenhagen high risk study, was not, at the time that it was started, concerned with the physiological state of the organism indexed by EDA, but rather, EDA was used as a measure of "arousal". As outlined in the report of a conference held in 1960, (Mednick, 1960), the work which was eventually started in Copenhagen was initially proposed as a project to be started in the Detroit area and was explicitly designed to test a model of the aetiology of schizophrenia which was proposed by Mednick in 1958,(Mednick, 1958). The theory of how an acute episode of schizophrenia might develop was based on three propositions; that an individual so disposed might show (1) low threshold for arousal, (2) **slow** recovery from arousal and (3) high generalization responsiveness. As measures of arousal level Mednick cited "GSR's EMG's Blood pressure, heart rate, I/E ratio etc", (Mednick, 1960),p89. These variables, (with the exception of blood pressure) were recorded in the 1962 Copenhagen study as levels and responses to stimuli in a classical conditioning paradigm (Mednick, 1967),p190, however, little has been published on the results of this data collection with the exception of the work on GSR (EDA). Thus at this point the collection of EDA data in this major high-risk study was based on a psychological theoretical position, with arousal as its central tenet, at a time when the concept of arousal was probably less under fire than it is to-day. The other crucial point to be noted was that Mednick's theory contained the notion of slow recovery from arousal, leading him to be one of the first investigators, in the field of psychopathology, to use skin conductance recovery as a measure. (As so often, in this field, acknowledgement of prior use of the variable must be given to Darrow, who described it in 1932, (Darrow, 1932) and concluded in 1937, (Darrow, 1937) that it was exponential in form. It is Edelberg, (Edelberg, 1970) however, who published the initial authoritative work, which lead to a major interest in the recovery limb of the skin conductance response (SCR).) Subsequently, several authors e.g (Ax & Bamford, 1970; Biswas, 1991; Gruzelier & Venables, 1972; Gruzelier & Venables, 1973; Zahn, Carpenter, & McGlashan, 1981) have reported faster SC recovery in schizophrenic patients, although Maricq & Edeleberg, (1975) , in contrast provided data showing longer recovery in schizophrenics.

Mednick and Schulsinger used an electrodermal conditioning paradigm in their work, specifically in order to test Mednick's 1958 theory of schizophrenic development. The outline of the paradigm used is presented in Table 1. Of particular relevance, the short CS-UCS interval is to be noted. With such a small CS-UCS interval there was no possibility of distinguishing the three types of responses in a conditioning paradigm, such as those later employed ( e.g. Prokasy and Kumpfer (1973)), in consequence, only single response data are reported for each trial, which in reinforced trials is effectively the response to the intense UCS.

The data reported in 1967 (Mednick, 1967), concern, *inter alia,* the comparison of the electrodermal responses of high-risk and low risk subjects who were of mean age 15 years at the time of testing. That any significant results were found is perhaps initially surprising, bearing in mind the low expectation of pathology in the high risk group. If only abnormality of EDA were to be expected in those subjects who were eventually to become schizophrenic, then we might expect that 15% of the high-risk as against 1% of the low-risk group might show that abnormality, an expectation that would hardly be likely to produce significant differences in response variables. However, if we take the point of view outlined above that perhaps a further 32% of the high risk group might exhibit some sort of schizotypic electrodermal characteristics and 6% of the control group might show such characteristics, then the proportions of subjects possibly showing electrodermal abnormality might be 47% in the high risk group as against 7% in the low risk group, giving a much greater likelihood of finding significant group differences. (This expectation, of course, depends on the possibility that schizotypic subjects show the same types of electrodermal characteristics as those shown by schizophrenics. Relevant data on this point will be reviewed below.)

The results of the initial (1967) analysis of the data from the Copenhagen High-Risk Study which concentrated on the latency, amplitude and recovery of SCRs were

TABLE 1
Stimulation paradigms used in
high-risk for schizophrenia studies

| Study | Habit-uation | CS | CS/USInt | UCS | General-ization |
|-------|----------|----|----------|-----|------------|
| Mednick & Schulsinger | 8 trials 1000 Hz 54dB | 14 trials 1000Hz 54dB | 0.5 sec | 9 pairings noise 96dB | 9 trials 3 of 1000Hz 3 of 1311Hz 3 of 1967Hz |
| Van Dyke et al | 8 trials 1000 Hz 54dB | 14 trials 1000Hz 54dB | 0.5 secs | 9 pairings noise 96dB | 9 trials 3 of 1000Hz 3 of 1311Hz 3 of 1967Hz |
| Erlenmeyer-Kimling (Note. One type of paradigm as example) | 8 trials 1000 Hz 8 trials 500 Hz 50 dB | 12 CS+ paired 6 CS+ unpaired 1000Hz 50dB | 5.0 secs | noise 96dB | 6 trials 2 of 1000Hz 2 of 1311Hz 2 of 1967Hz |
| Salzman & Klein | 20 trials 1000 Hz 75 dB | 20 trials 1000Hz 75dB | 8.0 secs | 14 pairs white noise 95dB | 10 trials 4 of 1000Hz 3 of 1300Hz 3 of 2000Hz |
| Kugelmass, Marcus & Schmueli | 10 trials 1000Hz 70dB followed by 1 trial 2000Hz and 3 trials 1000Hz. Finally, 1 trial 90dB loud rasping noise | | | | |

summarized by Mednick as follows: "The high risk subject then takes shape as an individual quick to react with vigorous autonomic responses....This very rapid, highly vigorous responding is balanced by an equally labile rate of recovery from autonomic imbalance. The quick recovery may explain why avoidant associates are so firmly and easily learnt by schizophrenics." However, examination of the data presented, while showing that there is fairly adequate support for the view that high risk subjects produce SCRs with faster latencies and larger amplitudes than low risk subjects, does not provide material which very strongly leads to the view that the SCR half recovery is faster in high risk than low risk subjects. The largest significant difference in recoveries between high and low risk subjects is, in fact shown, not in the regular stimulation series, but to the response where the headphones are placed on the subject. The emphasis on fast recovery in potentially pathological subjects is perhaps made because the findings of this first analysis tend to go against the proposals of Mednick's 1958 theory and this early rebuttal demanded a change in his theoretical position. What the finding does, however leave us with is the position that those subjects who may become schizophrenic, or schizoptypic, (possibly about half the sample, see above), would tend to be electrodermally hyper-responsive. The other point to be noted is that there is no indication from the data reported of non-responsivity or hypo-responsivity in this sample in spite of the fact that it was later to be shown, (Bernstein et al., 1982; Gruzelier & Venables, 1972; Öhman, 1981) that some 40% of adult schizophrenics tend to be non-responders.

In a second report, Mednick & Schulsinger (1968) provided data on the electrodermal characteristics of three groups from the 1962 project. These were (1) the members of the high risk group who had become psychiatrically ill; the sick group (2) the members of the high risk group who remained well; the well group and (3) the control group. This report is thus unique in the field in that it relates EDA measurements taken in the pre-morbid phase to actual psychiatric breakdowns. The sick group was distinguished from the well and control groups by SCRs with shorter latencies, higher amplitudes and greater recovery **rates** of SCRs to the UCS, a loud raucous noise. It was reported (p287) "The measure (recovery rate) separates the groups better than any other in our test battery." Unfortunately, as Edelberg (1970) has shown recovery **rate** is highly correlated with amplitude and is thus not an independent measure as half recovery time would be. This point is discussed at greater length in Venables (1974). The fact that recovery rate is not independent of amplitude should not, of course, be a reason for dismissing it as an empirically useful measure, however, it might be better if amplitude and recovery **time** were treated as independent measures which were combined, as for instance in multiple regression, in which case the contribution of each could be assessed.

Mednick addressed the need to revise his earlier (1958) theory in which it was proposed that schizophrenics should show a longer than normal recovery from arousal in light of the findings suggesting a **shorter** SCR recovery in those to become schizophrenic in Mednick & Schulsinger, (1968) (p288) and also in greater depth in Mednick, (1974) Briefly, Mednick's revised theory suggested that some of the aspects of schizophrenic behaviour exemplify learnt avoidance and this learnt avoidance is reinforced by fear reduction. "The faster and greater the reduction of fear, the greater the reinforcement value. The rate at which this fear is reduced depends in large part on the rate at which the autonomic nervous system recovers from a fear state to a normal level" (Mednick, 1974) p137.

The difficulty which arises, and which is addressed by Venables (1974), is concerned with the extent to which the phasic recovery of the SCR is an analogue of the recovery from fear or arousal which is the essence of the Mednick theory. Although the eccrine sweat glands are sympathetically innervated and the extent of activation of this innervation may be reflected by the latency and amplitude of the SCR, the speed and extent of the return of the response to baseline is not clearly related to the extent of decline in sympathetic activity. It is not immediately evident that the amplitude of response is maintained over time by continuing sympathetic innervation. What Mednick's theory would appear to be referring to is a maintenance of **tonic** arousal, whereas what may be measured by the time of recovery of the SCR is a mixture of diminution of tonic arousal and other local effects. (see Chapter by Edelberg, this volume) It is possible that very short recovery times may reflect only phasic effects whereas in the case of long recovery it is impossible to distinguish what might be long phasic recovery from maintenance of tonic arousal.

The emphasis given to the recovery of the skin conductance response in the Copenhagen study has been because it exemplifies a particular stage of work in the high risk field and shows up the difficulties of extrapolation from one level of analysis to another. The lack of later studies to support Mednick and Schulsingers' findings with regard to the theoretical centrality of the recovery of the SCR (see Table 3) has meant that SCR recovery has, in this field, become of less importance.

### The Copenhagen Adoptee Study

A study conducted in the same laboratory and with **exactly** the same techniques as the Mednick and Schulsinger high-risk study and which should have produced supportive data is that of Van Dyke, Rosenthal, & Rasmussen (1974). The subjects in this study were the adopted-away offspring of schizophrenic parents taken from the same sample as the well-known "adoptee" study of Rosenthal, Wender, Kety, Schulsinger, Welner, & Östergaard (1968). The control subjects were also adoptees but there was no record of psychiatric illness among their biological parents. The subjects of this study were of mean age 33 years at the time of testing. In contrast to the Mednick and Schulsinger study, in which there were no subjects exhibiting diagnosable mental illness at the time of testing at age 15, 23.4% of the index subjects and 4.4% of the control subjects were exhibiting one of the serious types of schizophrenia spectrum disorders when tested. There were no differences in latency, recovery, or frequency of non-specific responses between the two groups although the index group did produce significantly larger responses than the control group, the index subjects also responded more frequently.

Thus, although using exactly the same techniques as the Mednick and Schulsinger study, Van Dyke et al did not replicate the findings of the earlier study as far as the temporal EDA variables of latency and recovery time were concerned. Mednick (1978) suggested an explanation for this discrepancy. By obtaining access to data on the samples used he was able to show that the level of criminality among the index cases was higher than among the controls, and as SCR amplitudes have been shown to be smaller and SCR recoveries to be **longer** than normal in criminal subjects (see, for instance, review by Venables (1987), Mednick suggested that the hyper-responsivity to be expected in the index subjects was "diluted" by the opposite tendency, due their apparent greater level of criminality.

### The New York High-Risk Study

Another study which aimed, in general, to replicate the procedures of the Copenhagen study was that of Erlenmeyer-Kimling and her colleagues in New York, (Erlenmeyer-Kimling, Marcuse, Cornblatt, Friedman, Rainer, & Rutschmann, 1984). The stimulus procedure, while having major similarities to that of Mednick and Schulsinger, did have some notable differences (see Table 1). In particular, it is important to note the longer CS-UCS interval used, which could enable more than a single response to be scored. Nevertheless, the data reported refer to the response to the loud noise UCS and thus may be compared to the data reported by Mednick and Schulsinger. Data are available from Sample A of the project, which consisted of 205 subjects tested between the ages of

7 and 12 years. The high risk group consisted of children of schizophrenic parents. However, in contrast to the Copenhagen group which were all children of schizophrenic mothers, in some instances these were children of schizophrenic fathers and there was also an exceptionally high risk sub-group consisting of children of **two** schizophrenic parents. There were two control groups, one of normal parents and one of children of one or more parents psychiatrically hospitalised with diagnoses other than schizophrenia. In contrast to the Copenhagen study, high-risk subjects had significantly **longer** response latencies and non significantly **longer** recovery times than controls while the amplitude of their SCRs was the same. A sub-analysis was carried out on the same data to compare it with the data from Copenhagen by taking the children of schizophrenic fathers and mothers separately. In the case of children of schizophrenic mothers the mean recovery times to the UCS stimuli were shorter in the high risk than the control subjects, in line with the Copenhagen data, although this difference was not significant. However in the case of children of schizophrenic fathers the SCR recovery times were non-significantly **longer**. Mednick (1978) suggested that the difference between the findings of the New York and Copenhagen studies was that in the case of the Copenhagen study a larger number of the subjects were from non-intact homes, while in the New York study most were from intact homes. Mednick showed that there were few differences in electrodermal parameters distinguishing high- from low-risk groups, in the intact home children in the Copenhagen study and that it was high-risk children from non intact homes who showed faster latencies, higher amplitudes and faster recovery rates. Erlenmeyer-Kimling and colleagues (Erlenmeyer-Kimling, Friedman, Cornblatt, & Jacobsen, 1985) tested this proposition on their data. However, even with sex taken into account children living away from the parental home had **longer** SCR recoveries than those living at home, the opposite direction to that found in the Copenhagen study. In summary, the findings of the New York study do not appear to be in accord with those from Copenhagen and for that reason Erlemeyer-Kimling(Erlenmeyer-Kimling, 1987) dismisses electrodermal activity from a list of possible markers for schizophrenia.

There are however, other possible differences between the two studies which need

TABLE 2
Electrodermal measurement techniques used in
high-risk for schizophrenia studies

| Author | Electrode | Electrolyte | Placement | Hand | Rest period |
|---|---|---|---|---|---|
| Mednick & Schulsinger | Zn | ZnSO₄ Liquid on sponge | nk | nk | 15min |
| Van Dyke et al | Zn | ZnSO₄ Liquid on sponge | nk | nk | 15min |
| Erlenmeyer-Kimling | Beckman | Beckman paste | mid & index | L | 10min |
| Salzman & Klein | Beckman miniature | Unibase 0.5% KCl | mid & index | L | 10min |
| Venables | Beckman miniature | Agar-agar 0.5% KCl | mid & index | L | 5 min |

to be taken into account. The first is age, the mean age of testing of the New York group was 9.5 years while that of the Copenhagen group was 15.1 years. The second is the manner in which the tests were carried out. In the Copenhagen situation the subjects were rushed from test to test with little time for reassurance or acclimatization. In contrast, in the New York study the children were familiarised with the testing situation before assessment started. Finally, the details of the electrodermal measurement techniques were quite different in the two studies. Table 2 shows the details of the procedures used. In particular, it should be noted that the Copenhagen study used a non-biological electrolyte type and probably hydrated the skin surface maximally by the use of a wet sponge electrode/skin interface applied 15 minutes before stimulation. On the other hand, in the New York study Beckman electrode paste was used, which is a saturated electrolyte. It can be said that neither of these techniques would be considered optimal. Nevertheless it needs to be noted that it is not necessarily the measurement technique that is responsible for the difference between the New York and Copenhagen studies insofar as the Van Dyke study which used the same lab and techniques as the Mednick and Schulsinger study produced different results.

## The University of Rochester Child and Family Study

A third study, aiming to build on the Copenhagen study, is the University of Rochester Child and Family study. Details of the electrodermal procedures and findings are given in two papers, (Prentky, Salzman, & Klein, 1981; Salzman & Klein, 1978). In the introduction to the study it is stated "a decision was made to try and replicate as closely as possible, except where methodological improvements could be introduced, the experimental design and measurement strategies employed by Mednick". In the Salzman and Klein paper results from 42 ten year old children are reported. Of these, 12 were designated as high risk, while 30 were of low risk (for schizophrenia) status, insofar as they had parents with diagnosis of affective disorder, neurosis or personality disorder. The stimulation paradigm used is summarized in Table 1. During the habituation phase no differences were found between low and high risk groups in response magnitude, latency or numbers of spontaneous responses. However, analysis of responses to the UCS showed that initially high risk children showed larger responses than low risk children, although this difference disappeared later in the trial sequence. There were no other significant differences in response amplitude in the first and second response intervals, the measurement of these responses being made possible by the use of the longer CS-UCS interval in this study as compared to that of Mednick. No differences in latency or recovery time were found for the responses to the UCS. Later results are reported in the Prentky et al. paper. In this, analyses are based on the data from 99 children; 42 seven year olds and 57 ten year olds. In the case of the control group a division was made into two sub-groups, children of non-psychotics and children of affective psychotics. The methods used were the same as those shown under Salzman and Klein in Table 1. In the habituation phase no differences between groups were found for magnitude of SCR or numbers of spontaneous responses, nor were there any differences in numbers of trials to habituation. In the case of responses to the UCS the high risk group produced larger responses than the other two control groups taken together. There was no significant difference in recovery times between the groups.

## The Israeli High-Risk Study

Finally, data are available from the Israeli high risk study(Nagler & Mirsky, 1985) on the electrodermal reactivity to auditory stimuli in a habituation and dishabituation paradigm (Kugelmass, Marcus, & Schmueli, 1985). This, apparently, is the only high risk for schizophrenia study in which electrodermal techniques are employed, which does not emulate the paradigm originally used by Mednick and Schulsinger. The reports do not include details of recording methods except that a 20μA constant current was used. The sample consists of 100 subjects, nearly equally divided by sex. Fifty children were at high risk by reason of having a schizophrenic parent, the 50 control children had parents with no psychiatric diagnosis. The sample was further divided equally into those born on a Kibbutz and raised in a Kibbutz children's home, and those born in a town and raised in the usual family setting. The age range of the subjects when they were first studied was between 8 and 15 years with a mean of 11.3 and 11.4 years for boys and girls respectively. The one significant difference between index and control subjects is in recovery rate. In these data the index children had **longer** recovery times than the control children, a finding opposite to that of Mednick and Schulsinger. There are some few significant interactions between risk status and living type (Kibbutz v town). These show that the Kibbutz high-risk children exhibited fewer spontaneous fluctuations and longer latencies that the other sub-groups. On the whole, therefore, although weakly, the data tend to suggest hypo- rather than hyper- responsivity in the risk group.

## Summary

Table 3 attempts to summarize the results of the studies which have been reviewed. All the studies with the exception of the Israeli project, use an electrodermal conditioning paradigm and consequently results are reported which may be compared. This is because all studies effectively report responses to an intense stimulus, the UCS. There is a general tendency for high-risk subjects to show larger amplitude responses than low-risk subjects, although when temporal SCR variables are considered, the only general tendency which can be noted is that in all studies which follow the Copenhagen study, results are reported which are not in line with the Copenhagen findings.
With the exception of the Copenhagen study, there appears to have been little attempt to make further use of the electrodermal data gathered as part of the initial phases of the

TABLE 3
Summary of EDA findings of high-risk for schizophrenia
studies. (Response to UCS)
(DATA SHOW DIRECTION OF HIGH RISK GROUP)

| Study | Lev. | Lat. | Amp. | Rec. | Spont. |
|-------|------|------|------|------|--------|
| Copenhagen High-Risk | (nk) | shorter | larger | shorter | (nk) |
| Copenhagen Adoptee | (ns) | (ns) | larger | (ns) | (ns) |
| New York | (nk) | longer | (ns) | longer (ns) | (nk) |
| Rochester | inc less over trials | (ns) | larger | (ns) | (ns) |
| Israeli | (ns) | (ns) | (ns) | longer | (ns) |

studies. However, that such an exercise might be valuable is indicated by work subsequently carried out on the Copenhagen data.

### The Copenhagen High-Risk Study, a reprise

Although the original reports of the Copenhagen study (Mednick, 1967; Mednick & Schulsinger, 1968) made no mention of electrodermal non-responsivity among the population tested, later reports establish the existence of some subjects who were hypo- or non-responders (Cannon, Fuhrmann, Mednick, Machon, Parnas, & Schulsinger, 1988; Cannon & Mednick, 1990). The 1988 report showed that subjects with CT scans showing enlarged third ventricles had significant overall reductions in electrodermal responsiveness to orienting, conditioned and generalization stimuli. It should be noticed, in the context of the data presented in Table 3 that responses to the UCS were not significantly related to ventricle size. In the 1990 paper it was found possible to define 20.5% of the original high risk sample as electrodermal non-responders. When responder/non-responder status was related to large or small ventricle size, a very significant association showed that the non-responders were to be found in the large third ventricle group. Furthermore, those who were non-responders, who also suffered severe birth delivery problems and because of their high-risk status were at genetic risk, were patients who exhibited largely negative symptoms.

The importance of these findings lies not only in their intrinsic interest, but also in showing the value of continuing to use the early electrodermal data even after other studies, because of non-replication, have tended to dismiss the value of electrodermal measurement in the high-risk field. Also to be noted, is the need to take into account a variety of variables, other than simply those of EDA, in multivariate analyses of the total database before a useful outcome is produced.

In passing, it should also be noted that Cannon's finding of reduced responsiveness in those subjects with enlarged ventricles was not replicated by Schnur, Bernstein, Mukherjee, Loh, Degreef, & Reidel, (1989) who showed that, among their subjects, it was the responders rather than the non-responders who exhibited enlarged ventricles. Schnur et al. point out that the difference between the two studies may lie in the fact that in their study all the subjects were schizophrenic while in the Danish sample only nine of the 34 subjects involved were so diagnosed at the time.

A further complication is that Raine (see Chapter, this volume) and Raine, Reynolds, & Sheard (1991), using MRI techniques has shown that, in normal subjects, extent of SC orienting was related to left and right prefrontal area, are of the pons, and left but not right temporal/amygdala area. However, third ventricle size was **not** related to extent of SC orienting. The latter finding may, however, be a function of the orientation of the MRI cut used in measurement.

## ELECTRODERMAL ACTIVITY IN SCHIZOTYPIC SUBJECTS

Earlier, in the section on epidemiological concerns, the point was raised about the inclusion of schizotypic subjects in both high- and low- risk groups and the extent to which their electrodermal characteristics might bias results of high-risk studies. Nielsen & Petersen (1976) were the first to publish work in this field. They constructed a "schizophrenism" scale measuring characteristics derived from those described by Chapman (1966) as being typical of early schizophrenia. "Schizophrenism" may be considered to measure those aspects of schizotypy which are analogous to "positive symptom" schizophrenia (see Venables, Wilkins, Mitchell, Raine, & Bailes (1990) for a review of the area). Neilsen and Petersen also measured neuroticism, extraversion, fearfulness and anxiety. The subjects for the study were female psychology students age

19-25 years. Their measures of EDA included SCL, SCR amp, SCR recovery rate, numbers of responses and habituation. The stimulation paradigm included an orientation section with 60dB white noise and 70 Db 200 Hz pure tones which were to be used as CS+ and CS-, followed by a conditioning phase in which CS+ stimuli were followed **immediately** by a 105dB white noise.. This was followed by a test of conditioning period in which the CS+ and CS- were presented without reinforcement. There was thus some similarity with the paradigm used by Mednick and Schulsinger. The important results, as far as the present paper is concerned, are that schizophrenism was positively related to SCR amp and SCR recovery rate in the orientation condition but not to SCR amplitude or recovery as far as responses to the UCS were concerned.

The next study by Simons (1981) also used undergraduate students as subjects, whose mean age was 20 years. The Chapman scales of Physical anhedonia and Perceptual aberration (Chapman, Chapman, & Raulin, 1976; Chapman, Chapman, & Raulin, 1978) were use to define an Anhedonic, a Perceptual aberration and a control group. The first group might be considered to have parallels to patients with negative symptom schizophrenia while the second, like Neilsen and Petersens' with subject characteristics measured by "schizophrenism", might be thought to be analogous to patients with positive symptoms. An orienting stimulus paradigm was used, 15, 1000Hz 75dB pure tones being presented to the subjects. Findings showed that while there were no differences in SCR amplitude between controls and subjects with Perceptual aberration, the anhedonics displayed hyporesponsivness during early trials. Only SCR amplitude and no other SCR components were measured.

The final study to be reviewed is that by Bernstein & Riedel (1987). In this, the same scales as those used by Simons were used to identify groups of subjects drawn from a college population. The mean age of the subjects was 23 years. The stimulus paradigm employed was that of an initial orienting session, followed by one in which the tones used during orientation were given significance by requiring a foot press to some of the tones. Stimuli were either 1000 or 2000Hz at 60 or 58dB. As with the Simons study, Anhedonics showed smaller SCR amplitudes than controls during the orientation trials while aberrant subjects did not differ from controls. During the "significant" later trials the subjects' responses did not differ. Because Bernstein, Riedel, Graae, Seidman, Steele, Connolly & Lubowsky (1988) have shown that depressives tend to show "non-normalizing" responses to significant stimuli, while schizophrenics "normalize", the implication is that the pattern of results shown by the anhedonics is consistent with the group showing characteristics which are an attenuated form of schizophrenia rather than being allied to depression.

In considering the data from these three studies, the first point to note is that all use acceptable EDA measurement technology, in contrast to the variety of techniques used in the high-risk studies reviewed earlier (see Table 2). Secondly, the significant findings are derived from responses to orienting stimuli rather than more intense stimuli which would elicit defensive responses which was where, if any, results were found in the high-risk studies. Thirdly, only SCR amplitudes and habituation findings are reported in the Simons and Bernstein et al studies so that it is only in the Neilsen and Petersen study that the finding of short SCR response recovery is related to positive schizophrenic tendency, and that only to orienting stimuli.

The reason for reviewing these three studies is to gain some impression of the characteristics of schizotypic subjects who might be included in control or index groups in high risk studies. What is clearly the case is that there will be heterogeneity among these subjects and the balance which they contribute to the index or control high-risk groups will depend on the make up of the schizotypic population included. If the balance is towards the "positive" characteristic end as it is with the "schizophrenism" data of Neilsen and Petersen, then these subjects will add hyper-responsivity, with large amplitudes and short recovery, to the group characteristics. On the other hand, if the subjects are characterized by "negative" tendencies such as anhedonia, then the balance will tend toward hypo-responsivity.

## THE MAURITIUS HIGH-RISK STUDY

The Mauritius study which began in 1972, differed from those high-risk studies which preceded it in that risk for schizophrenia was to be assessed, not on the basis of familial factors, but rather on the basis of putative autonomic markers. The island of Mauritius has a population of just less than 1 million, and on an expectation of risk for schizophrenia of 1% in the general population, some 10,000 persons might be likely to develop schizophrenia at some time during their lives. (It should be noted that Murphy & Raman (1971), showed that although the incidence of schizophrenia in Mauritius is the same as in Western society, the chronicity of the disease is less.) There is only one mental hospital on the island with about 200 beds and consequently the expectation is that most schizophrenics might be found in the community. As a community survey was not possible, it was decided to start the study by testing a total population of three year old children in two towns on the island whose ethnic mix was representative of the total population. Data on 1795 children was obtained in one year of testing. Data collection has been continued to the present day, but the report in this chapter will concentrate on the relation between electrodermal data collected at age 3 and measurement of schizotypal characteristics at age 16/17 years. A clinical follow-up has since been conducted but has found too few schizophrenics to make a statistically satisfactory report possible at this stage.

The Mauritius study was originally to be seen as an extension of the Copenhagen study, described in the last section. As it was initiated by Mednick, Schulsinger and Venables in 1972 on the basis of the then available findings from Copenhagen it was expected that electrodermal **hyper**-responsivity would be an indication of risk status. However, as Gruzelier & Venables (1972) had just shown that among a population of schizophrenic patients almost half were non-responders, it was also thought that electrodermal non-responsivity would be a risk factor.

The electrodermal measurement technique was standard, employing a constant voltage system, Beckman miniature electrodes and 0.5% KCl electrolyte in an agar-agar base. Responses were identified as specific if they fell in a latency window of 1.0-3.0 sec. The minimum change in EDA scorable as a response was $.05\mu S$. Responses were recorded from the left hand although initial, pre-stimulus SCLs were available from both hands. The stimulation paradigm used in Mauritius was an attenuated version of that used in Copenhagen. It is described in detail in (Venables, 1978; Venables, Mednick, Schulsinger, Raman, Bell, Dalais, et al., 1978). A standard stimulus tape presented 6 orienting stimuli, 1000Hz, 75dB, followed by 12 stimuli or stimulus pairs in an SCR conditioning paradigm with 1000Hz or 500Hz, 60dB CS+ or CS- stimuli with a 90dB unpleasant noise as UCS, a 10sec CS-UCS interval was used, in a final section 6 further stimuli were used to test for extinction. The stimulus paradigm was thus short, but this was necessitated by the need to test the population within a year. The paradigm contained the conditioning section in order to allow some continuity with the Copenhagen study, but it should be noted at this point that it has not been possible to show any signs of conditioning in the data available. The material is thus used largely as a series of orienting responses, while the responses to the UCS are used as examples of defensive responses. The initial use of the electrodermal data was to select subgroups of subjects who might be at risk for schizophrenia, and their controls, and to place half of these subgroups in nursery schools. The result of this process is described, for instance, in Venables, Dalais, Mitchell, Mednick, & Schulsinger (1983). As, however, the selection for this process was made in some haste, as the nursery schools were open and had to be filled, it was thought useful to examine the data in more detail for the purpose of more extensive analyses. Furthermore, since the original selection

TABLE 4
FACTOR ANALYSIS OF SC DATA FROM MAURITIUS STUDY

| VARIABLE | FACTOR 1 | FACTOR 2 | FACTOR 3 | MEAN |
|---|---|---|---|---|
| INITIAL SCL LEFT HAND | .89 | | | 2.67 $\mu$S |
| INITIAL SCL RIGHT HAND | .81 | | | 2.86 $\mu$S |
| No. OF SPONT FLUCTUATIONS | .45 | .31 | -.30 | 3.4 /MIN |
| MEAN MAGNITUDE OF SCORS | .41 | .70 | | .12 LN$\mu$S |
| MEAN MAGNITUDE OF SCDRS | .60 | | .44 | .25 LN$\mu$S |
| FREQUENCY OF SCORS | | .73 | | 3.96 /6 |
| FREQUENCY OF SCDRS | | | .40 | 5.96 /6 |
| MEAN LATENCY OF SCORS | | -.60 | | 1.61 SECS |
| MEAN LATENCY OF SCDRS | | -.50 | | 1.41 SECS |
| MEAN HALF-RECOVERY OF SCORS | | | .53 | 2.31 SECS |
| MEAN HALF-RECOVERY OF SCDRS | | | .69 | 4.29 SECS |
| SUGGESTED FACTOR NAME | AROUSAL | ORIENT-ATION | DEFENSE | |

process, there had been publication of the data described in the first section of this chapter, which made it evident that basing selection entirely on the Copenhagen data, as had been originally the case, might require rethinking.

The large number of subjects on whom electrodermal data was available presented a unique opportunity for analysis of inter-relationships between variables. The data available were SCL, SCR lat, SCR amp, SCR half rec, and numbers of spontaneous responses, (NSF) in the minute before stimulation began. Mean magnitude of responses to the first 6 orienting responses was calculated and as the distribution was skewed the log magnitude was employed in further analyses. Similar calculations were employed for the responses to the 6 UCSs, and the log magnitude of defensive responses was calculated. Figures for mean latencies and mean half recoveries for the available responses to orienting and defensive stimuli were calculated, these were reasonably normally distributed. The other data used were numbers of responses elicited to orienting and defensive stimuli. Factor analysis of the data were carried out. Cattell's scree test(Cattell, 1966) indicated that a three factor solution was appropriate. Table 4 shows the results. The pattern of results appears reasonably interpretable. A first factor loading on SCL, NSF, and magnitudes of Ors and Drs might be termed "arousal". The second factor which loads on magnitude, latency and numbers of SCORs could be interpreted as a factor of "orientation" except for the fact that latency of Drs loads on this factor. The third factor loads on magnitudes, recovery and numbers of DRs and could be interpreted as a factor of "defensive" response were it not for the fact that recovery to orienting responses loads on this factor. What appears to be the case from this analysis is that latency of response appears to be an orienting feature while recovery is a feature which is more allied to the intensive aspect of the stimuli eliciting the response.

Thus, it appears that these data go some way to support the standard division into responses to intense and therefore "defensive" stimuli and responses to orienting, less intense stimuli. Furthermore, insofar as this division may be useful in attempting an understanding of the high-risk studies reviewed earlier, it is useful to analyze the Mauritian data on this basis.

As outlined above, the "ultimate" validation of the use of the electrodermal data collection at age 3 by relating it to the status of diagnosed schizophrenics is not possible at this stage. However, as data on a schizotypy questionnaire were collected on 570 subjects between the ages of 16 and 17 years it is possible to relate the electrodermal data to this material. Scores on the schizotypy questionnaire are of course continuous and there is no cut off between normality and abnormality, nevertheless, as has been reviewed earlier, there is a base rate likelihood of 6% of the population being diagnosable with schizotypal personality disorder and this group will score at the high end of the schizotypy scale. The scale used was one specially produced for this study, being as short as possible consistent with reliability and as innocuous as possible as it was to be given to a general population for survey purposes. The scale contains two subscales and measures "schizophrenism", analogous to positive symptom schizophrenia, and anhedonia, which may be thought of as a component of negative symptom schizophrenia. The scale and its use and validation are described in Venables (1990) and Venables, et al. (1990)

The subjects were divided into three groups on the basis of the magnitude of their responses to orienting and defensive stimuli. In each case one group, the non-responders consisted of those who gave no responses to the 6 orienting or defensive stimuli, another group, the hyper-responders had ORs and DRs which were more than $2\sigma$ above the mean, the third group, the median responders had ORs and DRs which were within $0.5\sigma$ of the mean for the group. Thus not all of the subjects on whom data are available were used in the analysis.

The first analysis concerns the relation between schizophrenism, the positive symptom aspect of schizotypy and orienting and defensive responses. The results are shown in Figure 1. Schizophrenism is higher in both the potential risk groups, the non-responders and the hyper-responders than in the median responder group. This result is however only significant in the case of responses to the defensive stimuli ($F(2,268) =$ 3.39 p $=0.035$). By *post hoc* testing of group differences by Tukey HSD both the non- and hyper-responders have significantly ( $p< .05$) higher levels of schizophrenism than the median responders.

The next analysis looks at the relation between electrodermal activity at age 3 and anhedonia, the negative symptom aspect of schizotypy. The result is shown in Figure 2. No significant difference by response type is shown in the case of defensive responses, however, in the case of the response to the orienting stimuli the hyper-responders show significantly ($p< .05$) decreased levels of anhedonia than the other two groups.

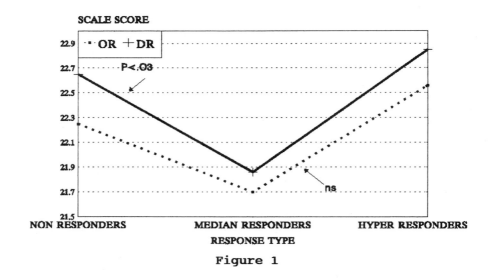

Figure 1

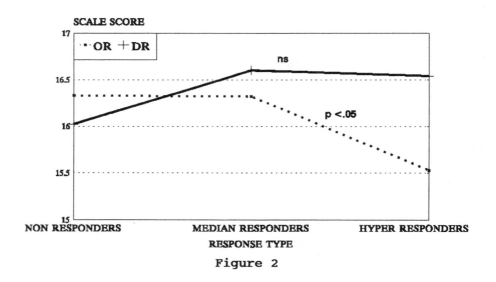

Figure 2

These results, while not at a very high level of significance, are noteworthy in that they show that electrodermal activity at age 3 is related to later schizotypal characteristics 13 years later. Later analyses, taking into account a wider range of variables, will no doubt sharpen up the findings presented here. Where the results are able to throw some light on the findings of other studies reviewed in the earlier section is that it appeared in these studies that it was responses to the UCS, called in this later section defensive responses, which were related either to high-risk status, or in the case of the Copenhagen studies were related to early breakdown with schizophrenia. This early breakdown is most likely to occur in those who manifest positive symptoms and consequently would be most likely to be those who would score highly on the schizophrenism scale. Thus the finding in the present study, that hyper-responders to intense stimuli score highly on the schizophrenism scale is in line with these earlier findings. What is, perhaps, less expected is that **non-responders** to intense stimuli also score highly on the schizophrenism scale. However, both Alm, Lindstom, Öst & Öhman (1984) and Green, Nuechterlein & Satz (1989) report the finding of positive symptomatology in schizophrenic patients who are non-responders. Less easy to relate to other findings is that scoring on the "negative symptom" anhedonia scale is not related to non-responding but rather to lower scoring on this scale is found in hyper-responders to orienting stimuli.

Thus, the data from the Mauritius study do suggest that, in spite of the variety of conflicting results reported from earlier high-risk studies, EDA may indeed be used as a vulnerability marker, (but probably in conjunction with others) for the development of later pathology. The fact that EDA activity at age 3 can be related to reflections of oncoming symptomatology at the beginning of the risk period for schizophrenia suggest that a degree of the predisposition to schizophrenia is laid down by infancy.

# REFERENCES

Alm, T., Lindström, L.H., Öst, L-G., and Öhman, A., 1984, Electrodermal non-responding in schizophrenia: Relationships to attentional, clinical,biochemical, computed tomographical and genetic factors. *International Journal of Psychophysiology* 1: 195-208.

Ax, A. F., and Bamford, J. L., 1970, The GSR recovery limb in chronic schizophrenia. *Psychophysiology* 7: 145-147.

Bagshaw, M. H., Kimble, D. P., and Pribram, K. H., 1965, The GSR of monkeys duringorientation and habituation and after ablation of the amygdala and infero-temporal cortex. *Neuropsychologia* 3: 111-119.

Baron, M., and Risch, N., 1987, The spectrum concept of schizophrenia: Evidence for agenetic-environmental continuum. *Journal of Psychiatric Research* 21: 257-267.

Bell, B., Mednick, S.A., Gottesman, I I. and Sergeant, J., 1977, Electrodermal parameters in male twins. In: *Biosocial basis of criminal behavior*, S.A. Mednick and K.O. Christiansen, Eds., (pp.217-228). New York: Gardner Press.

Bernstein, A. S., Frith, C. D., Gruzelier, J. H., Patterson, T., Straube, E., Venables, P.H., and Zahn, T. P., 1982, An analysis of skin conductance orienting response in samples of American, British and German schizophrenics. *Biological Psychology* 14: 155-211.

Bernstein, A. S., and Riedel, J. A., 1987, Psychophysiological response patterns in college students with high physical anhedonia: Scores appear to reflect schizotypy rather than depression. *Biological Psychiatry* 22: 829-847.

Bernstein, A. S., Riedel, J. A., Graae, F., Seidman, D., Steele, H., Connolly, J., and Lubowsky, J., 1988, Schizophrenia is associated with altered orienting activity; Depression with electrodermal (cholinergic?) deficit and normal orienting response. *Journal of Abnormal Psychology* 97: 3-12.

Biswas, P. K., 1991, Characteristics of galvanic skin response in schizophrenic patients and normal subjects. *Psychologia* 34: 266-271.

Cannon, T. D., Fuhrmann, M., Mednick, S. A., Machon, R. A., Parnas, J., and Schulsinger, F., 1988, Third ventricle enlargement and reduced electrodermal responsiveness. *Psychophysiology* 25: 153-156.

Cannon, T. D., Mednick, S. A. and Parnas, J., 1990, Antecedents of predominantly negative- and predominantly positive- symptom schizophrenia in a high-risk population. *Archives of General Psychiatry* 47: 622-632.

Cattell, R. B., 1966, The Scree Test for number of factors. *Multivariate Behavioral Research* 1: 245-266.

Chapman, J., 1966, The early symptoms of schizophrenia. *British Journal of Psychiatry* 112: 225-251.

Chapman, L. J., Chapman, J. P., and Raulin, M. L., 1976, Scales for physical and social anhedonia. *Journal of Abnormal Psychology* 85: 374-382.

Chapman, L. J., Chapman, J. P., and Raulin, M. L., 1978, Body-image aberration in schizophrenia. *Journal of Abnormal Psychology* 87: 399-407.

Darrow, C. W., 1932, The relation of the GSR recovery curve to reactivity, resistance level and perspiration. *Journal of General Psychology* 7: 261-272.

Darrow, C. W., 1937, The equation of the galvanic skin reflex curve: I, The dynamics of reaction in relation to excitation-background. *Journal of General Psychology* 16: 285-309.

Edelberg, R., 1970, The information content of the recovery limb of the electrodermal response. *Psychophysiology* 6: 527-539.

Erlenmeyer-Kimling, L., 1987, Biological Markers for the liability to schizophrenia. In: *Biological perspectives of schizophrenia*, H. Helmchen and F. A. Henn, Eds., (pp. 33-56). Chichester: John Wiley.

Erlenmeyer-Kimling, L., Friedman, D., Cornblatt, B., and Jacobsen, R., 1985, Electrodermal recovery data on children of schizophrenic parents. *Psychiatry Research* 14: 149-161.

Erlenmeyer-Kimling, L., Marcuse, Y., Cornblatt, B., Friedman, D., Rainer, J. D., and Rutschmann, J., 1984, The New York high-risk project. In: *Children at risk for schizophrenia*, N. F. Watt, E. J. Anthony, L. C. Wynne, and J. E. Rolf, Eds., (pp. 169-189). Cambridge: Cambridge University Press.

Green, M.F., Nuechterlein, K.H. and Satz, P., 1989, The relationship of symptomatology and medication to electrodermal activity in schizophrenia. *Psychophysiology* 26: 148-157.

Gruzelier, J. H., and Venables, P. H., 1972, Skin conductance orienting activity in a heterogenous sample of schizophrenics. *Journal of Nervous and Mental Disease* 155: 277-287.

Gruzelier, J. H., and Venables, P. H., 1973, Skin conductances responses to tones with and without attentional significance in schizophrenic and non-schizophrenic psychiatric patients. *Neuropsychologia* 11: 221-230.

Iacono, W. J., 1985, Psychophysiologic markers for psychopathology: A review. *Canadian Psychology* 26: 96-112.

Kimble, D. P., Bagshaw, M. H., and Pribram, K. H., 1965, The GSR of monkeys during orienting and habituation after selective partial ablations of the cingulate and frontal cortex. *Neuropsychologia* 3: 121-128.

Kotchubei, B.I., 1987, Human orienting reaction: The role of genetic and environmental factors in the variability of evoked potentials and autonomic components. *Acta Nervosa Superior* 29: 103-108.

Kugelmass, S., Marcus, J., and Schmueli, J., 1985, Psychophysiological reactivity in high-risk children. *Schizophrenia Bulletin* 11: 66-73.

Loeb, J., and Mednick, S. A., 1977, A prospective study of the predictors of criminality: 3. Electrodermal response patterns. In: *Biosocial basis of criminal behavior*, S. A. Mednick and K. O. Christiansen, Eds., (pp. 245-254). New York: Gardner Press.

Maricq, H. R., and Edelberg, R., 1975, Electrodermal recovery rate in a schizophrenic population. *Psychophysiology* 12: 630-641.

Mednick, S. A., 1958, A learning theory approach to research in schizophrenia. *Psychological Bulletin* 55: 316-327.

Mednick, S. A., 1960, The early and the advanced schizophrenic. In: *Current research in schizophrenia*, S. A. Mednick and J. Higgins, Eds, (pp. 69-95). University of Michigan: University of Michigan.

Mednick, S. A., 1967, The children of schizophrenics: Serious difficulties in current research methodologies which suggest the use of the "High-risk-group" method. In: *Origins of schizophrenia*, J. Romano, Ed, (pp. 179-200). Amsterdam: Excerpta Medica.

Mednick, S. A., 1974, Electrodermal recovery and psychopathology. In: *Genetics, environment and psychopathology*, S. A. Mednick, F. Schulsinger, J. Higgins, and B. Bell (Eds.), (pp. 135-146). Amsterdam: North-Holland.

Mednick, S. A., 1978, Berkson's fallacy and high-risk research. In: *The nature of schizophrenia: New approaches to research and treatment*, L. C. Wynne, R. L. Cromwell, and S. Matthysse, Eds., (pp. 442-452). New York: John Wiley.

Mednick, S. A., and Schulsinger, F., 1968, Some pre-morbid characteristics related to breakdown in children with schizophrenic mothers. In: *The transmission of schizophrenia*, D. Rosenthal and S. S. Kety, Eds., (pp. 267-291). New York: Pergamon Press.

Meehl, P. E., 1962, Schizotaxia, schizotypy and schizophrenia. *American Psychologist* 17: 827-838.

Murphy, H. B. M., and Raman, A. C., 1971, The chronicity of schizophrenia in indigenous tropical peoples: Results of a twelve-year follow-up survey in Mauritius. *British Journal of Psychiatry* 118: 489-497.

Nagler, S., and Mirsky, A. F., 1985, Introduction: The Israeli High-risk study. *Schizophrenia Bulletin* 11: 17-29.

Nielsen, T. C., and Petersen, K. E., 1976, Electrodermal correlates of extraversion, trait anxiety and schizophrenism. *Scandinavian Journal of Psychology* 17: 73-80.

Ohman, A., 1981, Electrodermal activity and vulnerability to schizophrenia: A review. *Biological Psychology* 12: 87-145.

Pearson, J. S., and Kley, I. B., 1957, On the application of genetic expectancies as age-specific base rates in the study of human behavior disorders. *Psychological Bulletin* 54: 406-419.

Prentky, R. H., Salzman, L. F., and Klein, R. H., 1981, Habituation and conditioning of skin conductance responses in children at risk. *Schizophrenia Bulletin* 7: 281-291.

Prokasy, W. F., and Kumpfer, K. L., 1973, Classical conditioning. In: *Electrodermal activity in psychological research*, W. F. Prokasy and D. C. Raskin, Eds., (pp. 197-202). New York: Academic Press.

Raine, A., Reynolds, G. P., and Sheard, C., 1991, Neuroanatomical correlates of skin conductance orienting in normal humans: A magnetic resonance imaging study. *Psychophysiology* 28: 548-557.

Rosenthal, D., Wender, P. H., Kety, S. S., Schulsinger, F., Welner, J., and Östergaard, L., 1968, Schizophrenics' offspring reared in adoptive homes. In: *The transmission of schizophrenia*, D. Rosenthal and S. S. Kety, Eds., (pp. 377-391). Oxford: Pergamon Press.

Salzman, L. F., and Klein, R. F., 1978, Habituation and conditioning of electrodermal responses in high risk children. *Schizophrenia Bulletin* 4: 210-222.

Schnur, D. B., Bernstein, A. S., Mukherjee, S., Loh, J., Degreef, G., and Reidel, J., 1989, The autonomic orienting response and CT scan findings in schizophrenia. *Schizophrenia Research* 2: 449-455.

Schulsinger, H., 1976, A ten-year follow-up of children of schizophrenic mothers: Clinical assessment. *Acta Psychiatrica Scandinavica* 53: 371-386.

Seidman, L. J., 1983, Schizophrenia and brain dysfunction: An integration of recent neurodiagnostic findings. *Psychological Bulletin* 94: 195-238.

Simons, R. F., 1981, Electrodermal and cardiac orienting in psychometrically defined high-risk subjects. *Psychiatry Research* 4, 347-356.

Van Dyke, J. L., Rosenthal, D., and Rasmussen, P. V., 1974, Electrodermal functioning in adopted-away offspring of schizophrenics. *Journal of Psychiatric Research* 10, 199-215.

Venables, P. H., 1974, The recovery limb of the skin conductance response in "high-risk" research. In: *Genetics, environment and psychopathology*, S. A. Mednick, S. F., J. Higgins, and B. Bell, Eds., (pp. 117-133). Amsterdam: North-Holland.

Venables, P. H., 1978, Psychophysiology and psychometrics. *Psychophysiology*, 15, 302-315.

Venables, P. H., 1987, Autonomic nervous system factors in criminal behavior. In: *The causes of crime: New biological approaches* S. A. Mednick, T. E. Moffitt, and S. A. Stack, Eds., (pp. 110-136). Cambridge: Cambridge University Press.

Venables, P. H., 1990, The measurement of schizotypy in Mauritius. *Personality and Individual Differences* 11: 965-971.

Venables, P. H., 1991, Autonomic activity. In: *Windows on the Brain*, R. A. Zappulla, F. F. LeFever, J. Jaeger, and R. Bilder, Eds., (pp. 191-207). New York: New York Academy of Sciences.

Venables, P. H., Mitchell, D. A., and Schulsinger, F., 1983, Outcome at age nine of psychophysiological selection at age three for risk of schizophrenia: A Mauritian study. *British Journal of Developmental Psychology* 1: 21-30.

Venables, P. H., Mednick, S. A., Schulsinger, F., Raman, A. C., Bell, B., Dalais, J. C., and Fletcher, R. P., 1978, Screening for risk of mental illness. In: *Cognitive defects in the development of mental illness*, G. Serban (Eds.), (pp. 273-303). New York: Brunner/Mazel.

Venables, P. H., Wilkins, S., Mitchell, D. A., Raine, A., and Bailes, K., 1990, A scale for the measurement of schizotypy. *Personality and Individual Differences* 11: 481-495.

Zahn, T. P., 1977, Autonomic nervous system characteristics possibly related to a genetic predisposition to schizophrenia. *Schizophrenia Bulletin* 3: 49-60.

Zahn, T. P., Carpenter, W. T., and McGlashan, T. H., 1981, Autonomic nervous system activity in acute schizophrenia I. Method and comparison with normal controls. *Archives of General Psychiatry* 38: 251-258.

# THE SKIN CONDUCTANCE ORIENTING RESPONSE,

# ATTENTION, AND SCHIZOPHRENIA

Anne M. Schell[1], Michael E. Dawson[2],
Erin Hazlett[2], Diane L. Filion[2],
and Keith H. Nuechterlein[3]

[1] Psychology Department
   Occidental College, 1600 Campus Road
   Los Angeles, CA 90041 USA

[2] Psychology Department
   University of Southern California
   SGM 501
   Los Angeles, CA 90089-1061 USA

[3] Dept. of Psychiatry and Biobehavioral Sciences
   University of California, Los Angeles
   300 UCLA Medical Plaza. Rm. 2251
   Los Angeles, CA 90024-6968 USA

## INTRODUCTION

This chapter reports a series of investigations of the relationships between the skin conductance orienting response (SCR OR) and measures of automatic and controlled information processing during basic information processing tasks that are of general interest to psychophysiologists. These have included a variety of orienting tasks and also classical conditioning. We have been particularly interested in studying the effect of manipulating attention to stimuli on the SCR OR and cognitive processing measures. We began by examining attentional processes and their psychophysiological correlates in normal college undergraduates, and then extended these studies to include a population of recent-onset schizophrenic patients, a population where fundamental mechanisms of attention and information processing are agreed to be abnormal.

When a stimulus impinges on an organism, a complex series of processes is initiated. The first stage of information processing, usually referred to as preattentive or automatic,

*Progress in Electrodermal Research*, Edited by
J.-C. Roy *et al.* Plenum Press, New York, 1993

involves an automatic filtering process in which stimuli are compared to representations in short term memory. Stimuli deemed novel or significant (perhaps because of an explicit attentional set toward them) are referred for further processing and a "call" is made for allocation from the limited pool of controlled processing resources (e.g. Kahneman, 1973; Öhman, 1979). The controlled resource pool has a limited capacity and its contents are sometimes considered to overlap greatly with conscious attention. Elicitation of the orienting response (OR) has been associated with the preattentively triggered call for these limited processing resources (Öhman, 1979), as well as with the actual allocation of resources (e.g. Dawson, Filion, & Schell, 1989; Dawson, Schell, Beers, & Kelly, 1982; Kahneman, 1973, Näätänen, 1990; Öhman, 1990; Spinks, 1989).

## THE SCR OR AND CONTROLLED PROCESSING IN NORMAL SUBJECTS

Techniques exist for probing both the early preattentive and the later controlled processes. In the studies reported here, controlled processing was assessed using the probe reaction time (RT) technique, and the startle blink modification technique was used to investigate a combination of automatic and controlled processes.

The secondary RT task technique has long been used to measure processing demands during a wide variety of primary tasks. The assumption underlying this technique is that processing the primary task, in these studies processing stimuli that are conditioned stimuli or to-be-attended or to-be-ignored orienting stimuli, will leave less resources available to process a concurrently presented secondary task, to process in these studies a reaction time imperative stimulus (Kerr, 1973; Posner & Boies, 1971). The degree of slowing of RT when the imperative stimulus is presented during the CS or orienting stimulus, compared to when it is presented alone during the intertrial interval, indexes the amount of controlled processing resources being allocated to the primary task.

The first studies in this series were of controlled processing during classical discrimination conditioning (Dawson et al., 1982). College student subjects were first practiced in a button-press RT task in response to a brief auditory (tone) stimulus and were then classically conditioned using different colored lights as CS+ and CS- with a 7.0 s CS - UCS interval and an electric shock UCS. Auditory RT probes were presented (across two studies) during some presentations of each visual CS both immediately after CS onset (at 300 or 500 ms after onset), during the middle of the ISI (at 3500 ms), near the point of UCS onset (at 6500, 7500, or 8000 ms), and during the intertrial interval (ITI) for comparison purposes. As would be expected, the skin conductance response immediately following CS onset was significantly greater to CS+ than to CS-.

Figure 1 shows the RT change scores (RT to probes during a CS minus RT to the probes presented during the ITI) for probes presented during CS+ and CS- at various points after onset. Overall, RT was faster during the CSs than during the ITI, but subsequent research has shown this to be due to a probability density effect: on a second-by-second basis, RT tones were more likely during the CS than during the ISI. We also see this density effect operating in the orienting studies described below. The points of interest are the greater resource allocation throughout the CS to the more significant CS+ than to CS-, and the very heavy allocation immediately after CS+ onset, with a second upswing near the point of UCS onset. These results demonstrated for the first time that human autonomic classical conditioning is accompanied by controlled cognitive processing and are contrary to the traditional view that classical conditioning occurs automatically without controlled processing.

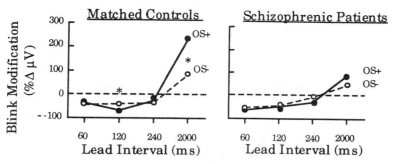

**Figure 1.** RT change scores during CS+ and CS-.

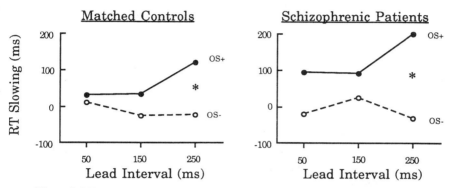

**Figure 2.** RT change scores during conditioning for Large and Small FIR Responders.

We next looked at the relationship between controlled processing and the SCR CR. We compared those subjects who gave large responses to the CSs with those who gave small responses in terms of their RT change scores. These data are shown in Figure 2.

As can be seen, controlled processing resource allocation is greater among large responders than among small responders immediately after CS+ onset and throughout the middle of the ISI, and differential resource allocation to CS+ and CS- is more consistent. Large responders also seem to finish processing the onset of the CS+ more rapidly than small responders. Note that RT to the 500 ms probe during CS+ is slower for small responders; large responders appear to have finished processing CS+ onset by the time that they must react to this probe. These results further suggest that the conditioned SCR is associated with, and possibly mediated by, controlled cognitive processes.

We next turned to the investigation of controlled processing during orienting tasks (Dawson, Filion, & Schell, 1989). In the series of studies summarized here, the primary task of the subject was to process an intermixed series of two stimuli, one of which was designated the to-be-attended orienting stimulus (OS+) and the other of which was designated the to-be-ignored orienting stimulus (OS-). These stimuli were easily discriminable tones or lights. The subject's task was to count the number of OS+s which were 7 s in duration rather than the standard 5 s. RT probes in a different modality from the

OSs were delivered at various times within the first 1000 ms of OS onsets and during the ITI for baseline comparison purposes.

When the discrimination between OS+ and OS- is an easy one, for instance when OS+ is a light and OS- is a tone and the RT probe is a vibrotactile stimulus, a pattern of resource allocation occurs that is consistent across studies. What is seen is greater resource allocation to OS+, particularly 150 ms post OS+ onset, with allocation being greater during early trials (typically the first 12 presentations of each OS) than during later trials (typically the second 12 presentations of each OS). (See Figure 3). The SCR OR is greater to OS+ than to OS-, and habituation of the SCR OR is associated with a decline in controlled processing. We also have found that introduction of a novel stimulus, such as a tone of a new frequency presented at the end of a series of familiar orienting stimuli, is reliably associated with increased resource allocation as indexed by even greater RT slowing.

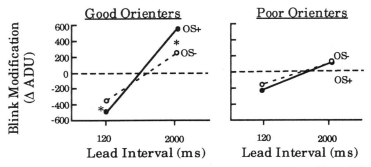

**Figure 3.** RT change scores during an orienting task. (Asterisks indicate significant differences between OS+ and OS-).

Furthermore, the degree of resource allocation to OS+ at 150 ms as indexed by the RT change score is positively correlated with the SCR OR to OS+ during the early trial block, with Pearson correlation coefficients ranging between .40 and .60 across studies. Large orienters to the attended stimulus are large resource allocators. Figure 4 illustrates the difference in controlled processing between good and poor orienters .

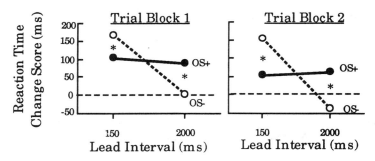

**Figure 4.** RT change scores during an orienting task for Good and Poor Orienters (Asterisks ind ate significant differences between OS+ and OS-).

Interestingly, this picture changes when the discrimination between OS+ and OS- becomes more difficult, for example a tone presented to the left ear versus the right ear or a high pitched versus a low pitched tone. In such situations, we have consistently found slower RTs immediately after presentation of the OS- than the OS+ on the early trials of these orienting tasks, indicating less availability of controlled processing resources following OS- than OS+, even though the SCR OR to OS+ is greater than to OS-. We have hypothesized that this is due to a switch in attention which occurs when a difficult to discriminate OS- is presented. That is, the subject maintains a focus of attention anticipatory of OS+, a focus of attention on the attended channel. When the OS- appears, it is rapidly identified by preattentive automatic processes as a probable target-mismatch, but then a switch of attention away from the task-relevant channel occurs to positively identify the task-irrelevant stimulus. Although the disengagement, movement, and reengagement of attention may not itself consume resources, it makes them temporarily unavailable for other tasks. Thus, the slowing of RT during OS- is primarily due to unavailability of resources due to the shift in focus of attention rather than to consumption of resources by processing of the OS-, while the slowing of RT after OS+ is due to the processing of the OS+. This interpretation is consistent with our finding that RT immediately after OS+ is positively correlated with the SCR OR to OS+, while the RT immediately after OS- is not significantly correlated with the SCR OR to OS-.

Evidence consistent with these findings, and with a controlled resource allocation view of orienting, also has been presented by Siddle and Packer (1987) using the secondary RT technique. They found increased SCR ORs and resource allocation to omission and then representation of an expected stimulus. In addition, Packer and Siddle (1989) reported increased orienting and allocation to miscued stimuli.

This research provides a picture of controlled processing resource allocation in discrimination classical conditioning and orienting tasks with simple stimuli and normal college student subjects. It is clear that this sort of information processing in humans involves considerable controlled processing, and that the magnitude of the SCR OR is related to the allocation of controlled processing resources to the attended stimulus. Stimuli that elicit larger ORs (CS+, OS+, stimuli presented early in a habituation series, unexpected novel or mis-cued stimuli) elicit heavy controlled processing as indexed by RT slowing. Moreover, individuals who give large SCR ORs are heavy processors.

## THE SCR OR AND PREATTENTIVE PROCESSING IN NORMAL SUBJECTS

Useful as it is in investigating controlled attentional processes, the secondary RT task technique cannot provide information about the earlier, more automatic, "preattentive" stages of information processing hypothesized to be involved in OR elicitation. Such information may be provided, however, by the use of the startle eyeblink modification technique.

The startle eyeblink modification technique involves presentation of startle-eliciting stimuli as probes in a manner similar to the secondary RT technique. It is based on the well-documented finding that the amplitude of the eyeblink component of the startle reflex is reliably modified when a nonstartling stimulus is presented just prior to the presentation of the startle-eliciting stimulus (see Anthony, 1985; Graham, 1975; Hoffman & Ison, 1980, for reviews).

When the interval between the presentation of the nonstartling prepulse and the startle-eliciting probe (the lead interval) is short (less than 250 ms), the typical result is a reliable reduction of blink magnitude compared to that elicited in the absence of a prepulse; in humans this inhibition has been found to be maximal at a lead interval of 120 ms (e.g., Graham & Murray, 1977). This early inhibition is referred to as "prepulse inhibition", is unlearned, requires only midbrain and lower structures (Leitner & Cohen, 1985), is evident during sleep (Silverstein, Graham, & Calloway, 1980), and is found in a variety of species (Hoffman & Ison, 1980). Short lead interval prepulse inhibition is thought to reflect the action of an automatic sensorimotor gating system, protective of preattentive processing, which allows the efficient management of rapidly presented information (e.g. Braff & Geyer, 1990; Graham, 1980).

Although the traditional view of prepulse inhibition is that it is a purely automatic process, several recent studies suggest that it may be modifiable by attentional sets. These studies demonstrated that prepulse inhibition in humans may be increased or decreased by instructions that direct attention toward or away from the prepulse (Acocella & Blumenthal, 1990; Delpezzo & Hoffman, 1980; Filion, Dawson, & Schell, in press; Hackley & Graham, 1987). In one such study, (Filion et al., in press) we used a modification of our selective attention orienting task (Dawson et al., 1989) in which subjects were presented with a series of high and low pitched tones and instructed to count the number of longer than usual tones of one pitch. The to-be-attended and to-be-ignored tones served as prepulses for an auditory startle-eliciting stimulus (noise burst) presented at lead intervals of 60, 120, and 240 ms, and occasionally during the intertone intervals.

Significant blink inhibition occurred during the prepulses, with maximum inhibition at 120 ms. Moreover, the attended prepulse produced significantly greater inhibition than the ignored prepulse. Thus, although prepulse inhibition can occur at a purely preattentive level, it may also reflect the modulation of preattentive sensory gating mechanisms by controlled cognitive processes.

Not only can blink inhibition be used to track early preattentive processes, it may also be useful in studying late sensory facilitation processes associated with the OR. When the lead interval is relatively long, greater than 1000 ms, the typical result is an increase in blink amplitude when the prepulse is in the same modality as the startle stimulus or when subjects are instructed to focus attention on the startle stimulus (Bohlin & Graham, 1977; Bohlin, Graham, Silverstein, & Hackley, 1981; Hackley & Graham, 1983). When attention is directed toward a prepulse in a different modality from the startle stimulus, blink magnitude is inhibited.

These findings have led to the suggestion that although startle blink is an automatic process, it can be modified by the sensory pathway enhancement or inhibition associated with controlled resource allocation (Anthony, 1985) and with the OR. When attention is directed toward stimuli in a particular modality, there is facilitation of processing of all stimuli in that modality, and inhibition of processing of stimuli in other modalities. Blinks elicited by stimuli in an attended modality should be particularly facilitated if the stimulus is presented during an OR. In the Filion et al. (in press) study, we found that at a lead interval of 2000 ms, attended prepulses, which elicited larger SCR ORs than ignored prepulses, also produced greater blink facilitation.

In a second study which directly compared probe RT and startle blink (Filion, Dawson, & Schell, 1992), subjects were presented with the tone length judging selective attention task using tones of two different pitches. RT probes were presented during some attended and ignored tones (at 150 and 2000 ms after tone onset), acoustic startle probes were presented on other trials (at 120 and 2000 ms), and other trials were unprobed to allow measurement of the SCR OR. As would be expected, the SCR OR was greater to attended than to ignored tones, with habituation over the two 24 trial blocks (12 OS+ and 12 OS- trials per block). (See Figure 5).

Figure 6 shows the startle modification scores (expressed as a difference between blink amplitude during the prepulse and amplitude of intertone interval blinks). As can be seen, blink amplitude was inhibited at 120 ms and facilitated at 2000 ms, with modification effects decreasing over trial blocks, particularly the late facilitation.

When the prepulse-modified blinks were compared with the intertone interval baseline blinks, we found that both the attended and the ignored prepulse produced significant inhibition at 120 ms during both trial blocks, and both prepulses produced significant facilitation at 2000 ms only during the first trial block. Moreover, the attended prepulse produced greater modification than did the ignored prepulse. Significantly greater inhibition was observed following OS+ than OS- during both trial blocks and greater facilitation following OS+ than OS- during the early block.

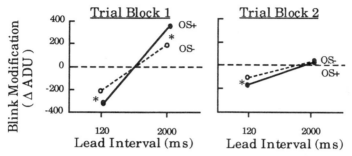

**Figure 5.** SCR ORs to Attended and Ignored orienting stimuli, normal subjects. (Asterisks indicate significant differences between OS+ and OS-).

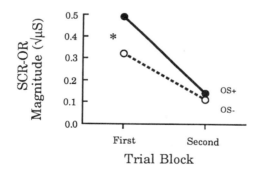

**Figure 6.** Blink modification during Attended and Ignored orienting stimuli, normal subjects. (Asterisks indicate significant differences between OS+ and OS-).

The RT change scores (expressed as a difference between RT during a prepulse and intertrial interval RT) for these same subjects are shown in Figure 7. RT was, as expected, slower during the tones than during the ITI, particularly at the 150 ms point, with the degree of slowing decreasing over trial blocks. During both blocks, RT was slower to the ignored than to the attended tone at 150 ms, presumably due to the need to switch the focus of attention to the ignored tone. But at 2000 ms during both trial blocks, RT is slower during the attended tone.

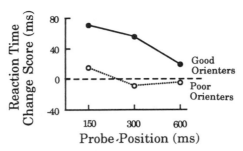

**Figure 7.** RT change scores during Attended and Ignored orienting stimuli, normal subjects. (Asterisks indicate significant differences between OS+ and O-).

Correlations were computed on a between-subjects basis for the first trial block among the magnitude of the SCR OR and the attentional measures provided by blink modification and RT change. These correlations for the attended prepulse are shown in Table 1.

**Table 1.** Pearson product moment correlations among skin conductance orienting response magnitude (SCOR), blink inhibition at 120 ms (Blink-120), blink facilitation at 2000 ms (Blink-2000), secondary reaction time at 150 ms (RT-150), and secondary reaction time at 2000 ms (RT-2000). *indicates significant correlations for two-tailed tests, p<.05. (Critical r = .374).

| | ATTENDED PREPULSE, TRIAL BLOCK 1 | | | |
| | SCOR | Blink-120 | Blink-2000 | RT-150 |
| --- | --- | --- | --- | --- |
| SCOR | ---- | | | |
| Blink-120 | -.68* | ---- | | |
| Blink-2000 | +.67* | -.47* | ---- | |
| *RT-150 | +.53* | -.49* | +.27 | ---- |
| RT-2000 | -.01 | -.14 | -.12 | +.21 |

For the attended prepulse (and for the ignored prepulse as well) SCR OR magnitude was negatively correlated with blink magnitude at the 120 ms lead interval; subjects who showed the greatest amount of blink inhibition also produced the largest SCR ORs. Also noteworthy are the negative correlations between blink magnitude at 120 ms and at 2000 ms; subjects who show the greatest early inhibition also show the greatest late facilitation. For the attended tone only, consistent with earlier findings, RT at 150 ms is correlated with the SCR OR; large orienters exhibit greater RT slowing. Blink amplitude at 2000 ms is also positively correlated with the SCR OR; large orienters exhibit greater blink facilitation. It is also interesting to note that RT at 2000 ms does not correlate with any of the other attentional or orienting measures; in this task paradigm controlled processing at 2000 ms seems to reflect subjects' monitoring of the length of the attended tone rather than processes associated with stimulus recognition and orienting (Filion, Dawson, & Schell, 1992).

These correlations suggest that those subjects who produce large SCR ORs allocate more controlled attentional resources to the attended tone, show greater attentional modulation of automatic processing, and produce greater sensory facilitation during the attended tone than subjects who produce small SCR ORs. The blink modification data for the third of the subjects giving the largest SCR ORs to the attended tone on the first trial block and those giving the smallest SCR ORs are shown in Figure 8. As can be seen, there is markedly greater early inhibition and late facilitation of blink amplitude among the good orienters, as well as better attentional modulation of both processes, that is, better discrimination between attended and ignored stimuli.

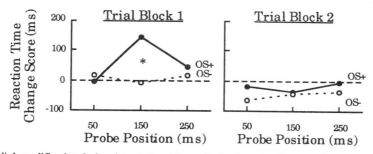

**Figure 8.** Blink modification during Attended and Ignored orienting stimuli among Good and Poor Orienters. (Asterisks indicate significant differences between OS+ and OS-).

All of these studies, taken together, indicate reliable relationships between the SCR OR and measures of attentional processing in normal human subjects. Stimuli which elicit large ORs, such as novel stimuli, those early in a habituation series, or those made significant by an instructional set, are those which receive greater protection of preattentive processing and greater allocation of controlled processing resources. Viewed from an individual difference perspective, subjects who exhibit large ORs are also those whose attentional processes are more closely tuned to the demands of the environment; they show greater protection of preattentive processing, greater controlled processing, and greater sensory facilitation in attended sensory pathways.

These data are also suggestive of where in the flow of information processing the OR may be elicited. Inspection of Figures 5, 6, and 7 indicates that by the second trial block differential orienting to the attended and ignored stimuli is no longer occurring; neither the SCR OR nor the blink facilitation at 2000 ms discriminates between the two stimuli. The stimuli are familiar to the subjects at this point and subjects have the task well practiced. However, short lead interval blink inhibition is still significant in the second trial block (being an automatic process) and, more important, the attended stimulus continues to receive greater protection of preattentive processing than the ignored stimulus. Thus, the automatic processing mechanisms continue to respond to the designated significance of the attended stimulus even when the SCR OR has habituated. This suggests that the automatic processor, during the second trial block, continues to call for greater allocation of controlled resources to process the onset of the attended stimulus than the ignored stimulus, but, since the controlled processor does not respond to that differential call, there is no differential OR (Filion et al., 1992).

Having observed these relationships among normal subjects, we next turned our attention to the schizophrenic spectrum .

## ELECTRODERMAL ABNORMALITIES IN SCHIZOPHRENIA

Electrodermal activity and particularly the SCR OR have long been of interest to researchers in the field of schizophrenia, due to their hypothesized relationship to processes which have been considered dysfunctional in schizophrenia, most notably arousal, attention, information processing, and emotion. Although in the early research literature (and to some extent in the later research literature) results varied from study to study, in the last decade some consensus has emerged about the nature of two electrodermal abnormalities typically seen in this disorder (Bernstein et al., 1982; Dawson & Nuechterlein, 1984; Holzman, 1987; Öhman, 1981: Spohn & Patterson, 1979). First, it is generally agreed that there is a large subgroup of schizophrenic patients who are SCR OR nonresponders. In most studies, between 40% and 50% of patients fail to give SCR ORs to novel innocuous non-task stimuli, as compared to only 5% to 10% of the normal population. Second, tonic electrodermal arousal among the SCR OR nonresponder subgroup is low to moderate, while tonic arousal among the responder subgroup is abnormally high.

If the SCR OR does indeed reflect controlled cognitive processing, as data from normal subjects seem to suggest, then one might reasonably expect that a disorder in which attentional processes are dysfunctional would be characterized by SCR OR dysfunction. As Bernstein (1987) appropriately asked, "What does it cost the schizophrenic nonresponder to be nonresponsive"? We have begun to approach this question, and the question of cognitive processing abnormalities in schizophrenia in general.

Because it is probable that many of the inconsistancies in findings about the psychophysiology of schizophrenia come from differences in patient populations, it is important to be specific about the population to be discussed here. These were patients with a recent first onset of psychosis who were tested on several occasions as part of a longitudinal study of the early stages of schizophrenia, "Developmental Processes in Schizophrenic Disorders" (Keith Nuechterlein, Principal Investigator). Criteria for patient entry into the study included a diagnosis by Research Diagnostic Criteria (Spitzer, Endicott, & Robins, 1978) of schizophrenia or schizoaffective disorder (Nuechterlein et al., 1992). Approximately 70% of these patients entered the study during their first psychotic episode and within six months of the onset of their first psychotic symptoms. The remainder were in a first psychotic episode that had lasted more than six months or had experienced their first episode within the last two years. Thus, this is a young (average age in the early twenties), recent onset population, without a long prior history of institutionalization or medication. It is also a predominantly (80%) male population. The control population in this study was matched to the patient population for age, sex, ethnicity, and education level.

We have compared the patient and control groups at a number of points in the course of treatment for the patients, including at entry into the study, when the patients were still for the most part in a psychotic episode and were hospitalized. To determine if this group initially exhibited the electrodermal abnormalities usually reported in the recent literature, we compared a group of 98 patients who exhibited psychotic symptoms at the time of their first test occasion with 40 control subjects (Dawson, Nuechterlein, & Schell, 1992). Nonspecific skin conductance responses (NS-SCRs) and skin conductance level (SCL) were measured during a 5 min rest period, then SCR ORs were measured during a series of innocuous non-task tones, a series of task-significant tones, and a series of brief loud noises.

For the innocuous tones, 43% of the patients were SCR OR nonresponders, similar to the findings from other studies (Bernstein et al., 1982). However, unexpectedly, in this control group, 40% were nonresponders, unlike the typically reported 5% to 10%. We are at present unable to account for this difference in the control group. However, Iacono, Fichen, and Beiser (this volume) also report a 40% level of nonresponding to innocuous tones among a community-based control sample having approximately the same demographic characteristics as their patient group, suggesting that demographic matching may be an important factor. Group differences in nonresponsiveness did occur during the task-significant tones (36% of the patients versus 8% of the controls) and in response to the loud noises (16% of the patients versus 3% of the controls) .

We divided both the patients and controls into their responder and nonresponder subgroups based on their responses to the innocuous tones, to determine if our responder subgroup showed the often-reported tonic electrodermal hyperarousal. As predicted, the frequency of NS-SCRs was significantly greater among responder patients than responder controls, but not among nonresponder patients and their controls. SCL was only marginally higher among responder patients than among their controls (perhaps due to the anticholinergic effects of antipsychotic and antiparkinsonian medications), while SCL was significantly lower among nonresponder patients than among their controls. Thus, the electrodermal abnormalities in this population are generally consistent with the consensus reported in the literature.


## SCR OR AND ATTENTIONAL ANOMALIES IN SCHIZOPHRENIA

We next undertook to examine information processing anomalies, particularly those which relate to attentional processes, in these patients using the probe RT and reflex blink modification techniques.

The subjects were 15 schizophrenic outpatients and 14 demographically matched controls. Most subjects participated in two test sessions. During these test occasions patients were either off all psychoactive medication or were stabilized on a low dose of injectable fluphenazine decanoate. The patients were all outpatients in a state of relative clinical remission at the time of testing.

During the first session the subject was given practice in a reaction time task and was then presented with a series of lights and tones and asked to perform our length-judging task, attending to either the lights or the tones and ignoring the other stimulus. Probe RT stimuli were presented at 50, 150, and 250 ms after OS onset during some of the tones and during the intertrial intervals. During the second session one week later, the subject performed the length-judging task while listening to a series of tones of two different pitches, being instructed to attend to one tone and to ignore the other. Startle blink probe stimuli were presented at 60, 120, 240, and 2000 ms after tone onset on some trials and during the intertone intervals.

### Skin Conductance ORs

We examined the SCR ORs elicited by the attended and nonattended stimuli during both test sessions, from trials on which no RT or startle probes had been presented. On the first test occasion we observed a significant difference in overall responsiveness between the patient group and the control group, with the controls being more responsive. Although there was significant SCR OR habituation across trial blocks in both groups, during both the first and the second trial blocks (the first and last 12 presentations of each OS), there was significant discrimination in SCR OR magnitude between the OS+ and OS- in both the control group and the patient group. However, there was greater decline in discrimination among the patients.

During the second test session, during which startle blink was measured, electrodermal responsiveness was lower in both groups, perhaps because of adaptation to the laboratory and perhaps because the effortful RT task was not required during the second session. Only the control group exhibited significant SCR OR discrimination between OS+ and OS-, and that only during the first trial block.

## Information Processing Differences

The probe RT data, which measure differences in controlled processing of attended and ignored stimuli, did not indicate differences between patients and controls (see Figure 9). Both groups showed greater processing of the attended than the ignored stimulus. However, the groups did not differ at any probe position in the amount of differential processing that occured.

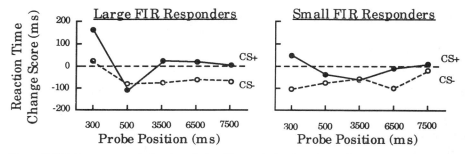

**Figure 9.** RT change scores during Attended and Ignored orienting stimuli, Schizophrenic Patients and Normal Controls. (Asterisks indicate significant differences between OS+ and OS-).

The startle modification data exhibited more striking differences between the groups (see Figure 10; Dawson, Hazlett, Filion, Nuechterlein, & Schell, 1992). The matched controls showed results very similar to those of the college students; there was greater inhibition of blink amplitude at the 120 ms lead interval during the attended than during the ignored tone (hypothetically reflecting greater protection of preattentive processing), and there was greater facilitation of blink amplitude at the 2000 ms lead interval (hypothetically reflecting greater enhancement of sensory processing in the auditory modality). At both lead intervals, the normal group demonstrated attentional modulation of startle blink. However, the patient group showed neither differential early inhibition nor differential late facilitation. There was no significant attentional modulation of either process among the schizophrenic patients.

In this paradigm in which subjects are actively engaged in a task, the basic startle blink process and simple prepulse inhibition appear to be normal in the patient group. (It should be noted that patients perform this task almost as accurately as controls). The degree of prepulse inhibition during OS- could be taken as an approximate measure of inhibition produced by the presence of a nonsignificant stimulus. (Processing of an OS- in a

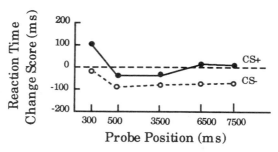

**Figure 10.** Blink modification during Attended and Ignored orienting stimuli, Schizophrenic Patients and Normal Controls. (Asterisks indicate significant differences between OS+ and OS-).

discrimination paradigm may differ in some respects from processing stimuli in a passive attention paradigm). Prepulse inhibition during the OS- at the 120 ms lead interval, where we would generally expect to see such inhibition maximize, is significant in both groups, and the amount of inhibition does not differ between groups.

The results of the startle blink modification data suggest that, at least with respect to tasks of this nature, early, automatic information processing mechanisms appear to be operating normally in these relatively remitted young patients, in that basic prepulse inhibition appears to be normal. What is abnormal is the attentional modulation of prepulse inhibition. The attentional set produced by the instructions to attend to one tone and to ignore the other, which produces greater protection of preattentive processing of the attended than the ignored tone in the normal group, does not do so in the patient group. Attentional modulation also fails to affect the later sensory facilitation process associated with the OR among the schizophrenic patients. Patients do not show greater blink facilitation during the attended than during the ignored stimulus as controls do, and controls show significantly greater late blink facilitation during the attended stimulus than do patients.

These data suggest that perhaps the basic mechanisms of early, automatic information processing are normal in these patients, and that what appears to create anomalies in early processing is actually a deficit in modulation by controlled information processing mechanisms. In terms of neural substrates, the brain stem and midbrain structures thought to mediate the startle blink and its prepulse inhibition may not themselves be dysfunctional; the primary dysfunction may lie in higher (including cortical) centers hypothesized to mediate attentional modulation of the lower structures.

In considering the possibility raised above, one should note that Braff and his colleagues (Braff & Geyer, 1990) did find impaired short lead interval prepulse inhibition in a heterogeneous population of hospitalized, medicated, acute and chronic schizophrenic patients using nontask stimuli. They theorized that the reduced inhibition reflected a deficit in inhibitory sensorimotor gating. The difference between our results with respect to prepulse inhibition at 120 ms during the nonattended tone and those of Braff and his colleagues may lie in differences in the patient populations; our patients were more recent in onset and in relative remission. Important differences in functioning among the patients may also have been created by our imposition of a task, even with respect to processing of a non-attended stimulus. Basic early, automatic information processing mechanisms might be normalized when a task is required, but not otherwise. Bernstein and others (Bernstein et al., 1982) have reported that the proportion of schizophrenic patients who are SCR OR nonresponders compared to the proportion of controls drops when stimuli are given task significance, which is consistent with this interpretation.

These data, taken as a whole, indicate relationships between the SCR OR and measures of early and late attentional processes which exist in both normal and schizophrenic populations. On an individual difference basis, subjects who produce large SCR ORs show other evidence of heavy processing of stimuli. Schizophrenics, who suffer from a disorder generally thought to involve attentional processes, show both SCR OR deficits and processing abnormalities. Concurrent measurement of the SCR OR and independent measures of attentional processing such as startle blink modification and probe RT can add much to our understanding of both the basic nature of these attentional mechanisms and their dysfunctions in psychopathology.

## REFERENCES

Acocella, C.M., & Blumenthal, T.D. (1990). Directed attention influences the modification of startle reflex probability. *Psychological Reports,66*, 275-285.

Anthony, B.J. (1985). In the blink of an eye: Implications of reflex modification for information processing. In P.J. Ackles, J.R. Jennings, and M.G.H. Coles (Eds.), *Advances in Psychophysiology, Vol.1,* (pp. 167-218). Greenwich, CN: JAI Press.

Bernstein, A.S. (1987). Orienting response research in schizophrenia: where we have come and where we might go. *Schizophrenia Bulletin,* 13, 623-641.

Bernstein, A.S., Frith, C.D., Gruzelier, J.H., Patterson, T., Straube, E., Venables, P.H., & Zahn, T.P. (1982). An analysis of the skin conductance orienting response in samples of American, British, and German schizophrenics. *Biogical Psychology,* 14, 155-211.

Bohlin, G., & Graham, F.K. (1977). Cardiac deceleration and reflex blink facilitation. *Psychophysiology,* 14, 423-430.

Bohlin, G., Graham, F.K., Silverstein, L.D., & Hackley, S.A. (1981). Cardiac orienting and startle blink modification in novel and signal situations. *Psychophysiology,* 15, 339-343.

Braff, D.L., & Geyer, M.A. (1990). Sensorimotor gating and schizophrenia: Human and animal studies. *Archives of General Psychiatry,* 47, 181-188.

Dawson, M.E., Filion, D.L., & Schell, A.M. (1989). Is elicitation of the autonomic orienting response associated with allocation of processing resources? *Psychophysiology,* 26, 560-572.

Dawson, M.E., & Nuechterlein, K.H. (1984). Psychophysiological dysfunctions in the developmental course of schizophrenic disorders. *Schizophrenia Bulletin,* 10, 204-232.

Dawson, M.E., Nuechterlein, K.N., & Schell, A.M. (1992). Electrodermal abnormalities in recent-onset schizophrenia: Relationships to symptoms, prognosis, and processes. *Schizophrenia Bulletin,* 18, 295-311.

Dawson, M.E., Schell, A.M., Beers, J.R., & Kelly, A. (1982). Allocation of cognitive processing capacity during human autonomic classical conditioning. *Journal of Experimental Psychology: General,* 111, 273-295.

Delpezzo, E.M., & Hoffman, H.S. (1980). Attentional factors in the inhibition of a reflex by a visual prestimulus, *Science,* 210, 673-674.

Filion, D.L., Dawson, M.E., & Schell, A.M. (in press). Modification of the acoustic startle-reflex eyeblink: a tool for investigating early and late attentional processes. *Biological Psychology.*

Filion, D.L., Dawson, M.E,, & Schell, A.M, (1992). Probing the orienting response with startle modification and secondary reaction time. Submitted to *Psychophysiology.*

Graham, F.K. (1975). The more or less startling effects of weak prestimulation. *Psychophysiology,* 12, 238-248.

Graham, F.K. (1980). Control of reflex blink excitability. In R.F. Thompson, L.H. Hicks, & V.B. Shvyrkov (Eds.), *Neural Mechanisms of Goal-Directed Behavior and Learning* (pp. 511-519). New York: Academic Press.

Graham, F.K., & Murray, G.M. (1977). Discordant effects of weak prestimulation on magnitude and latency of the reflex blink. *Physiological Psychology, 5*, 108-114.

Hackley, S.A., & Graham, F.K. (1983). Early selective attention effects on cutaneous and acoustic blink reflexes. *Physiological Psychology, 11*, 235-242.

Hackley, S.A., & Graham, F.K. (1987). Effects of attending to the spatial position of reflex-eliciting and reflex modulating stimuli. *Journal of Experimental Psychology: Human Perception and Performance, 13*, 411-424.

Hoffman, H.S., & Ison, J.R. (1980). Reflex modification in the domain of startle: I. Some empirical findings and their implications for how the nervous system processes sensory input. *Psychological Review, 87*, 175-189.

Holzman, P.S. (1987). Recent studies of psychophysiology in schizophrenia. *Schizophrenia Bulletin, 13*, 49-75.

Kahneman, D. (1973). *Attention and Effort.* Englewood Cliffs, NJ: Prentice Hall.

Kerr, B. (1973). Processing demands during mental operations. *Memory and Cognition, 1*, 401-412.

Leitner, D.S., & Cohen, M.E. (1985). Role of the inferior colliculus in the inhibition of acoustic startle in the rat. *Physiology and Behavior, 34*, 65-70.

Näätänen, R. (1990). The role of attention in auditory information processing as revealed by event-related potentials and other brain measures of cognitive function. *Behavioral and Brain Sciences, 13*, 201-288.

Nuechterlein, K.N., Dawson, M.E., Gitlin, M., Ventura, J., Goldstein, M.J., Snyder, K., Yee, C., & Mintz, J. (in press). Developmental processes in schizophrenic disorders: The UCLA longitudinal studies of recent-onset schizophrenia. *Schizophrenia Bulletin.*

Öhman, A. (1979). The orienting response, attention, and learning: An information processing perspective. In H.D. Kimmel, E.H. van Olst, & J.F. Orlebeke (Eds.) *The Orienting Reflex in Humans* (pp. 443-471). Hillsdale, NJ: Lawrence Erlbaum.

Öhman, A. (1981). ELectrodermal activity and vulnerability to schizophrenia: A review. *Biological Psychology, 12*, 87-145.

Öhman, A. (1985). Face the beast and fear the face: Animal and social fears as prototypes for evolutionary analyses of emotion. *Psychophysiology, 23*, 123-145.

Öhman, A, (1990). Orienting and attention: Preferred preattentive processing of potentially phobic stimuli. In B.A. Campbell (Ed.) *Attention and information processing in infants and adults:Perspectives from Human and Animal Research.* Hillsdale, N.J.: Lawrence Erlbaum.

Packer, J.S., & Siddle, D.A.T. (1989). Stimulus miscuing, electrodermal activity, and the allocation of processing resources. *Psychophysiology, 26*, 192-200.

Posner, M.I., & Boies, S.J. (1971). Components of attention. *Psychological Review, 78*, 391-408.

Siddle, D.A.T., & Packer, J.S. (1987). Stimulus omission and dishabituation of the electrodermal orienting response: The allocation of processing resources. *Psychophysiology, 24*, 181-190.

Silverstein, L.D., Graham, F.K., & Bolllin, G. (1981). Selective attention effects on the reflex blink. *Psychophysiology, 18*, 240-247.

Silverstein, L.D., Graham, F.K., & Calloway, J.M. (1980). Preconditioning and excitability of the human orbicularis oculi reflex as a function of state. *Electroencephalography and Clinical Neurophysiology, 48*, 406-417.

Spinks, J.A. (1989). The orienting response in anticipation of information processing demands. In N.W. Bond and D.A.T. Siddle (Eds.) *Psychophysiology: Issues and Applications* (Proceedings of the 24th International Conference of Psychology, Sydney, AU, Vol.6). Amsterdam: Elsevier, pp. 138-150.

Spohn, H.E., & Patterson, T. (1979). Recent studies of psychophysiology in schizophrenia. *Schizophrenia Bulletin, 5*, 581-611.

Spitzer, R.L., Endicott, J., & Robins, E. (1978). Research Diagnostic Criteria: Rationale and reliability. *Archives of General Psychiatry, 35*, 773-782.

# ELECTRODERMAL ACTIVITY AND ANTISOCIAL BEHAVIOR:
# EMPIRICAL FINDINGS AND THEORETICAL ISSUES

Don C. Fowles

Department of Psychology
University of Iowa
Iowa City, IA 52242

## INTRODUCTION

A common finding in psychophysiological approaches to psychopathology has been that of electrodermal hyporeactivity among individuals variously described as psychopathic, sociopathic, antisocial, delinquent, hyperactive, or aggressive. The present chapter will review this literature. Special attention will be given to the conditions under which electrodermal hyporesponsivity is seen and the potential theoretical interpretations of the hyporesponsivity.

Electrodermal activity (EDA) refers collectively to all of the common measurements of the electrical activity across the epidermis on the palms of the hands: skin conductance (SC), its reciprocal skin resistance (SR), and skin potential (SP). All three measurements yield information about both *tonic level* (EDL) and *phasic responses* (EDRs). SP is rarely used and SR is usually converted to SC. In view of the dominance of SC in this literature, the measures of greatest interest are SC level (SCL) and SC responses (SCRs).

The primary phenomenon of psychological interest in electrodermal measurements is activity of the sweat glands, which are innervated solely by the sympathetic nervous system (SNS). SCRs are primarily influenced by sweat gland responses, whereas SCL reflects a complex mixture of sudorific (i.e., sweat gland) and nonsudorific components (see Edelberg, this volume; Fowles, 1986). True resting SCLs, influenced largely or totally by nonsudorific components, have little or no psychological significance. Consequently, differences in resting SCL are of psychological significance only if they reflect sweat gland responses to participation in the experiment. As Hare (1970, p. 40) suggested, the experimental situation itself constitutes a complex stimulus and in "resting" conditions we are observing a response to the experimental situation.

Except for intense or painful stimuli, the SCRs to discrete stimuli are usually called orienting responses (ORs). They are ORs to neutral stimuli (tones or lights without meaning or significance) and signal ORs to stimuli with meaning or significance (e.g., the CS in a classical conditioning paradigm, the warning and imperative stimuli in a reaction time paradigm, or any stimulus that is to be detected by the subject).

*Progress in Electrodermal Research,* Edited by
J.-C. Roy *et al.* Plenum Press, New York, 1993

Another aspect of the SCR is sometimes quantified: the speed of recovery. Neither of the two popular theoretical interpretations of this measure can be considered valid. Mednick (1975) proposed that rate of the peripheral recovery mirrors the course of fear reduction in the central nervous system. There is no basis for this hypothesis, since the complexity of the peripheral mechanism affecting recovery rate (e.g., Fowles, 1986) precludes a simple reflection of central states. Edelberg (1970, 1972) proposed that slow recovery SCRs reflect a defensive orientation, that rapid recovery SCRs reflect a goal-directed orientation, and that different peripheral mechanisms with separate neural innervation underlie the two types of responses. This hypothesis appeared to enjoy good empirical support at the time and stimulated a considerable amount of research, but it was subsequently rejected by Edelberg and Muller (1981), who found that prior EDA exerts a strong influence on recovery time. It now appears that slow recovery SCRs reflect less prior EDA (Edelberg, this volume; Fowles, 1986).

Due to the complexity of the peripheral mechanism, SCL, SCR amplitude and frequency, and SCR recovery times are noisy, imperfect reflections of the underlying sweat gland activity. This noise--as well as the sensitivity of EDA to subtle experimental conditions--probably contributes to the difficulty of precisely replicating findings from one study to the next and to findings that different aspects of electrodermal activity are associated with antisocial behavior from study to study. One can, at least, state the direction of effects to be expected from electrodermal hyporeactivity: lessened sweat gland activity is associated with lower SCL, fewer nonspecific SCRs, smaller amplitude SCRs, and slow recovery SCRs.

## A REVIEW OF EMPIRICAL FINDINGS

As noted above, a large literature has examined EDA in antisocial individuals. Many of these studies have selected "primary psychopaths" on the basis of Cleckley's (e.g., 1950, 1964) concept of psychopathy from among adult prison inmates or adolescent delinquents. An important alternative has been the Gough and Peterson (1952) Delinquency (De) scale or its later version, the Gough Socialization Scale (So), which was incorporated into the California Psychological Inventory (Gough, 1960; Megargee, 1972). Schalling, Lidberg, Levander, and Dahlin (1973) pointed out that many of the So scale items overlap criteria used by Cleckley to select primary psychopaths. However, Blackburn (1983) commented that the intercorrelations among various approaches to diagnosing psychopathy in this literature fall in the region of 0.4 to 0.5--leaving considerable room for diagnostic variation.

Several reviews of EDA and antisocial behavior have been published, almost all of which have found some aspects of EDA to distinguish antisocial groups from controls. One of the most comprehensive was Hare's (1978) chapter, which will be cited when possible with more recent studies added where appropriate.

### SCL and Nonspecific SCRs

**Resting Conditions.** Under resting conditions Hare (1978) reported that six studies found lower tonic SC levels while ten did not, but that even in the negative studies the differences were in the direction of lower SCLs for psychopaths. Pooling resting level data from eight of his own experiments, the comparison yielded a highly significant difference between psychopathic and nonpsychopathic inmates. Siddle (1977) also reviewed data on resting SCL and, although acknowledging that some of Hare's studies showed significant differences, found that "no firm conclusions can be drawn."

Differences for nonspecific fluctuations in phasic responses, if any, have been even weaker than for SCL. Again, Hare (1978) reported that four studies found small differences (fewer for psychopaths), while three did not. When Hare pooled data from several (apparently four) of his own experiments, the results were not significant. Siddle (1977) also reached a negative conclusion.

Since these reviews, Schmidt, Solanto, and Bridger (1985) using conduct disordered children vs. normal controls and Delameter and Lahey (1983) using learning disabled children further subdivided on the basis of conduct disorder and tension-anxiety (from the Conners Teacher Rating Scale) both failed to find resting differences for either SCL or for nonspecific fluctuations. Raine, Venables, & Williams (1990b) found no differences in resting SCL among 15-year-old school boys as a function of antisocial behavior or among a subgroup who became criminals by age 24, but the criminal-to-be subgroup did show fewer nonspecific SCRs.

It appears, therefore, that differences in the direction of less sweat gland activity among psychopaths may occasionally be found under resting conditions for SCL, but that the effect size is small. There is even weaker evidence of differences in nonspecific fluctuations during rest, although such a difference probably should not be ruled out entirely. It appears that most experiments are not seen as stressful enough to bring out differences between the two groups during the initial rest period.

**Monotonous/Repetitive Stimulation.** Somewhat more positive results have been obtained during prolonged periods of repetitive stimulation. Hare (1968) found that psychopathic subjects showed declining SCL during repetitive stimulation (simple tones), compared with a slight increase in levels for nonpsychopathic subjects. Unfortunately, nonspecific fluctuations were not reported during the tone series. Schalling et al. (1973) reported that psychopathic subjects (criminals with high De scores) showed a smaller increase in SCL from rest than the nonpsychopathic criminals. Similarly, Schalling et al. (1973) reported differences in nonspecific SCRs during a tone series with psychopathic subjects showing rather dramatically fewer responses. In contrast, Borkovec (1970) did not find differences in SCL during a series of tones. Although the number of studies is small, there has been at least a suggestion of somewhat stronger results with minimal stimulation than under resting conditions.

**Stimulating/Stressful Conditions.** More challenging experimental conditions have yielded still more positive results. One study involving injection of adrenalin (Hare, 1972) showed increases in SCL during the experiment in nonpsychopaths compared with stable records for psychopathic subjects. A second study (Dengerink & Bertilson, 1975) involving administration of shocks to other subjects showed increases in SCL over trials in nonpsychopathic controls, contrasted with stable records for psychopathic subjects.

Even more to the point are eight studies (Hare, 1965b; Hare & Craigen, 1974; Hare, Frazelle, & Cox, 1978; Lippert & Senter, 1966; Schalling & Levander, 1967; Schalling, Levander, & Dahlin-Lidberg, 1975; Schmauk, 1970; Sutker, 1970) cited in Hare's review that showed smaller increases in EDA (levels, nonspecific fluctuations, or smaller anticipatory phasic responses) during a time period prior to an *anticipated* stressor. The anticipated stressor usually was electric shock (Hare, 1965b; Hare & Craigen, 1974; Lippert & Senter, 1966; Schalling & Levander, 1967; Schalling, et al., 1975; Schmauk, 1970), but also included a 120 dB fast-onset tone (Hare et al., 1978), mental arithmetic (Schalling et al., 1975), social disapproval (Schmauk, 1970) and shock to another subject (Sutker, 1970). In the Hare et al. (1978) study, differences were not obtained when inmates were defined as psychopaths by ratings on Cleckley's criteria, but were obtained when the psychopathic and nonpsychopathic groups were further subdivided on the basis of So scores. Only the subjects that were rated as Cleckley psychopaths *and* had low So scores showed lower SCL increases and fewer nonspecific SCRs in anticipation of the aversive tones. After Hare's review, Tharp, Maltzman, Syndulko, & Ziskind (1980) reported similar results using noninstitutionalized psychopathic subjects recruited from Gamblers Anonymous in a countdown procedure with a 95 dB 1,000 Hz tone as the mildly aversive stimulus. Compared with normal controls, the anticipatory increase in SCL for the psychopathic gamblers began later and was smaller in magnitude.

## SCRs to Discrete Stimuli

**Signal Stimuli.** Classical aversive conditioning studies are often viewed as parallel to those just reviewed that include anticipation of punishment, yet the dependent measures differ. Whereas nonspecific EDRs and changes in SCL are of interest in the previous studies, in classical conditioning paradigms it is the SCR to the conditioned stimulus (CS) that is of interest. This SCR is said to be a signal OR, because the CS acquires signal value through its pairing with the UCS.

In the seminal study in this literature, Lykken (1957) assessed conditioned anxiety with SR responses (SRRs) as the conditioned response (CR) and electric shock as the unconditioned stimulus (UCS). Prison inmates selected on the basis of Cleckley's criteria for psychopathy were termed primary sociopaths. Those who did not meet the Cleckley criteria in certain respects were termed neurotic sociopaths. Normal (non-inmate) controls were roughly matched on age, IQ, and socioeconomic background. The SRRs of the primary sociopaths to the CS during conditioning were significantly smaller than those of the normal controls. The SRRs of the neurotic sociopaths during conditioning resembled those of the primary psychopaths, but this group showed a perseveration of responding during extinction that was significantly greater than even the normal controls. Lykken suggested the prolonged SRRs during extinction indicated perseveration of the anxiety response in the neurotic group and concluded that only the primary sociopaths were defective in conditioning anxiety responses.

Lykken's conditioning results have been replicated by other investigators. Hare (1965a) found that psychopathic inmates produced fewer SCRs to the CS during conditioning than did nonpsychopathic inmates. He also reported that the conditioning was more narrowly defined by the psychopathic subjects, in the sense that they showed less response generalization from the 1,000 Hz CS to a 153 Hz generalization stimulus. Similarly, the psychopathic inmates in Hare and Quinn's (1971) study produced only very small SCRs and failed to show differential conditioning to the CS+ (associated with shock) versus the CS- (not followed by anything), whereas the nonpsychopathic inmates gave much larger SCRs to the CS+ than to the CS-. Hare and Craigen (1974) found that psychopaths gave smaller SCRs to the onset of 10 second tones signalling shock at tone offset. Ziskind, Syndulko, and Maltzman (1977) reported deficient classical conditioning for psychopaths in two experiments: they either failed to establish differential conditioning (Experiment 1) or showed rapid habituation of a conditioned electrodermal response in spite of continued pairing with the aversive UCS. In a study of patients discharged from a state institution for dangerous or violent mental defectives, many or most of whom "could fit a legal definition of the psychopath" (p. 936), Tong (1959) reported that poor classical conditioning was associated with relapse within one year. The UCS consisted of a brush on the closed eyelid with a piece of cotton and the CS was a simultaneous auditory click. Specific diagnoses of psychopathy were not reported.

Raine & Venables (1981) examined classical conditioning among a representative sample of 15-year-old male school children. Antisocial behavior, assessed by teacher ratings and by a self-report measure (derived from a factor analysis of 18 standardized self-report scales), was not related to conditioning in the initial analysis with the entire sample. However, when they divided the sample into high vs. low social class, the expected association between poor conditioning and low socialization was found among high social class boys for both self-report and teacher ratings. The authors proposed that biological influences are stronger in the higher social classes where environmental influences toward antisocial behavior are minimized. The effect of high social class may have been to exclude subcultural delinquents.

Delameter and Lahey (1983) induced signal value by a reaction time paradigm in which learning disabled children (average age approximately 10 years) pressed a telegraph key as quickly as they could following high frequency tones but not low frequency tones. Subdivision into four groups on the basis of tension-anxiety and conduct problem scales on the Conners (1969) Teacher Rating Scale yielded a conduct problem x tension-anxiety crossover interaction for both high and low frequency tones. Among low tension-anxiety children conduct problems were associated with smaller SCRs to the tones, whereas among high tension-anxiety children conduct problems were associated with larger SCRs. The differences between high and low conduct problem children appeared to be greater among low tension-anxiety children. Even though the selection for learning disability differs from the other studies reviewed here, the finding that the association of antisocial behavior with electrodermal hyporeactivity may be restricted to low tension-anxiety children is of interest, as is the use of a reaction time paradigm.

Some stimuli have pre-existing signal value to the subject. In a rare study with negatively-valenced stimuli, psychopaths showed smaller SCRs to pictures of severe facial injuries (Mathis, 1970). In contrast, slides of female nudes (presumably having a positive valence) did not produce a significant difference in the Hare and Quinn (1972) study, although there was a trend toward smaller responses to the slides of nudes for the psychopaths (0.73 microsiemens) than the nonpsychopaths (4.10 microsiemens). In the discussion of his paper, Borkovec (1970) comments that he found normal SCR reactivity in psychopaths to repeated pictures of a nude female, but he does not report details of the results. Schmauk (1970) reported normal SCRs among psychopaths in anticipation of the loss of money. Although the loss of money is technically a punishment condition, perhaps the positive valence quality of money was critical. Using the eyeblink startle paradigm rather than EDRs, Patrick found diminished reactivity to aversive stimuli but normal reactivity to positively-valenced stimuli among psychopaths (Lang, Bradley, Cuthbert, & Patrick, 1993). These studies suggest the possibility of a selective deficit to stimuli with negative valence, although clearly more studies are needed to exclude a generalized hyporeactivity hypothesis.

**Comment.** In spite of the differences in electrodermal measures and temporal parameters, studies involving changes in SCL and/or counts of nonspecific SCRs in the anticipation of aversive stimulation and those employing SCR amplitude in classical aversive conditioning appear to yield parallel, moderately reliable results. The specific electrodermal measure and the temporal aspects appear to be less important than the presence of an aversive stimulus. In addition, there is slight evidence that stimuli involving signal value other than being paired with shock or noxious noise may also reveal hyporeactivity among antisocial subjects. These findings are in sharp contrast with the weak and unreliable findings in conditions of minimal stimulation. As Hare (1978) noted, the hyporeactivity in anticipation of painful stimuli is consistent with the traditional hypothesis that psychopaths show very little anticipatory fear to cues associated with painful stimuli.

**Nonsignal Stimuli.** Many studies, especially those with children, employ a series of tones of low to moderate intensity to elicit SC ORs. Discussion of this paradigm has been delayed to this point, because the issues involved represent a digression from the relatively simple picture presented above.

Borkovec (1970) found smaller SCRs to the first tone for psychopathic than for subcultural delinquents but no differences thereafter. Siddle, Nicol, and Foggitt (1973) also reported a smaller response to the first tone in a series for their most psychopathic group among male prison inmates. Schmidt, Solanto, and Bridger (1985) exposed undersocialized aggressive conduct disordered children (approximately 10 years of age) and normal controls to a series of eight 75-dB tones followed (after a rest period) by eight

90 dB bell sounds. No differences were found to the tones (failing to replicate the two studies just cited), but the conduct disordered group did show a smaller SCR to the first bell. Prior to the bell series the experimenter told the subject that the sounds "will not be really scary, but loud," instructions intended to "induce mild anticipatory anxiety" (p. 655) and possibly creating anxiety that facilitated a larger SCR among the controls but not the conduct disordered children. In their study of learning disabled children Delameter and Lahey reported a trend ($\underline{p}$ < .06) for a main effect of conduct problem during a series of ten nonsignal tones, with conduct problem associated with smaller SCR amplitudes. On the other hand, there were no group differences in the response to two novel tones that followed the ten identical tones--a negative finding inconsistent with the positive results for the initial tone (the most novel) in the studies of Borkovec (1970) and Siddle et al. (1973).

Raine and Venables (1984a) rejected the hypothesis that antisocial behavior is associated with a smaller response to the first tone in a habituation series. Although acknowledging the positive results reported by Borkovec (1970) and Siddle, Nicol, & Foggitt (1973), they cite 6 experiments (Blackburn, 1979; Hare, 1968; Hinton, O'Neil, Dishman, & Webster, 1979 - two failures; Hinton, O'Neil, Hamilton, & Burke, 1980; Lippert & Senter, 1966) plus their own with negative results, all of which examined the SCR to the first tone in a series of repetitive auditory orienting stimuli. Three additional studies (Goldstein, 1965; Hare, 1978; Ziskind, Syndulko, & Maltzman, 1978) used somewhat different stimulation paradigms or scoring methods and also found no differences. To this latter list might be added Hare, Frazelle, & Cox as reported in Hare (1978), who found no differences to 80 dB tones embedded in a series of varying intensity .

In their own study, Raine and Venables (1984a) found an association between antisocial behavior and number of SCRs to all nine tones. Their subjects were those described for Raine and Venables (1981) above. The canonical correlation between the frequency of SCORs to the tones and the pooled assessments of antisocial behavior was 0.44 (p < .001) with antisocial boys showing fewer SCRs. In a further analysis, Raine and Venables dichotomized subjects as electrodermal responders/nonresponders and as Antisocial/Prosocial. Eighty percent of nonresponders were Antisocials, indicating a strong association, but this was such a small group that the majority (78%) of Antisocials were electrodermal responders. In view of this result, they subdivided the Antisocials into "Antisocial Responders" and "Antisocial Nonresponders" and compared them with "Prosocials" (not subdivided on SCR responding). The Antisocial Nonresponders were higher than the Prosocials (but not the Antisocial Responders) on a composite of Introversion and Psychoticism scores on the Junior Eysenck Personality Questionnaire. The authors concluded that 'it is specifically a "schizoid" group of antisocials who are characterized by nonresponding' (p. 430) and argued for a link between antisociality and psychosis-proneness.

A nine-year follow-up of the Raine and Venables (1981) sample by Raine, Venables, and Williams (1990a, 1990b) found that 17 of the 101 subjects had a criminal record. Looking backward to the original electrodermal data, the 17 criminals showed fewer SCORs to tones and a higher proportion of nonresponders to tones (Raine et al., 1990a) and fewer nonspecific SCRs during rest (Raine et al., 1990b) at age 15 than did the remaining subjects. Differences on "schizoid" scores were not reported for the criminals.

Raine (1987) failed to find a relationship between psychopathic criminals rated with Hare's (1980) Checklist among inmates in a top-security prison and frequency of SCRs to a series of 12 tones. A positive relationship (r = -.43) for SCR frequency was found with "Anhedonia-Psychoticism" (a composite of four scales that were orthogonal to one another: Social Anhedonia, Physical Anhedonia, Psychoticism, and Hallucinatory Predisposition) but not with "Schizphrenism" (a composite of four scales that did intercorrelate significantly: Schizophrenism, Disordered Thinking, Withdrawn-Disturbed Relationships and Perceptual Abberation). When the subjects were subdivided on the basis of whether before the age of ten they had lived in broken vs. intact homes, the correlation between SCR frequency and Anhedonia-Psychoticism was a significant -.51 for the intact homes sample and a nonsignificant -.26 for the broken homes sample. The author did not report whether these two correlations were significantly different. On the basis of results with WAIS digit span and arithmetic subtests, Raine concluded that an attentional disturbance in schizoid antisocials is responsible for the smaller number of SCRs to tones and accounts for the association between antisociality and psychosis-proneness. He rejected the notion that psychopathy is related to reduced orienting or shows autonomic hyporesponsivity, although he did not consider the many positive findings with threats of aversive stimulation reviewed above.

**The SCR Recovery Limb.** A few investigators have reported that antisocial subjects show a slower return of their SCRs to baseline conductance levels (e.g., see Blackburn, 1983; Hare, 1978). For example, Siddle (1977) found slower recovery for a high antisocial group compared to low antisocial inmates. Levander, Schalling, Lidberg, Bartfai, and Lidberg (1980) reported that, among criminals, slow EDR recovery time during responses to (moderately aversive) 93 dB tones was associated with high scores on De and, to a lesser extent, with a measure of impulsivity. As argued in the introduction, these results can be attributed to diminished EDA.

**EDR Hyporeactivity in Noncriminal Populations.** Waid and Orne have found electrodermal hyporeactivity among college students who score low on the So scale. This was found for noxious (98 dB) noise bursts by Waid (1976) and to an unexpected loud hand clap by Waid, Orne, and Wilson (1979). Waid, Orne, and Wilson (1979) reported significant correlations between So scores and the mean SCR accompanying deception across four different lie detection tests and across all test questions in the four tests for innocent subjects (r = .56). Waid and Orne (1982) found smaller SCRs for low So subjects in a verbal response conflict task modified from the Stroop Color-Word Interference Test.

Crider (this volume) called attention to two important studies: Jones (1950) and Block (1957). In a longitudinal study of one hundred adolescents, Jones (1950) obtained EDRs in a series of 11 experiments "in the mild stress situation of a free association test" (p. 164). The 20 high and 20 low reactive subjects were then compared on independent ratings of overt behavioral characteristics. The low EDR responders were rated by psychologists (who studied them for years) as easily excited, irritable, impulsive, irresponsible, more talkative, more attention-seeking, more animated, more assertive, and extremely uninhibited, and they were rated by peers as more attention-seeking, talkative, restless, and bossy. In terms of motivational bases of behavior, psychologists rated them as showing drives for aggression, dominance, recognition, and escape. The latter is described as a tendency to avoid tension, to project failures on others or on circumstances, and to embrace immediate pleasures rather than sacrifice pleasures for future goals. Jones suggested that these characteristics within a normal sample are mild versions of the "impulse neurotic" who discharges tensions immediately and emphasized that the low EDR responders showed more overt emotional expression.

Jones' results inspired Block (1957) to study 70 applicants for medical school who were observed during an 18-hour assessment. On the basis of overall EDR reactivity in a lie detection test, the 20 most reactive and 20 least reactive subjects were compared on psychologists' ratings. He described the highly reactive subjects as "withdrawing, worrying individuals who turn their anxieties toward internal routes of expression" and the least reactive subjects as "independent, aggressively direct, and relatively nonconforming, all of these being visible rather than inward or covert expressions of impulses" (p. 13). Block concluded that the dimension underlying his results was a version of that described by Jones, but argued that EDR reactivity is simply an index of anxiety or affect in a given situation and has no implications for whether tension is discharged in motor activity.

These studies combine to suggest that EDA hyporeactivity is not limited to criminal populations and provide some indication as to the nature of this dimension. Hyporeactive individuals are impulsive and uninhibited, whereas reactive individuals are withdrawing and worrying. In the theoretical discussion below, it is proposed that worry and withdrawal (behavioral inhibition) mark the high anxiety end of the dimension of anxiety that is deficient in psychopathy--further supporting the relevance of these studies to psychopathy. Finding this dimension among normal subjects implies that it is not related to criminality per se, but rather may constitute a temperament risk factor for criminality that interacts with environmental factors.

## THEORETICAL INTERPRETATIONS

### The Anxiety Hypothesis

Although space does not permit a comprehensive review of theoretical interpretations of the electrodermal data, it is possible to address some of the major theories and current issues. The dominant approach has been to view electrodermal activity as an index of conditioned anticipatory anxiety (e.g., Hare, 1970; Hare & Quinn, 1971; Lykken, 1957). By way of illustration, Hare (1970, Chapter 6) cited Mowrer's two-factor theory of avoidance learning, in which fear responses are acquired through classical conditioning and then, in turn, serve to motivate and reinforce both active and passive avoidance. Passive avoidance (the avoidance of a response-contingent punishment by not making the response) is particularly important in this theory: the psychopath's impulsivity is viewed as a form of poor passive avoidance with regard to future (response-contingent) punishments. In approach-avoidance conflict situations, in which both rewards and punishments may be expected as a result of some action, this poor passive avoidance hypothesis accounts for the psychopath's inability to resist temptation--e.g., cashing bad checks, abusing credit. It is of importance to the discussion below that the anxiety in question involves *anticipatory* fear responses and feelings of *apprehension*.

The early studies (reviewed above) showing electrodermal hyporeactivity in the anticipation of punishment were consistent with the anxiety conditioning/passive avoidance hypothesis. Data on heart rate changes, on the other hand, were not supportive. By the time of Hare's (1978) review, it was clear that cardiac responses to simple stimuli such as tones and shock do not differ between psychopaths and controls (p. 130). In studies involving the anticipation of punishment, Hare and Quinn (1971) found normal cardiovascular responses in a classical conditioning paradigm, but Hare (1978) cited other studies in which cardiac acceleration in the anticipation of noxious stimuli was greater for criminal psychopaths than controls (Hare & Craigen, 1974; Hare et al., 1978) and for non-criminal subjects scoring low on the So scale (Hare, 1978, Note 6; Schalling, 1975) or on the anxiety scale used in Lykken's (1957) study (Lykken, MacIndoe, & Tellegen, 1972). These results precluded a simple autonomic hyporesponsivity hypothesis and required an explanation for the specificity of heart rate and electrodermal activity.

Hare's (1978) solution was to apply Lacey's (1967) intake-rejection hypothesis. In this hypothesis, cardiac deceleration lowers blood pressure in the carotid sinus which, in turn, increases cortical arousal and makes the brain receptive to sensory intake, whereas cardiac acceleration has the opposite effect--increased blood pressure, decreased cortical arousal, and sensory rejection. Hare argued that psychopaths have an efficient coping response that promotes cardiac acceleration in anticipation of aversive stimulation with beneficial results (reduced responsiveness to pain) and that "electrodermal activity gives some indication of how successful the attempts are" (p. 136). The psychopath's difficulty in avoiding punishments was attributed to a reduction in anticipatory fear because the relevant cues are 'tuned out.' This model emphasizes an attentional consequence of the efficient coping mechanisms, rather than a direct effect of poor anxiety conditioning as in his earlier view. Hare (1978) also cited Obrist's (1976) active coping hypothesis, in which Obrist argued that attempts to actively cope with an impending aversive stimulus (by making some response) will produce cardiac acceleration, whereas passively accepting the punishment is associated with cardiac deceleration, or at least an absence of acceleration. Hare then commented that the psychopath's cardiac acceleration possibly is "a reflection of active attempts to cope with the impending stressor" (p. 138).

It is not clear from Hare's comments whether he intended the active coping hypothesis as an alternative to Lacey's intake-rejection or as an extension of it. Further, it is not entirely clear whether Hare fully intended to embrace the Lacey hypothesis, in which cardiac acceleration is a critical component of the *causal* pathway to controlling the brain's response to sensory input, or whether he thought of the cardiac response more as an *index* of a central coping process. It should be noted that Obrist's active coping hypothesis was presented in the context of criticizing Lacey's intake-rejection hypothesis and as representing an alternative, making it difficult to integrate the two. Further, the Lacey hypothesis involves the assumption that the brain takes a circuitous causal pathway via the cardiovascular system in order to control its own sensitivity to stimulation, and it makes the cardiac acceleration the primary causal factor. Even assuming the validity of the carotid sinus pressure mechanism, using it to explain all of psychopathic behavior places a heavy demand on a peripheral mechanism. Finally, this hypothesis encounters difficulty explaining findings of electrodermal hyporeactivity that are not accompanied by differences in cardiac acceleration--e.g., Tharp et al. (1980).

Fowles (1980) adopted an alternative approach to explaining the dissociation between heart rate and electrodermal activity--one based on an integration of Obrist's active coping hypothesis with Gray's motivational theory. Gray (e.g., 1987) argued that two major motivational systems respond to conditioned stimuli, one concerned with behavioral activation and one with behavioral inhibition. The behavioral activation system (BAS) activates behavior in response to CSs for response-contingent reward (simple reward paradigm) or for relieving nonpunishment (active avoidance paradigm). The behavioral inhibition system (BIS) inhibits behavior in response to CSs for response-contingent punishment (approach-avoidance conflict paradigm) or frustrative nonreward (extinction paradigm). Activity in the BAS is associated with positive affect (hope, relief), whereas that in the BIS is associated with negative affect (fear or anxiety, frustration). The various anxiolytic drugs (alcohol, barbiturates, minor tranquilizers) reduce the efficacy of the BIS. Gray argued that the BIS is the neurophysiological substrate for anxiety. Several authors (Gray, 1970; Fowles, 1980; see especially Trasler, 1978; Quay, 1990) have proposed that psychopathic behavior can be seen as reflecting a quantitative weakness of the BIS (and possibly a strong BAS, as well). This hypothesis accounts for (1) impulsivity in the form of poor passive avoidance and poor extinction, (2) reduced anxiety in response to CSs for punishment or failure, and (3) normal active avoidance of punishment.

Drawing on the work of Obrist and others, as well as the widely-accepted cardiac-somatic coupling hypothesis, Fowles (1980) proposed that heart rate is more strongly tied to the BAS (reward incentives, active avoidance) than to the BIS. At the same time, he argued that EDA appears to reflect the emotional response to threats of punishment and, at least in that sense, could be used to assess the BIS reaction to such threats. Thus, the diminished EDA seen in psychopaths faced with threats of punishment were consistent with the weak BIS hypothesis, and the failure of heart rate to follow this pattern was attributed to its independence of the BIS. The greater cardiac acceleration in anticipation of punishment was attributed to a dominance of active avoidance tendencies (BAS) over inhibitory processes associated with passively accepting the punishment. The attractive features of this proposal were that it accounted for the divergent electrodermal and heart rate patterns while retaining the original link between deficient anxiety and impulsivity--albeit in the context of a somewhat different theory of motivation. The post hoc quality of the explanation for the cardiac acceleration is a weakness, although it is not unreasonable in view of data on animals and humans facing an impending punishment, where both cardiac acceleration and deceleration can be seen, with deceleration emerging as animals stop struggling to escape and as human subjects become resigned to the punishment.

## Additional Hypotheses

**The Attentional Deficit Hypothesis.** Other theories have focused on attentional factors. Possibly the most salient of these is the suggestion by Raine and Venables (Raine, 1987; Raine & Venables, 1984a) that their finding of an association between nonresponding to tones and a schizoid antisocial personality primarily reflects an attentional deficit. Since it is common to view the OR as reflecting attentional processes (e.g., Bernstein, Frith, Gruzelier, Patterson, Straube, Venables, & Zahn, 1982; Filion, Dawson, Schell, & Hazlett, 1991), this theory is particularly suited to the OR paradigm. On the other hand, Raine and Venables have not explained how the attentional hypothesis would account for the results for the larger literature reviewed above. One possibility is to suggest two deficits--one to nonsignal stimuli, the other in anticipation of punishments-- that apply to different subtypes of antisocial individuals. This possibility is of interest in connection with Schalling's proposal of schizoid and impulsive subtypes (see below). A second possibility would be to attribute the attentional deficits to motivational factors, although Raine (1987, p. 285) rejects both motivational and arousal explanations. At present, it is unclear how to evaluate the attentional hypothesis. It should also be noted that the definitions of schizoid personality employed in these studies are somewhat unusual and that the results need replication, not to mention positive evidence for a genetic link to schizophrenia.

A second line of research on attentional correlates of EDA is the literature on lability-stability among normal college students. Lability-stability is defined jointly in terms of the number of nonspecific EDRs at rest and the number of trials to habituation for electrodermal ORs to a series of tones, with stabiles being hyporeactive on both. Lability-stability has been related to attentional factors (Schell, Dawson, & Filion, 1988) and to a personality dimension of antisociality (Crider, this volume). Crider's stimulating review, in particular, seems to indicate a relevance to psychopathy and, as mentioned above, he cites the studies by Jones (1950) and Block (1957). On the other hand, it is not clear how strong is the connection between lability-stability and psychopathy in view of the very weak findings for psychopaths on the two electrodermal indices that define lability-stability.

**Two Types of Anxiety.** A substantial modification of the anxiety deficit hypothesis may be in order. In an extensive review of the literature on the anxiety disorders, Barlow (1988) argues forcefully for two types of anxiety, one preparatory and one acute. "Anxiety" or "*anxious apprehension*" prepares the organism to cope with the challenges and stresses of everyday life. Barlow views this preparatory anxious apprehension as the process underlying *Generalized Anxiety Disorder*. It consists of a diffuse cognitive-affective structure including negative affect, high arousal, perceptions of helplessness or uncontrollability of future events, and worry (pp. 235, 247). "Fear" is a massive "*alarm reaction*" to potentially life-threatening situations. The most frequent alarm reaction involves strong behavioral and cardiovascular activation, which Barlow equates with Cannon's well-known "fight or flight" response (pp. 3-4, 158). *Panic attacks* are viewed as alarm reactions. In contrast to the traditional view of the fight/flight response as a reaction only to a life-threatening event (a "true alarm"), Barlow concludes that this same reaction can occur without such an event, in which case the uncued panic attack is a "false alarm." Thus, false alarms or panic attacks include a sudden burst of anxiety accompanied by somatic symptoms and by a fear of dying and/or losing control.

Fowles (1992a) proposed that Barlow's anxious apprehension is parallel to Gray's BIS and that Barlow's alarm reaction parallels Gray's fight/flight system. Gray's fight/flight system has heretofore been neglected, because according to Gray it responds to unconditioned stimuli for punishment--a rationale response rather than the irrational forms of anxiety seen in a clinical context. With Barlow's concept of false alarms, it is reasonable to consider that the fight/light system may go awry and is clinically relevant.

In the context of antisocial behavior, this perspective lends considerable importance to Schalling's (1978) review of her own work, in which she distinguished two kinds of anxiety. On the basis of a cluster analysis of ratings of psychiatric patients, Schalling contrasted *psychic anxiety* with *somatic anxiety*. Following additional studies, she described psychic anxiety as including "worry, anticipatory anxiousness, slow recuperation after stress, sensitivity, insecurity, and social anxiety" (p. 88)--a description remarkably similar to Barlow's anxious apprehension. Somatic anxiety consists of "autonomic disturbances, vague distress and panic attacks, and distractability" (p. 88). The reference to panic attacks, the autonomic disturbances, and the vagueness of the stimulus for distress all link somatic anxiety to Barlow's alarm reaction. Schalling's work shows that psychopaths "tend to have more vague distress and panic, more cardiovascular symptoms and muscular tenseness, but less worry and anticipatory concern than non-psychopaths have" (p. 89)-- i.e., they are *high* on somatic anxiety and *low* on psychic anxiety. This juxtaposition of Schalling's work with Barlow's theory supports the deficient BIS hypothesis of psychopathy, but it underscores the need to differentiate somatic anxiety, which will be high in some psychopaths. Additionally, Schalling reported that somatic anxiety is positively correlated with impulsivity--a finding consistent with the old idea that a state of arousal (from somatic anxiety) might energize behavior, and thereby increase impulsivity in some individuals. This analysis is certainly more complex than the traditional view that low anxiety is related to impulsivity. Perhaps this hypothesis could help to clarify the orthogonality of scales that appear to measure behavioral inhibition and scales that measure neuroticism/anxiety or negative affect (see Fowles, 1983, 1992b; Tellegen, 1985). It may well be that the scales measuring neuroticism are more strongly tied to somatic anxiety/alarm than to the psychic anxiety/anxious apprehension dimension underlying psychopathy (see also Lykken, 1957).

**Possible Subtypes.** Schalling (1978) cited Mayer-Gross, Slater, & Roth (1954) for the existence of two subgroups within the psychopaths identified by Cleckley ratings or low So scores: (1) the Unstable Drifters or *impulsiveness syndrome*, characterized by impulsiveness, stimulus-seeking, high somatic anxiety, an easy-going style, leading aimless lives, inability to learn from experience, and indifference to their own future and past; and (2) the Cold and Emotionally Callous or *detachment syndrome*, characterized by low empathy, detachment (a lack of close, warm interpersonal relations), a lack of concern for others, poverty of affect and suspiciousness, and high scores on the Eysenck Psychoticism Scale. Following Mayer-Gross et al., Schalling suggests that the detachment syndrome is related to a *schizoid personality* type that is found in excess among the relatives of schizophrenics. Finally, Schalling calls attention to developmental theories that argue that the development of conscience does not depend solely on anxiety-mediated avoidance learning. Rather, internalization of social norms is strongly facilitated by warm attachments (perhaps especially with the same-sexed parent).

The present author was unable to follow completely Schalling's application of these subtypes to her own research on EDA hyporeactivity. Consequently, the following comments are entirely speculative. What is interesting, nevertheless, is a possible etiologic pathway that has a basis in a lack of early attachments. The implication appears to be that the absence of warm attachments could happen to a perfectly normal child as a result of external factors or could happen as a result of a child's inability to form warm attachments due to genetic loading for a schizoid personality. Such individuals might not show the

EDA deficit in the anticipation of punishment discussed above, and a schizoid subset of them might show a different deficit. On the other hand, there are problems with this train of thought. First, the clinical description of poverty of affect might suggest limited anxiety reactions to potential punishment. Second, it is not at all clear how mutually exclusive are these clinically-based subtypes. For example, Fowles (1980) suggested that poor attachments might be secondary to impulsivity, reflecting conflict with the social environment as a result of impulsivity--a suggestion consistent with the impact of impulsive behavior on parents and peers and consistent with peer rejection secondary to impulsivity. Similarly, there may be an impulsivity component associated with the detachment syndrome, especially in view of its association with high scores on the Eysenck Psychoticism scale. Tellegen (1985, p. 699) notes that impulsivity is a strong component of this scale. Additionally, Schalling (1978, Table 6.3) reported that both Psychoticism and So loaded 0.83 on the same factor and were the only scales with a loading above 0.5. In view of this apparent association with impulsivity and the broad application of the So scale in studies of antisocial behavior, it is not clear that the detachment syndrome is as distinct as the above hypothesis suggests. Nevertheless, this is an interesting subtype distinction and etiological hypothesis to pursue, if only because it might reduce the heterogeneity of psychopathic groups with respect to impulsivity and EDA hyporeactivity.

## SUMMARY

At an empirical level, there are many findings that support an inference of electrodermal hyporeactivity among psychopaths. At present, the strongest findings seem interpretable as reflecting a weak response to the anticipation of punishment--consistent with the weak behavioral inhibition system hypothesis--but studies are needed that compare equally stimulating positive versus negative stimuli to preclude a more general hyporeactivity hypothesis.

Other questions have been raised in the present review. These include the implications of the two anxiety hypothesis for both the diagnosis of psychopathy and the measurement of electrodermal reactivity, the relationship of responding to simple tones to the hyporeactivity seen in anticipation of punishment and in other stimulating conditions, the possible contribution of a schizoid psychopathic subtype, the relationship of the personality dimension of Socialization to criminality and the concept of psychopathy, and the role of attentional as opposed to motivational factors in antisocial behavior.

## REFERENCES

Barlow, D. H., 1988, "Anxiety and its Disorders: The Nature and Treatment of Anxiety and Panic," Guilford Press, New York.

Bernstein, A. S., Frith, C. D., Gruzelier, J. H., Patterson, T., Straube, E., Venables, P. H., and Zahn, T. P., 1982, An analysis of the skin conductance orienting response in samples of American, British, and German schizophrenics. *Biol. Psychol.*, **14,** 155-211.

Blackburn, R., 1979, Cortical and autonomic arousal in primary and secondary psychopaths. *Psychophysiol.*, **16,** 143-150.

Blackburn, R., 1983, Psychopathy, delinquency and crime, *in:* "Physiological Correlates of Human Behavior, Vol. 3," A. Gale and J. A. Edwards, eds., Academic Press, New York.

Block, J., 1957, A study of affective responsiveness in a lie-detection situation. *J. Abnorm. Soc. Psychol.*, **55,** 11-15.

Borkovec, T. D., 1970, Autonomic reactivity to sensory stimulation in psychopathic, neurotic, and normal juvenile delinquents. *J. Consult. Clin. Psychol.*, **35,** 217-222.

Cleckley, H., 1950, "The Mask of Sanity (2nd Ed.)," St. Louis: Mosby.

Cleckley, H., 1964, "The Mask of Sanity (4th Ed.),' St. Louis: Mosby.

Conners, C. A., 1969, A teacher rating scale for use in drug studies with children. *Am. J. Psychiat.*, **127**, 884-888.

Delamater, A. M., and Lahey, B. B., 1983, Physiological correlates of conduct problems and anxiety in hyperactive and learning-disabled children. *J. Abnorm. Child Psychol.*, **11**, 85-100.

Dengerink, H. A., and Bertilson, H. S., 1975, Psychopathy and physiological arousal in an aggressive task. *Psychophysiol.*, **12**, 682-684.

Edelberg, R., 1970, The information content of the recovery limb of the electrodermal response. *Psychophysiol.*, **6**, 527-539.

Edelberg, R., 1972, Electrodermal recovery rate, goal-orientation, and aversion. *Psychophysiol.*, **9**, 512-520.

Edelberg, R., and Muller, M., 1981, Prior activity as a determinant of electrodermal recovery rate. *Psychophysiol.*, **18**, 17-25.

Filion, D. L., Dawson, M. E., Schell, A. M., and Hazlett, E. A., 1991, The relationship between skin conductance orienting and the allocation of processing resources. *Psychophysiol.*, **28**, 410-424.

Fowles, D. C., 1980, The three arousal model: Implications of Gray's two-factor learning theory for heart rate, electrodermal activity, and psychopathy. *Psychophysiol.*, **17**, 87-104.

Fowles, D., 1983, Motivational effects on heart rate and electrodermal activity: Implications for research on personality and psychopathology. *J. Res. Person.*, **17**, 48-71.

Fowles, D., 1986, The eccrine system and electrodermal activity, *in:* "Psychophysiology: Systems, Processes, and Applications, Vol. 1," M. G. H. Coles, S. W. Porges, and E. Donchin, eds., Guilford Press, New York.

Fowles, D., 1992a, A motivational approach to anxiety disorders, *in:* "Anxiety: Recent Developments in Self-appraisal, Psychophysiological, and Health Research," D. G. Forgays, T. Sosnowski, and K. Wrzesniewski, eds., Hemisphere/Taylor and Francis, London.

Fowles, D., 1992b, Schizophrenia: Diathesis-stress revisited. *Ann. Rev. Psychol.*, **43**, 303-336.

Goldstein, I. B., 1965, The relationship of muscle tension and autonomic activity to psychiatric disorders. *Psychosom. Med.*, **27**, 39-52.

Gray, J. A., 1970, The psychophysiological basis of introversion-extraversion. *Behav. Res. Therapy*, **8**, 249-266.

Gray, J. A., 1987, "The Psychology of Fear and Stress (2nd Ed.)," Cambridge University Press, Cambridge.

Gough, H. G., 1960, Theory and measurement of socialization. *J. Consult. Psychol.*, **24**, 23-30.

Gough, H. G., and Peterson, D. R., 1952, The identification and measurement of predispositional factors in crime and delinquency. *J. Consult. Psychol.*, **16**, 207-212.

Hare, R. D., 1965a, Acquisition and generalization of a conditioned fear response in psychopathic and non-psychopathic criminals. *J. Psychol.*, **59**, 367-370.

Hare, R. D., 1965b, Temporal gradient of fear arousal in psychopaths. *J. Abnorm. Psychol.*, **70**, 442-445.

Hare, R. D., 1968, Psychopathy, autonomic functioning, and the orienting response. *J. Abnorm. Psychol.*, Monogr. Suppl. **73**, no. 3, 1-24.

Hare, R., 1970, "Psychopathy," Wiley, New York.

Hare, R. D., 1972, Psychopathy and physiological responses to adrenalin. *J. Abnorm. Psychol.*, **79**, 138-147.

Hare, R. D., 1978a, Electrodermal and cardiovascular correlates of psychopathy, *in:* "Psychopathic Behavior: Approaches to Research," R. D. Hare and D. Schalling, eds., Wiley, New York.

Hare, R. D., 1978b, Psychopathy and electrodermal responses to nonsignal stimulation. *Biol. Psychol.*, **6**, 237-246.

Hare, R. D., 1980, A research scale for the assessment of psychopathy in criminal populations. *Person. Indiv. Diff.*, **1**, 111-119.

Hare, R. D., and Craigen, D., 1974, Psychopathy and physiological activity in a mixed-motive game situation. *Psychophysiol.*, **11**, 197-206.

Hare, R. D., Frazelle, J., and Cox, D. N., 1978, Psychopathy and physiological responses to threat of an aversive stimulus. *Psychophysiol.*, **15**, 165-172.

Hare, R. D., and Quinn, M. J., 1971, Psychopathy and autonomic conditioning. *J. Abnorm. Psychol.*, **77,** 223-235.

Hinton, J., O'Neil, M., Dishman, J., and Webster, S., 1979, Electrodermal indices of public offending and recidivism. *Biol. Psychol.*, **9,** 297-310.

Hinton, J., O'Neil, M., Hamilton, S., and Burke, M., 1980, Psychophysiological differentiation between psychopathic and schizophrenic abnormal offenders. *Brit. J. Soc. Clin. Psychol.*, **19,** 257-269.

Jones, H. E., 1950, The study of patterns of emotional expression, *in*: "Feelings and Emotions: The Mooseheart Symposium," M. L. Reymert, ed., McGraw-Hill, New York.

Lacey, J. I., 1967, Somatic response patterning and stress: Some revisions of activation theory, *in*: "Psychological Stress: Issues in Research," N. H. Appley and R. Trumbell, eds., Appleton-Century-Crofts, New York.

Lang, P. J., Bradley, M., Cuthbert, B. N., and Patrick, C. J., 1993, Emotion and psychopathology: A startle probe analysis, *in:* Models and Methods of Psychopathology, L. J. Chapman, J. P. Chapman, and D. C. Fowles, eds., Springer Publishing Company, New York.

Levander, S. E., Schalling, D. S., Lidberg, L., Bartfai, A., and Lidberg, Y., 1980, Skin conductance recovery time and personality in a group of criminals. *Psychophysiol.*, **17 ,** 105-111.

Lippert, W. W., and Senter, R. J., 1966, Electrodermal responses in the sociopath. *Psychon. Sci.*, **4,** 25-26.

Lykken, D. T., 1957, A study of anxiety in the sociopathic personality. *J. Abnorm. Soc. Psychol.*, **55,** 6-10.

Lykken, D. T., MacIndoe, I., and Tellegen, A., 1972, Autonomic response to shock as a function of predictability in time and locus. *Psychophysiol.,* **9,** 318-333.

Mathis, H. I., 1970, "Emotional Responsivity in the Antisocial Personality," Ph.D. dissertation, George Washington University, Washington, D.C.

Mayer-Gross, W., Slater, E., and Roth, M., 1954, "Clinical Psychiatry," Cassel, London.

Mednick, S. A., 1975, Autonomic nervous system recovery and psychopathology. *Scand. J. Behav. Therapy*, **4,** 55-68.

Megargee, E. I., 1972, "The California Psychological Inventory Handbook," Jossey-Bass, San Francisco.

Obrist, P., 1976, The cardiovascular-behavioral interaction--as it appears today. *Psychophysiol.*, **13,** 95-107.

Peterson, D. R., Quay, H. C., and Tiffany, T. L., 1961, Personality factors related to juvenile delinquency. *Child Devel.*, **32,** 355-372.

Quay, H. C., 1990, Electrodermal responding, inhibition, and reward-seeking in undersocialized aggressive conduct disorder. Paper presented at the annual meeting of the American Academy of Child Adolescent Psychiatry, Chicago, Illinois, October 14.

Raine, A., 1987, Effect of early environment on electrodermal and cognitive correlates of schizotypy and psychopathy in criminals. *Int. J. Psychophysiol.*, **4,** 277-287.

Raine, A. and Venables, P. H., 1981, Classical conditioning and socialization--a biosocial interaction. *Person. Indiv. Diff.*, **2,** 273-283.

Raine, A. and Venables, P. H., 1984a, Electrodermal nonresponding, antisocial behavior, and schizoid tendencies in adolescents. *Psychophysiol.*, **21,** 424-433.

Raine, A. and Venables, P. H., 1984b, Tonic heart rate level, social class and antisocial behaviour in adolescents. *Biol. Psychol.*, **18,** 123-132.

Raine, A., Venables, P. H., and Williams, M., 1990a, Autonomic orienting responses in 15-year-old male subjects and criminal behavior at age 24. *Am. J. Psychiat.*, **147,** 933-937.

Raine, A., Venables, P. H., and Williams, M., 1990b, Relationships between central and autonomic measures of arousal at age 15 and criminality at age 24 years. *Arch. Gen. Psychiat.*, **47,** 1003-1007.

Schachter, S., and Latane, B., 1964, Crime, cognition, and the autonomic nervous system, *in:* "Nebraska Symposium on Motivation (Vol. 12)," M. R. Jones, ed., University of Nebraska Press, Lincoln.

Schalling, D., 1975, The role of heart rate increase for coping with pain as related to impulsivity. Unpublished manuscript, University of Stockholm. Cited by Hare (1978) as Note 8.

Schalling, D., 1978, Psychopathy-related personality variables and the psychophysiology of socialization, *in:* "Psychopathic Behavior: Approaches to Research," R. D. Hare and D. Schalling, eds., Wiley, New York.

Schalling, D., and Levander, S., 1967, Spontaneous fluctuations in skin conductance during anticipation of pain in two delinquent groups differing in anxiety proneness. Reports from the Psychological Laboratories, The University of Stockholm, No. 306. Cited by Schalling (1978).

Schalling, D., Levander, S., and Dahlin-Lidberg, Y., 1975, A note on the relation between spontaneous fluctuations in skin conductance and heart rate, and scores on the Gough Delinquency scale. Unpublished manuscript, University of Stockholm. Cited by Hare (1978) as Note 5 and by Schalling (1978) as Note 9.

Schalling, D., Lidberg, L., Levander, S. E., and Dahlin, Y., 1973, Spontaneous autonomic activity as related to psychopathy. *Biol. Psychol.*, **1**, 83-97.

Schell, A. M., Dawson, M. E., and Filion, D. L., 1988, Psychophysiological correlates of electrodermal lability. *Psychophysiol.*, **25**, 619-632.

Schmauk, F. J., 1970, Punishment, arousal, and avoidance learning in sociopaths. *J. Abnorm. Psychol.*, **76**, 325-335.

Schmidt, K., Solanto, M. V., and Bridger, W. H., 1985, Electrodermal activity of undersocialized aggressive children: A pilot study. *J. Child Psychol. Psychiat.*, **26**, 653-660.

Siddle, D. A. T., 1977, Electrodermal activity and psychopathy, *in:* "Biosocial Bases of Criminal Behavior," S. A. Mednick and K. O. Christiansen, eds., Gardner Press, New York.

Siddle, D. A. T., Nicol, A. R., and Foggitt, R. H., 1973, Habituation and over-extinction of the GSR component of the orienting response in anti-social adolescents. *Brit. J. Soc. Clin. Psychol.*, **12**, 303-308.

Sutker, P. B., 1970, Vicarious conditioning and sociopathy. *J. Abnorm. Psychol.*, **76**, 380-386.

Tellegen, A., 1985, Structures of mood and personality and their relevance to assessing anxiety, with an emphasis on self-report, *in:* "Anxiety and the Anxiety Disorders," A. Tuma and J. Maser, eds., Lawrence Erlbaum, Hillsdale, New Jersey.

Tharp, V. K., Maltzman, I., Syndulko, K., and Ziskind, E., 1980, Autonomic activity during anticipation of an aversive tone in noninstitutionalized sociopaths. *Psychophysiol.*, **17**, 123-128.

Tong, J. E., 1959, Stress reactivity in relation to delinquent and psychopathic behaviour. *J. Ment. Science*, **105**, 935-956.

Trasler, G., 1978, Relations between psychopathy and persistent criminality--methodological and theoretical issues, *in:* "Psychopathic Behavior: Approaches to Research," R. D. Hare and D. Schalling, eds., Wiley, New York.

Waid, W. M., 1976, Skin conductance response to both signalled and unsignalled noxious stimulation predicts level of socialization. *J. Person. Soc. Psychol.*, **34**, 923-929.

Waid, W. M., and Orne, M. T., 1982, Reduced electrodermal response to conflict, failure to inhibit dominant behaviors, and delinquency proneness. *J. Person. Soc. Psychol.*, **43**, 769-774.

Waid, W. M., Orne, M. T., and Wilson, S. K., 1979, Effects of level of socialization on electrodermal detection of deception. *Psychophysiol.*, **16**, 15-22.

Ziskind, E., Syndulko, K., and Maltzman, I., 1978, Aversive conditioning in the sociopath. *Pavlovian J. Biol. Science*, **13**, 199-205.

Ziskind, E., Syndulko, K., and Maltzman, I., 1977, Evidence for a neurologic disorder in the sociopath syndrome: Aversive conditioning and recidivism, *in:* "Psychopathology and Brain Dysfunction," C. Shagass, S. Gershon, and A. I. Friedhoff, eds., Raven Press, New York.

# ELECTRODERMAL NONRESPONDING IN FIRST-EPISODE PSYCHOSIS AS A FUNCTION OF STIMULUS SIGNIFICANCE

William G. Iacono,[1] John W. Ficken,[1] and Morton Beiser[2]

[1] Department of Psychology
University of Minnesota
Minneapolis, MN 55455
USA

[2] Clarke Institute of Psychiatry
Toronto, Ontario M5T 1R8
Canada

## INTRODUCTION

Although electrodermal activity has been studied in psychiatric patients since the turn of the century, it has only been during the last two decades that specific electrodermal deviations associated with functional psychosis have been reliably identified. The most well established of these is the failure to emit an electrodermal response when presented with innocuous stimuli of moderate intensity, usually within the context of an orienting response-habituation paradigm. In this chapter, we have reviewed the literature on electrodermal nonresponding (EDNR) in schizophrenia and the mood disorders. Because the signal value or meaningfulness of stimuli may differentially affect the likelihood of observing EDNR in individuals with these types of disorders, we have paid special attention to how nonresponding in these diagnostic groups varies with stimulus meaningfulness. We have also presented the results of a large-scale investigation of EDNR in first-episode psychotic patients with these disorders. Finally, we have shown that although EDNR may be common among psychotic individuals, it may have special significance when it appears in schizophrenic patients because it is only in these patients that EDNR appears to be associated with being born during the winter. This finding raises the possibility that schizophrenics with EDNR suffer from a perinatal insult or viral infection leading to electrodermal dysregulation.

### Nonresponding in Schizophrenia and Mood Disorders

One of the most fundamental forms of information processing involves habituation of the orienting response (OR). Usually, when an organism is presented with

*Progress in Electrodermal Research,* Edited by
J.-C. Roy *et al.* Plenum Press, New York, 1993

**Table 1.** Electrodermal Nonresponding to Nonsignal and Signal Stimuli

| Study | Patient | | Control | | Percent Not Responding | | | |
| | | | | | Nonsignal | | Signal | |
| | N | Description | N | Description | Patient | Control | Patient | Control |
|---|---|---|---|---|---|---|---|---|
| SCHIZOPHRENIA | | | | | | | | |
| Gruzelier & Venables (1972) | 80 | Mostly Chronic | 20 | Normals (source unknown) & nonpsychotics | 54 | 0 | -- | -- |
| Gruzelier & Venables (1974) | 47 | Mostly Chronic | 20 | Nonpsychotics | 68 | 30 | -- | -- |
| Patterson (1976) | 52 | Chronic | 10 | Hospital Staff | 46 | 10 | -- | -- |
| Patterson & Venables (1978) | 73 | Chronic | 20 | Hospital Staff | 42 | 10 | -- | -- |
| Rubens & Lapidus (1978) | 40 | Chronic inpatients and outpatients | 20 | Religious institution employees, no psychiatric history | 22 | 0 | -- | -- |
| Straube (1979) | 50 | Mostly first admissions | 32 | Mostly clinical staff | 40 | 3 | -- | -- |
| Bernstein et al. (1981) | 40 | Chronic | 40 | Normals (source unknown), no psychiatric history | 50 | 13 | 13 | 10 |
| Gruzelier et al. (1981) | 33 | Mostly nuclear | 31 | Hospital Staff | 30 | 10 | 4 | 0 |
| Zahn et al. (1981) | 46 | Acute | 118 | Demographically matched twins | 26 | 5 | -- | -- |
| Iacono (1981) | 28 | Remitted outpatients | 22 | Healthy medical clinic volunteers, no psychiatric history | 46 | 18 | -- | -- |
| Bartfai et al. (1983) | 13 | Median 2 yrs. since onset | 18 | Hospital staff and others | 0 | 5 | -- | -- |
| Bernstein et al. (1985) | 40 | Chronic | 40 | Mostly hospital staff, no psychiatric history | 60 | 25 | 15 | 10 |

| Study | n | Patients | n | Controls | | | | |
|---|---|---|---|---|---|---|---|---|
| Sommer (1985) | 26 | Mostly chronic | 22 | Hospital staff | 42 | 19 | -- | -- |
| Zahn et al. (1987) | 13 | Total hospitalization less than 1 year | 19 | Normals (source unknown), screened for psychopathology | 15 | 0 | -- | -- |
| Bernstein et al. (1988) | 50 | From 4 hospitals | 50 | Primarily hospital staff, screened for psychopathology | 64 | 21 | 20 | 19 |
| Öhman et al. (1989) | 37 | Heterogeneous | 14 | Hospital staff | 59 | 7 | -- | -- |
| Levinson et al. (1991) | 36 | Acute inpatients & recent discharges | 25 | Community volunteers & hospital stafff, screened for psychopathology | 39 | 36 | 40 | 0 |
| Roth et al. (1991) | 31 | Primarily veterans | 23 | Age & education matched, screened for pschopathology | 26 | 17 | -- | -- |
| Öhlund et al. (1991) | 26 | Consecutive admissions | 14 | Hospital staff | 42 | 7 | -- | -- |
| Dawson et al. (1992) | 98 | Recent onset | 40 | Demographically matched | 43 | 40 | 16 | 0 |
| WEIGHTED AVERAGE | 43 | | 30 | | 43 | 14 | 24 | 9 |
| MOOD DISORDERS | | | | | | | | |
| Iacono et al. (1983) | 50 | Remitted outpatients | 46 | Healthy medical clinic volunteers | 56 | 24 | -- | -- |
| Iacono et al. (1984) | 44 | Remitted outpatients | 26 | Healthy medical clinic volunteers | 82 | 65 | 25 | 4 |
| Bernstein et al. (1988) | 50 | Drawn from 4 hospitals | 50 | Primarily hospital staff | 79 | 21 | 64 | 19 |
| Levinson (1991) | 24 | Inpatients & recent discharges | 25 | Community volunteers & staff | 46 | 36 | 16 | 0 |
| WEIGHTED AVERAGE | 42 | | 37 | | 68 | 32 | 40 | 10 |

a novel stimulus, an OR, indexed in part by an electrodermal response, is elicited. If the stimulus is irrelevant to the ongoing activity of the organism (i.e., is low in signal value), the repetition of the stimulus leads to habituation of the OR. If the stimulus is meaningful, because it is intense and thus disruptive or because it requires a behavioral response (i.e., is high in signal value), the OR will be pronounced and slow to habituate. The OR to both nonsignal and signal stimuli has been examined in psychopathology research. In this section, we have reviewed the orienting-habituation literature for schizophrenia and affective disorders, paying special attention to how stimulus significance affects EDNR.

**Studies Using Nonsignal Stimuli.** Gruzelier and Venables (1972) were the first to demonstrate that a substantial fraction of schizophrenic patients fail to respond to innocuous auditory stimuli in studies of electrodermal habituation. Since their ground breaking work, this basic finding has been replicated in over 20 investigations carried out in over a dozen independent laboratories in Europe and North America. The results of studies that have examined EDNR in schizophrenia, that included a control group, and that provided data on EDNR rates are summarized in Table 1. A total of 859 schizophrenics have been studied across 20 investigations. On average, 43% of these individuals were electrodermal nonresponders. This rate contrasts sharply with the average of 14% observed in the 598 nonschizophrenic subjects who composed comparison groups. Frequent nonresponding does not appear to be associated with chronicity or clinical state; it is evident in chronic cases, recent onset patients, and remitted schizophrenics.

Nonresponding to nonsignal stimuli does not appear specific to schizophrenia; it is also evident in patients with mood disorders. As a glance at Table 1 reveals, however, the evidence supporting an association between EDNR and these disorders is not nearly as overwhelming as it is for schizophrenia. There have been no published studies to date of EDNR in acutely disturbed patients with bipolar disorder. Only remitted bipolar patients have been assessed and these individuals have shown high rates of nonresponding (Iacono et al., 1983,1984). All four of the mood disorder studies listed in Table 1 found high rates of nonresponding in depressed patients whether these individuals were acutely ill or remitted.

**Studies Using Signal Stimuli.** Different approaches have been adopted to test the effects of stimulus significance on EDNR. In some studies, stimulus significance was enhanced by making the stimuli more intense, in others, by requiring a behavioral response to the stimulus, such as having subjects press a button in response to stimuli or move their eyes to a designated fixation point following stimulus presentation. The results to date seem to be independent of the method used to attach significance to the stimuli.

The first study to examine the effects of signal stimuli on EDNR was that of Gruzelier and Venables (1973). They had subjects press a button each time they heard a tone that they had previously failed to respond to when it had no special signal value. Of 20 schizophrenic nonresponders, 95% responded to these signal stimuli. Intermixed with the signal tones were nonsignal tones of identical intensity and duration but different frequency. The nonresponders continued to be nonresponsive to these neutral stimuli. The act of manipulating the button alone, in the absence of the stimulus, was shown not to elicit electrodermal responses. Thus, the results clearly demonstrated that the attentional significance of the signal tone was responsible for the elicited response.

Bernstein and his colleagues extended this line of research in a series of studies in which different methods were used to attach meaning to nonsignal stimuli. Bernstein et al. (1985), using a design similar to that of Gruzelier and Venables (1973), had subjects press a foot pedal to the presentation of target tones which were alternated with neutral tones that differed only in frequency. The high rate of EDNR evident in schizophrenics to the neutral stimuli was eliminated with the signal stimulus. In another study, Bernstein et al. (1980) presented recorded words that, for some subjects, required them to orally repeat a word that had been associated with previously designated target words. When the words were presented without the response requirement, schizophrenic patients were underresponsive. With the addition of the association task, the electrodermal responding of the schizophrenic patients was similar to that of the normal comparison subjects.

Increasing stimulus intensity also normalizes the frequency of EDNR in schizophrenia. Bernstein et al. (1981) showed that the disproportionately high rate of nonresponding in schizophrenics compared to normal subjects could be eliminated by increasing stimulus intensity from 60dB to 90dB. Gruzelier et al. (1981) achieved similar results by increasing stimulus intensity from 70dB to 90dB while simultaneously increasing stimulus duration from 1 sec to 5 sec. Of the nonresponders to the weaker stimuli, 90% responded to the loud tones.

Öhman et al. (1986) also examined the effects of stimulus significance on the electrodermal OR. Unlike other researchers, Öhman and his colleagues concluded that the skin conductance responses of schizophrenics did not differentiate signal from nonsignal stimuli. The schizophrenics were less responsive than the normal controls to both types of stimuli. Although such findings appear to contradict the results of Bernstein and others, they do not for several reasons. Öhman et al. (1986) did not examine EDNR per se. Instead, they looked at the level of responding present across three blocks of 20 trials each. Bernstein et al. (1981, 1985) showed that although enhancing the signal value of stimuli reduced the frequency of EDNR, their schizophrenics habituated more rapidly than normal to the signal stimuli and thus could be expected to be less responsive than normal across all the trials taken together. Moreover, Öhman et al. (1986) found that on the first block of trials, schizophrenics did respond like normal subjects and evidenced response differentiation to the two types of stimuli. Hence, the work from these two laboratories is consistent in demonstrating hyporesponsivity to signal stimuli blocked across many trials and by showing that initial responding to signal stimuli is indeed enhanced.

The effect of manipulating stimulus significance on EDNR in mood disorders has received less attention. The one study that specifically addressed this issued used as subjects remitted patients with an extensive history of prior episodes who were tested on two occasions one year apart. Both patients with unipolar depression and bipolar disorder were examined. At the first assessment, EDNR in the two affective disorder groups to 86dB tones was more than twice the rate evident in normal subjects (Iacono et al., 1983). At the time of the second assessment, this tone series was repeated followed by a second series of conspicuously loud (105dB) tones. Unlike the situation observed in other studies for schizophrenics, the addition of the loud tones did not normalize the EDNR rate: the mood disorder patients were three times as likely as the normal subjects to be nonresponsive to these intense stimuli. Following the presentation of the 105dB tones, subjects were presented with a series of "mystery sounds" (e.g., newsroom teletype, emergency buzzer) at a peak intensity of 105dB. They were instructed to attend to the sounds so they could answer questions about them later. Once again, however, these signal stimuli did not normalize the EDNR rate of the mood patients: they were still over three times more likely to be nonresponders than normal subjects.

These mood disorder findings, coupled with those regarding schizophrenia summarized above, indicating that enhancement of stimulus significance remedies EDNR in schizophrenia but not mood disorders, led Iacono et al. (1984) to hypothesize that different mechanisms determine the likelihood of EDNR in these two types of disorders. A somewhat similar position was presented by Bernstein et al. (1985) who noted that the normalizing effect of explicit significance seen in schizophrenics was not observed in a small subgroup of depressed patients they examined.

The most thorough investigation of this hypothesis was provided by Bernstein et al. (1988,1990) who carried out the first investigation in which the effects of stimulus significance were examined in relatively large groups of schizophrenic and depressed subjects tested using the same experimental protocol. Stimulus significance was manipulated by requiring subjects to press a foot pedal when they heard target tones that were intermixed with nontarget tones. As expected, both schizophrenic and depressed patients showed high rates of EDNR to the nonsignal stimuli. Also consistent with prior studies, schizophrenics were responsive to signal stimuli and were not differentiable from normal subjects. Depressed patients, by contrast, were nonresponsive to both types of stimuli.

Bernstein et al. (1988) also recorded a cardiovascular component of the OR, the finger pulse volume response. For the schizophrenics, the results for this variable paralleled those seen with skin conductance responses to the two types of stimuli. For the depressives, however, the finger pulse volume response to nonsignal and signal tones was normal. These findings were interpreted to reflect a CNS orienting deficit for the schizophrenics that can be offset by maneuvers that enhance the attentional value of stimuli. The depressives do not appear to possess dysfunctional orienting; instead, the peripheral electrodermal system appears to be deficient, perhaps reflecting a cholinergic deficit. The validity of this interpretation for depression is buttressed by other studies of depressed patients indicating that even physiological stimuli, such as demanding respiratory maneuvers, fail to normalize electrodermal activity in these individuals (Iacono et al., 1983; Storrie et al., 1981).

**Studies Using Nonpatient Samples.** These findings with clinical populations have been buttressed by the study of those with subsyndromal mood disorder and those at psychometric risk for schizophrenia. Lenhart (1985) found that college students identified as cyclothymic using Depue et al.'s (1981) General Behavior Inventory showed electrodermal hyporesponsivity. Other investigators have obtained similar results for high scorers on Chapman et al.'s (1976) physical anhedonia scale (Bernstein & Riedel, 1987; Simons, 1981), a scale designed to assess a trait indicating possible vulnerability to schizophrenia. Bernstein and Riedel (1987) documented that the EDNR rate seen in the anhedonics was sharply reduced when the auditory stimuli were given signal value by requiring a pedal press to some of them. The finger pulse volume response of these subjects paralleled the electrodermal response pattern, thus indicating that these two OR components behaved just as they did for the schizophrenics in Bernstein et al. (1988).

**Summary.** The decades of the seventies and eighties produced a remarkably consistent body of research on the association between EDNR and severe psychopathology. Many studies demonstrated that EDNR is characteristic of schizophrenia, although its prevalence among those with this disorder varies widely across reports. A smaller number of investigations suggest that mood disorders, especially major depression, also show high rates of EDNR. These reports are supported by work with nonclinical study samples of individuals putatively at risk for developing severe psychopathology. The mechanisms governing EDNR in these two types of disorder may be different. For schizophrenia this literature suggests that EDNR reflects an orienting deficit that can be brought out by comparing electrodermal responses to nonsignal and signal tones. For mood disorders, the corresponding research suggests that the OR seems to be intact; EDNR appears to reflect a dysfunction specific to electrodermal activation. Such findings led Iacono (1991b) to speculate that electrodermal assessments, using nonsignal and signal stimuli, could aid in the differential diagnosis of these disorders.

**Recent Studies of EDNR.** Two very recent studies challenge Iacono's (1991b) proposition by providing data that undermine the foundation on which it is based (Dawson et al., 1992; Levinson, 1991). These investigations carry special weight for several reasons. The Levinson (1991) study is the only one besides Bernstein et al. (1988) that includes large groups of both schizophrenic and depressed patients evaluated with a single experimental protocol. Both the Dawson and Levinson investigations used a relatively large patient sample with diagnoses assigned according to specified criteria, employed control subjects demographically matched to the patients, and included nonsignal as well as signal stimuli. Interestingly, these two reports presented findings not only at variance with those reviewed above, but also in disagreement with each other.

Levinson (1991) examined schizophrenic, schizoaffective (mainly schizophrenic) depressed, and psychiatrically well individuals as they were exposed in succession to 70dB tones, 103dB tones, 75dB tones requiring a manual response, and a 100dB white noise burst. His results showed that EDNR to the nonsignal tones was substantially reduced for the schizoaffective and control subjects when signal stimuli were used. For the schizophrenic and depressed patients, the opposite of the expected pattern (based on past research) was obtained. The EDNR rate of about 40% for the schizophrenic patients was essentially invariant across stimulus conditions. For the depressives, it dropped from a high of 46% to the neutral tones to a low of 10% during the button-press task.

Dawson et al. (1992) examined EDNR among 98 recent-onset schizophrenic patients and 40 normal individuals while they listened to 78dB tones; tones of this same intensity but varying in frequency, with some of the tones requiring a motoric response; and 98dB white noise bursts. The schizophrenic and normal subjects did not differ in their EDNR rate to the moderately loud tones. In addition to this unexpected result, Dawson et al. (1992) found that rather than the task-significant and white noise stimuli increasing the similarity of the two groups, the introduction of these procedures enhanced group differences, with the schizophrenics much less likely to respond to the stimuli than the normal subjects.

## THE MAP PROJECT

It is against this backdrop that we present EDNR findings from the Markers and Predictors of First-Episode Psychosis Project (MAP for short). Because it was initiated over a dozen years ago, the MAP study was not designed to resolve the discrepancies introduced by the recent findings in this area. Nevertheless, the MAP project possesses a number of significant strengths and introduces innovations in research design that are likely to make our findings illuminating.

Unlike prior studies which have used primarily chronic or repeatedly hospitalized patients, the MAP project recruited only first-episode cases. All the psychiatric subjects, including the nonschizophrenic cases, had psychotic features. None had received prior treatment with antipsychotic, antidepressant, or antimanic drugs. Although we could not control medication use, because the psychotic symptoms of these patients were often the focus of treatment, our psychiatric subjects were often treated with similar drug regimens regardless of their diagnosis. Perhaps the major innovation of the MAP project was the marriage of epidemiological and psychophysiological research methodology. Because this study was designed to identify and recruit every case of first-episode psychosis in a large city, the study samples are more broadly representative than those employed in investigations that rely on admissions to a single hospital. These various design features allowed us to obtain samples of psychotic subjects displaying more intergroup homogeneity than is typical in psychophysiological research. Our patient groups differed in diagnosis, but not in treatment history or the presence of psychotic features. Our samples are also relatively large, with 141 psychotic participants and 104 normal subjects drawn from the same community as the patients. The MAP investigation provides for the first examination of EDNR in schizophreniform disorder, a controversial diagnostic category that may not be distinct from schizophrenia. It also is the first study to include acutely ill bipolar subjects.

Finally, although it is beyond the scope of this chapter to consider all the possible correlates of EDNR, we will examine one possible correlate, the relationship of this variable to season of birth. Many studies have shown that schizophrenics are disproportionately more likely to be born during the winter (Bradbury & Miller, 1985), but few investigations have examined how this might be of significance to understanding schizophrenia's correlates. Because of the representative nature of the MAP sample, each of our diagnostic groups can be expected to characterize the relationship between EDNR and season of birth in a manner that makes the results broadly generalizable. Moreover, we can examine whether the relationship between these variables is the same or different across diagnoses.

### Method

**Subjects**. The strategy for recruiting subjects has been thoroughly outlined elsewhere (Iacono & Beiser, 1989, 1992a). Briefly, the study was carried out by drawing subjects from a catchment area centered on Vancouver, Canada. To be eligible for inclusion, subjects had to be between the ages of 16 and 54, have lived in the catchment area for at least six months, and not have an organic cerebral disorder, mental retardation, or a history of chemical dependence. All subjects gave written informed consent to participate in the study.

Psychiatric subjects were referred through a community-wide network consisting of psychiatric hospitals and services of general hospitals, private practice psychiatrists and general practitioners, and community counseling and mental health centers. Subjects were considered as prospects if they satisfied the inclusion and exclusion criteria listed above, were believed to be in their first episode, and were experiencing symptoms typically associated with psychosis, such as hallucinations, delusions, thought disorder, and grossly disorganized behavior. Each individual was interviewed with the Present State Exam (Wing et al., 1974). Information from this structured interview, a chart review, and interviews of friends and relatives was pooled at a case conference attended by project staff, including at least two experienced clinical diagnosticians with doctoral degrees. Prospective subjects were retained if this comprehensive review of clinical material established that the subject was indeed psychotic and experiencing a first episode, defined as not having been treated previously with neuroleptics, antidepressants, or lithium. Diagnoses were assigned without knowledge of the electrodermal data, according to DSM-III criteria, using the "best estimate" approach of Leckman et al. (1982).

As can be seen from Table 2, the psychotic subjects were almost evenly split between schizophrenia-related disorders (schizophrenia and schizophreniform disorder) and mood disorders. These participants were largely young and mostly male. Although it is conceivable that the preponderance of males in the sample reflects a recruitment bias, data we have presented in detail elsewhere (Iacono & Beiser, 1992a, 1992b) suggest that psychosis generally, and especially schizophrenia, shows a higher incidence in men than women. Table 2 also describes the medication status of the subjects. A majority of

**Table 2.** Characteristics of MAP Subjects

| Diagnosis | n M/F | Age M (SD) | Medication Status (%) | | | |
|---|---|---|---|---|---|---|
| | | | None | Neuro-leptic | Anti-Park. | Anti-dep. |
| Schizophrenia | 38/11 | 23 (5.4) | 20 | 80 | 48 | 9 |
| Schizophreniform | 21/7 | 21 (4.4) | 14 | 79 | 64 | 11 |
| Major Depression | 21/11 | 26 (7.2) | 22 | 53 | 34 | 50 |
| Bipolar | 17/15 | 27 (7.2) | 0 | 66 | 25 | 6 |
| Normal | 58/46 | 27 (9.2) | 100 | 0 | 0 | 0 |

Note: Anti-Park. = Anti-Parkinsonian drugs; Antidep. = antidepressants.

subjects in each diagnostic group was taking neuroleptics. Patients with major depression were more likely than others to be receiving antidepressants. The lithium status of subjects is not listed in the table because other than the 15 bipolar subjects on this drug, only one other subject (who had major depression) was on lithium.

Normal subjects were recruited from community agencies (e.g., employment centers, union halls, the Young Men's Christian Association), a family practice clinic, and vocational, technical and community colleges. Prospective volunteers with a history of mental health treatment, either for themselves or for their first-degree relatives, were excluded.

**Electrodermal Recording**. Skin conductance was recorded using Beckman silver-silver chloride 1 cm-diameter electrodes filled with the Unibase-saline electrolyte recommended by Fowles et al. (1981). The electrodes were attached to the medial phalanges of the first two fingers of each hand with two adhesive electrode collars, one attached to the finger (to control the exposed skin area) and the other to the electrode (to insure secure adhesion). Skin conductance was recorded using the constant voltage technique with a Sensor Medics R612 Dynograph and Type 9844 Skin Conductance couplers. The electrodermal activity from the two hands was averaged; skin conductance responses were counted as increases in conductance of at least .05 microsiemans occurring between one and four seconds of stimulus onset. Nonresponding was defined as a failure to respond to the first two tone stimuli presented. For the sound effect stimuli described below, nonresponding was characterized as a failure to generate any skin conductance response during the duration of the sound.

**Procedure**. Subjects were exposed in succession to three types of stimuli. First, they listened to 8 85dB (SPL) tones, each lasting .5 sec., with a frequency of 1000 Hz and 40 msec rise and fall times. The interstimulus interval was pseudorandomized, ranging from 25-70 sec and averaging 50 sec. These stimuli were followed by 12 105dB tones with otherwise identical physical properties. Finally, subjects heard two tape-recorded sound effects (identical to those used in Iacono et al., 1984) that lasted 45 sec and had a peak intensity of 95dB. All stimuli were presented against a background of 55dB pink noise.

Prior to each tone series, subjects were instructed to concentrate on becoming completely relaxed so they could ignore the meaningless, distracting tones. These instructions were intended to ensure that subjects understood that the tones were irrelevant by giving them a task to focus on (Iacono & Lykken, 1979). In contrast, subjects were told to pay special attention to the loud sound effects because they would be queried about them at the conclusion of the session.

## Results

Preliminary analyses revealed that the proportion of nonresponders was unrelated to gender in any subject group and for all three types of stimuli. Age was also unrelated to EDNR status. Medication effects were evaluated by comparing the EDNR rate for subjects on and off lithium and the types of medications listed in Table 2. None of these analyses yielded a significant result.

For the remaining group comparisons of the EDNR rate, chi square tests with Yates correction were carried out using a set of planned orthogonal contrasts that appear reasonable given the literature to date plus our hypotheses. These contrasts involved the following group comparisons: a) schizophrenic vs. schizophreniform, b) major depression vs. bipolar, schizophrenia related disorders (i.e., the groups contrasted in step "a") vs. mood disorders (i.e., the groups contrasted in step "b"), and c) all psychiatric subjects combined vs. the normal group.

**Moderate Intensity Tone Series**. The proportion of nonresponders in each group to the 85dB tones is presented in Figure 1A. The planned orthogonal contrasts revealed that the two schizophrenia-related groups did not differ, nor did the two mood disorder groups. Collapsing the schizophrenia-related and mood subjects into two groups and comparing them failed to yield a significant result. However, when all the patients were compared to the normal subjects, the patients were found to have a significantly elevated rate of nonresponding, $\chi^2(1)=14.43$, p<.001.

**Loud Tone Series and Sounds**. The pattern of statistical significance for the 105dB tones and the sound effect stimuli were identical to those evident for the moderate intensity tones (see Figure 1B). The only significant contrasts were those comparing all the psychotic subjects to the normals, $\chi^2(1)=9.10$, p<.01, for the loud tones, $\chi^2(1)=17.35$, p<.001, for the sounds.

**The Effect of Signal Value on Nonresponding**. Figure 1 indicates that the increased signal value contributed by the loud tones and sound effects reduced the EDNR rate for all subject groups. Of special importance is whether or not there was a differential reduction in the EDNR rate across groups. The work of Bernstein et al. (1988) favors the prediction that nonresponding subjects with schizophrenia-related disorders should be more likely than the mood disorder patients to respond to the stimuli as their significance is enhanced. To evaluate this possibility, the proportion of nonresponders to the 85dB tones who responded to the 105dB tones and sounds was determined (see Figure 1C). Chi square tests revealed only that when all the psychotic nonresponders were combined, as a group they were less likely than the controls to become responders to the sound effect stimuli, $\chi^2(1)=6.23$, p<.05. Inspection of Figure 1C indicates that the trend in the data was in the opposite of the expected direction. Mood disorder nonresponders were more likely than schizophrenia spectrum nonresponders to become responsive to the stimuli with greater signal value.

**Season of Birth**. Our results indicate that EDNR is a general feature of psychosis, one that does not differentiate diagnostic groups. An interesting question, however, concerns the possibility that the nonresponding evident in patients with different diagnoses stems from different underlying processes. As a first step toward tackling this issue, we attempted to replicate and extend Öhlund etal. (1990, 1991) who found an association between EDNR and winter births. A thorough presentation of our findings regarding the relationship of electrodermal activity to birth month can be found elsewhere (Katsanis et al., 1992). Here, we have focused on the likelihood that EDNR to the 85dB tones is associated with being born during the high risk winter season, defined as the months of January through April. A glance at Figure 2 reveals that there were differences across groups in the likelihood that EDNR was associated with birth during the season of excess risk. The figure indicates that those with mood disorder were likely to be nonresponsive whether they were born in the winter or seasons of nonexcess risk. Very different patterns were evident for the two types of schizophrenia-related disorders. Schizophreniform patients were more apt to be nonresponsive if born during the nonwinter months. For schizophrenic patients, the reverse seems to be true. The nonresponding rate in schizophrenics born during the low risk part of the year is essentially identical to that of the normal subjects. Indeed, to the extent that the schizophrenics were more nonresponsive than the normal control subjects, their higher rate of nonresponding seems to be attributable almost entirely to schizophrenic individuals born during the winter.

To determine whether or not these differences were significant, we compared the proportion of nonresponders in each group born during the winter with the proportion of nonresponders in the control group (the EDNR rate did not differ between controls born during the two parts of the year). As Figure 2 indicates, schizophrenics born during the winter had a rate of EDNR that was significantly higher than that of the normal subjects, $\chi^2(1)=3.97$, p<.05. Nonwinter born schizophrenics did not differ from normal. Schizophreniform patients differed from the normal subjects only if they were born during months of nonexcess risk, $\chi^2(1)=9.44$, p<.01. The bipolar and depressed patients produced similar data so they are considered here as a single group. Regardless when they were born, these individuals showed higher rates of nonresponding than the nonspychiatric comparison group, $\chi^2(1)=10.00$, p<.01, for nonwinter births, $\chi^2(1)=3.23$, p<.07, for winter births.

### Discussion

Our results are consistent with the large body of literature on EDNR in schizophrenia and depression in that we found that patients with these disorders show excessive rates of nonresponding. They also extend this literature by showing that schizophreniform and bipolar patients also demonstrated this anomaly. Our findings thus indicate that EDNR is probably a feature associated with functional psychosis in general rather then being specific to one or two disorders.

## A) Proportion of Nonresponders to 85 dB Tones

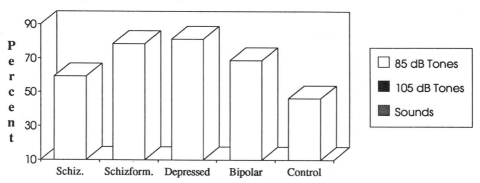

## B) Proportion of Nonresponders to Signal Stimuli

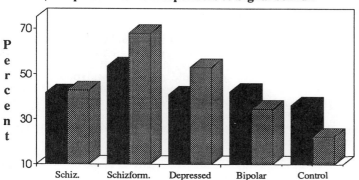

## C) Proportion of 85 dB Nonresponders Who Responded to Other Stimuli

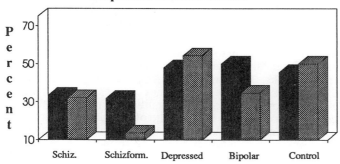

**Figure 1. Electrodermal Nonresponding of Each Diagnostic Group to Different Types of Stimuli**

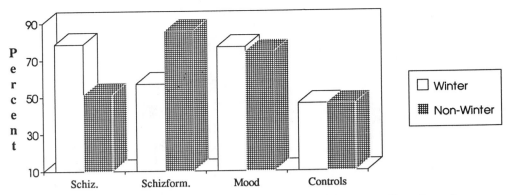

**Figure 2. Proportion of Nonresponders to 85 dB Tones as a Function of Birth Season**

We found that increasing the signal value of stimuli, although decreasing the overall rate of EDNR, did not normalize nonresponding in schizophrenia. These results are thus similar to those of other recent investigations that reported that increasing the intensity or task demands associated with stimuli did not cause schizophrenics to be similar to normal subjects (Dawson et al., 1992; Levinson, 1991). We also found that enhancing the signal significance of stimuli did not normalize the responding of mood disorder patients, a finding that affirms the results of prior reports (see Table 1). Taken in the aggregate, our data indicate that psychotic patients are generally nonresponsive, regardless of stimulus meaningfulness.

With respect to schizophrenia, our results, together with those of Dawson et al. (1992) and Levinson (1991), showing that increasing stimulus significance does not remedy EDNR, are discordant with those of Bernstein et al. (1981, 1985, 1988). The reasons for this discordance remain obscure. It is unlikely that medication differences across the studies could account for the inconsistencies. The present investigation and the Levinson (1991) and Dawson et al. (1992) studies obtained similar results despite the very different medication status of their subjects. Our study allowed medication status to vary naturalistically, Levinson used drug-free subjects, and Dawson et al. examined patients while on a standardized medication protocol. Moreover, Bernstein et al. (1988) found that medicated and drug-free schizophrenics did not differ electrodermally. Differences in the chronicity of schizophrenia across studies are also unlikely to be responsible for the discrepant results. Using the same procedures adopted in the present report, we found the EDNR rate of chronic schizophrenics to be essentially the same as that of our first-episode patients across all stimulus conditions (Ficken, 1991). It also seems unlikely that differences across studies in the nature of the stimuli employed could account for the findings. Bernstein et al. (1981, 1988) found normalized responding in schizophrenics to 90dB stimuli or to stimuli requiring a motor response. Our investigation and those of Levinson and Dawson et al. failed to generate this result despite using stimuli as loud as 105dB. Both Levinson and Dawson et al. also used stimuli requiring overt behavioral responses without success.

Another possible explanation centers on differences in the nature of the nonpsychiatric control groups used in these studies. However, although it is the case that the nonresponding rates among the normal groups in the Bernstein et al. vs. the other studies were very different, it is the change in the EDNR rate evident in schizophrenics, and not the change evident in these patients relative to the controls, that accounts for interstudy variability. For example, in the present report and that of Levinson, the lowest nonresponding rates evident in the schizophrenics, regardless of stimulus signal value, was 39%. For the current investigation and those of Levinson and Dawson et al., in the schizophrenic groups, the changes in EDNR rate between exposure to stimuli with the least signal value to those with the most was about 18%, 6%, and 28%, respectively. The lowest EDNR rate for schizophrenics in Bernstein at al. (1988) was about 15% (to stimuli requiring a pedal press), and the change in EDNR rate from innocuous to signal stimuli was about 63%, more than twice the change seen in the other reports.

**Nonresponding and Season of Birth.** The work of Bernstein et al. (1988) offered an interesting hypothesis regarding the mechanisms underlying EDNR in functional psychosis, namely, that schizophrenics possess an information processing deficit manifest in part by deficient orienting to neutral stimuli and that depressives have a dysfunctional electrodermal system reflecting possible cholinergic hypoactivity. Our data, together with those of Levinson (1991) and Dawson et al. (1992), undermine this hypothesis, at least as it pertains to schizophrenia. However, the findings we have presented may offer some insight into the mechanisms underlying EDNR in these disorders.

We found that excess nonresponding in schizophrenia occurred only in patients born during the winter. For mood disorder patients, season of birth was unrelated to EDNR. These results represent a replication and extension of the work of Öhlund et al. (1990, 1991) who also found that winter-born schizophrenics were disproportionately represented among schizophrenic nonresponders. Our findings, along with those of Öhlund and colleagues, suggest that winter birth is associated with some prenatal occurrence that increases the likelihood of EDNR in schizophrenia.

Because the prevalence of schizophrenia appears to be elevated among winter born people, it has been conjectured that individuals born during this season may be exposed to seasonally varying environmental circumstances that contribute to CNS damage (Watson et al., 1984; Torrey et al., 1988; Pulver et al., 1981). These include nutritional deficiencies, obstetrical complications, bacterial infections, and viral diseases. For instance, Watson et al. (1984) found that prenatal exposure to various infectious diseases was associated with increased likelihood of having process schizophrenia. Mednick et al. (1988) found that individuals who were in the second trimester of fetal development during an influenza epidemic had an increased risk of developing schizophrenia. Torrey (1991) has postulated that a viral infection in the upper respiratory tract of infants could lead to temporal lobe brain dysfunction because the nerves innervating this chest area lie near temporal lobe structures. Because temporal lobe structures play a role in electrodermal orienting and habituation (e.g. Bagshaw et al., 1965; Yokata et al., 1963), it is possible to speculate that the season of birth-EDNR association arises through perinatal factors that ultimately compromise temporal lobe functioning.

Additional support for such speculation derives from recent work in our laboratory (Katsanis & Iacono, 1992). We administered a neuropsychological test battery to 63 chronic schizophrenics who were evaluated using the electrodermal paradigm of the MAP project. We found that electrodermal hyporesponding was associated only with tests putatively tapping temporal lobe functioning.

Although patients with schizophreniform disorder had a high rate of EDNR, these subjects were unlike the schizophrenics in that the association between EDNR and season of birth was reversed. Although it is difficult to account for such a finding, it is worth noting that we have found the schizophreniform patients to differ from the schizophrenics on a number of important variables. Ventricular enlargement was evident in the first-episode schizophrenic patients. In contrast, the schizophreniform subjects had ventricular spaces that were nonsignificantly smaller than that of normal comparison subjects (Iacono et al., 1988). Smooth-pursuit eye tracking dysfunction was prominent in the schizophrenics, but the eye tracking performance of the schizophreniform subjects was virtually identical to that of normals (Iacono et al., 1992). We have also found that about 20% of the MAP schizophrenic patients were left handed, a rate of left-handedness that has often been associated with schizophrenia (Clementz et al., 1992; Katsanis & Iacono, 1989). The schizophreniform patients show a rate that is much lower (11%) and that is not different from the base rate of sinistrality in the general population. Finally, the schizophreniform patients had appreciably better outcomes than the schizophrenics nine and 18 months following episode onset (Beiser et al., 1988; Iacono & Beiser, 1989). All of these findings suggest that schizophrenia and schizophreniform disorder, although symptomatically similar, differ in important ways that may reflect different pathophysiologic mechanisms. They also point to the need to evaluate independently the correlates of these two DSM-III disorders.

**Choice of Control Group.** Psychopathology studies, in general, and schizophrenia research, in particular, are notorious for their inability to replicate. It is difficult to execute well studies in this field; there are a large number of reasons why replication failures are common. One often neglected but perhaps very significant factor contributing to this problem centers on the choice of the normal comparison group. Iacono and colleagues have shown that the choice of subjects for the control group seems to determine whether or not schizophrenics are found to have ventricular enlargement on computerized tomography (CT) scans (Iacono, 1991a; Smith & Iacono, 1986; Smith et al., 1988). A similar situation exists for the CT literature on mood disorders (Depue and Iacono, 1989). What these various CT studies show is that measured ventricular size in psychiatric patients is fairly constant across studies. The ventricle size of controls, however, varies across investigations such that studies that report ventriculomegaly have controls with small ventricles while those failing to find significant group differences employ control subjects with large ventricles. Iacono (1991a) noted that while the characteristics of patients who serve as subjects in psychopathology research are often described in detail, rarely is the characterization of control subjects either comparable or adequate. A review of 92 recent schizophrenia studies published in four major psychopathology journals revealed that in 40% of the reports, the source of the control group was unspecified. Hence, it should be no surprise that it remains a mystery as to why the outcome of CT studies appears to depend on control group choice.

Iacono (1991a) also argued that the choice of control group in EDNR studies of schizophrenia may affect the outcome because studies that use as controls hospital staff obtain lower EDNR rates in the normal subjects than those using nonstaff volunteers. As can be seen from careful inspection of Table 1, it is becoming evident that control differences in EDNR rates are a function of whether or not these comparison subjects are drawn from clinic personnel.

Although there is a wide range in the distribution of EDNR rates for schizophrenics across studies, the distribution seems to be continuous and unimodal. A very different picture emerges for the control subject EDNR rates. Most studies report EDNR rates of 10% or less, but some report rates over 35%. For studies relying primarily on hospital staff, the median EDNR rate is 10%. Investigations that select nonpsychiatric comparison subjects from other sources have a median EDNR rate of 18%. Three recent studies (the present report, Dawson et al., 1992; Levinson, 1991), which attempted to recruit community-based normal groups likely to be demographically similar to the psychiatric patients, found the highest normal EDNR rates (all over 35%). Whether or not community volunteers comprise an ideal control group is a complex question (Meehl, 1970), but it seems likely that community based, matched controls, who are likely to differ from the patients on only one major variable (presence or absence of psychopathology), comprise a more desirable control group than staff who, other than being affiliated with the same hospital that is treating the patients, are likely to have little in common with them.

Unlike the situation for the CT scan studies, the choice of controls in electrodermal investigations, while obviously having an effect, cannot be used to explain discordant results across studies. When weak stimuli are used, the control and schizophrenic EDNR rates are more similar when nonstaff serve as controls. In some cases, group differences are nonsignificant (e.g. Dawson et al., 1992). However, when stronger or more meaningful stimuli are employed, schizophrenics are still clearly hyporesponsive even with a nonstaff comparison group. EDNR thus remains a strong correlate of schizophrenia.

## Summary

EDNR is a common feature of schizophrenia and mood disorders. There are now over 20 studies examining this association. With few exceptions, all point to this conclusion.

The present investigation extended the literature by examining EDNR in a large sample of first-episode psychotic individuals divided among schizophrenic, schizophreniform, bipolar, and major depressive groups. Subjects with schizophrenia-related and mood-related disorders were found to be similar. Compared to a community based sample of normal subjects, all psychotic patients displayed a high rate of EDNR.

A disproportionately high rate of EDNR may exist in these diagnostic groups for different reasons. The plausibility of this notion is derived from our data on the relationship of season of birth to EDNR. Only schizophrenics showed an association between EDNR and winter birth. Schizophreniform subjects, by contrast, were more apt to be nonresponders if they had nonwinter births. Season of birth was unrelated to EDNR in patients with mood disorders.

How the presentation of signal stimuli affects EDNR in schizophrenic and affective disorders remains uncertain. The work of Bernstein and others suggests that signal stimuli can be used to differentiate these disorders. According to these investigators, nonresponding schizophrenics become normoresponsive when presented with signal stimuli while nonresponding depressed patients are relatively unaffected by this manipulation. Data we have presented here coupled with findings from other recent studies suggests that signal stimuli do not normalize the responding of schizophrenics, but in fact may enhance the differences between these patients and normal subjects.

Finally, our review of the literature suggests caution must be exercised in the conduct and interpretation of EDNR studies because the results may be influenced by control group choice. Normal response rates are considerably higher when hospital staff are employed as a comparison group then when nonstaff volunteers are used.

# References

Bagshaw, M.H., Kimble, D.P., & Pribram, K.H. (1965). The GSR of monkeys during orienting and habituation and after ablation of the amygdala, hippocampus, and inferotemporal cortex. *Neuropsychologia, 3,* 111-119.

Bartfai, A., Levander, S., Edman, G., Schalling, D., & Sedvall, G. (1983). Skin conductance responses in unmedicated recently admitted schizophrenic patients. *Psychophysiology, 20,* 180-187.

Beiser, M., Fleming, J.A.E., Iacono, W.G., & Lin, T-Y, (1988). Refining the diagnosis of schizophreniform psychosis. *Am J Psychiatry, 145,* 695-700.

Bernstein, A.S., & Riedel, J.A. (1987). Psychophysiological response patterns in college students with high physical anhedonia: Scores appear to reflect schizotypy rather than depression. *Biol Psychiatry, 22,* 829-847.

Bernstein, A. S., Riedel, J. A., Graae, F., Seidman, D., Steele, H., Connolly, J., & Lubowsky, J. (1988). Schizophrenia is associated with altered orienting activity; Depression with electrodermal (cholinergic?) deficit and normal orienting response. *J Abnorm Psychol, 97,* 3-13.

Bernstein, A. S., Riedel, J. A., Pava, J., Schnur, D., & Lubowsky, J. (1985). A limiting factor in the "normalization" of schizophrenic orienting response dysfunction. *Schizophren Bull, 11,* 230-254.

Bernstein, A. S., Schneider, S. J., Juni, S., Pope, A. T., & Starkey, P. W. (1980). The effects of stimulus significance on the electrodermal response in chronic schizophrenia. *J Abnorm Psychol, 89,* 93-97.

Bernstein, A. S., Taylor, K. W., Starkey, P., Juni, S., Lubowsky, J., & Paley, H. (1981). Bilateral skin conductance, finger pulse volume, and EEG orienting response to tones of differing intensities in chronic schizophrenics and controls. *J Nerv Ment Dis, 169,* 513-528.

Bradbury, T.N. & Miller G.A. (1985). Season of birth in schizophrenia: A review of evidence, methodology, and etiology. *Psychol Bull, 98,* 569-594.

Chapman, L.J., Chapman, J.P., & Raulin, M.L. (1976). Scales for physical and social anhedonia. *J Abnorm Psychol, 85,* 374-382.

Clementz, B.A., Iacono, W.G., & Beiser, M. (1992). Handedness in first-episode psychotic patients and their first-degree biological relatives. Unpublished manuscript.

Dawson, M.E., Nuechterlein, K.H., & Schell, A.M. (1992). Electrodermal anomalies in recent-onset schizophrenia: Relationships to symptoms and prognosis. *Schizophren Bull, 18,* 295-311.

Depue, R.A., & Iacono, W.G. (1989). Neurobehavioral aspects of affective disorders. *Annual Rev Psychol, 40,* 457-492.

Depue, R.A., Slater, J.F., Wolfstetter-Kausch, H., Klein, D., Goplerud, E., & Farr, D. (1981). A behavioral paradigm for identifying persons at risk for bipolar depressive disorder: A conceptual framework and five validation studies. *J Abnorm Psychol, 90*, 381-437.

Fowles, D.C., Christie, M.J., Edelberg, R., Grings, W.W., Lykken, D.T., & Venables, P.H. (1981). Publication recommendations for electrodermal measurements. *Psychophysiology, 18*, 232-239.

Ficken, J.W. (1991). *A comprehensive study of electrodermal activity in first-epsiode psychotic patients and their relatives.* Unpublished doctoral dissertation, University of Minnesota, Minneapolis.

Gruzelier, J., Eves, F., Connolly, J., & Hirsch, S. (1981). Orienting, habituation, sensitisation, and dishabituation in the electrodermal system of consecutive, drug free, admissions for schizophrenia. *Biol Psychol, 12*, 187-209.

Gruzelier, J. H., & Venables, P. H. (1972). Skin conductance orienting activity in a heterogeneous sample of schizophrenics: Possible evidence of limbic dysfunction. *J Nerv Ment Dis, 18*, 277-287.

Gruzelier, J. H., & Venables, P. H. (1973). Skin conductance responses to tones with and without attentional significance in schizophrenic and nonschizophrenic psychiatric patients. *Neuropsychologia, 11*, 221-230.

Gruzelier, J. H., & Venables, P. H. (1974). Bimodality and lateral asymmetry of skin conductance orienting activity in schizophrenics: Replication and evidence of lateral asymmetry in patients with depression and disorders of personality. *Biol Psychiatry, 8*, 55-73.

Iacono, W. G. (1981). Bilateral electrodermal habituation-dishabituation and resting EEG in remitted schizophrenics. *J Nerv Ment Dis, 170*, 91-101.

Iacono, W.G. (1991a). Control groups in schizophrenia research: A neglected source of variability. In D. Cicchetti & W.M. Grove (Eds.), *Thinking clearly about psychology: Essays in honor of Paul Everett Meehl, Vol 2*, (pp. 430-450). Minneapolis, MN: University of Minnesota Press.

Iacono, W.G. (1991b). Psychophysiological assessment of psychopathology. *Psychol Assess: J Consult Clin Psychol, 3*, 309-320.

Iacono, W.G. & Beiser, M. (1989). Age of onset, temporal stability, and eighteen-month course of first episode psychosis. In D. Cicchetti (Ed.), *The emergence of a discipline: Rochester symposium on developmental psychopathology.* (Vol. 1). (pp. 221-260). Hillsdale, N.J.: Lawrence Erlbaum.

Iacono, W.G., & Beiser, M. (1992a). Are males more likely than females to develop schizophrenia? *Am J Psychiatry, 149*, 1070-1074.

Iacono, W.G., & Beiser, M. (1992b). Where are the women in first-epsiode studies of schizophrenia? *Schizophren Bull, 18*, 471-480.

Iacono, W. G., Lykken, D. T., Haroian, K. P., Peloquin, L. J., Valentine, R. H., & Tuason, V. B. (1984). Electrodermal activity in euthymic patients with affective disorders: One-year retest stability and the effects of stimulus intensity and significance. *J Abnorm Psychol, 93*, 304-311.

Iacono, W. G., Lykken, D. T., Peloquin, L. J., Lumry, A. E, Valentine, R. H., & Tuason, V. B. (1983). Electrodermal activity in euthymic unipolar and bipolar affective disorders. *Arch Gen Psychiatry, 40*, 557-565.

Iacono, W.G., Moreau, M., Beiser, M., Fleming, J.A.E., & Lin, T-Y. (1992). Smooth pursuit eye tracking in first-epsiode psychotic patients and their relatives. *J Abnorm Psychol, 101*, 104-116.

Iacono, W.G., Smith, G.N., Moreau, M., Beiser, M., Fleming, J.A.E, Lin, T-Y., & Flak, B. (1988). Ventricular and sulcal size at the onset of psychosis. *Am J Psychiatry, 145*, 820-824.

Katsanis, J., & Iacono, W.G. (1989). Association of left-handedness with ventricular size and neuropsychological performance in schizophrenia. *Am J Psychiatry, 146*, 1056-1058.

Katsanis, J., & Iacono, W.G. (1992). Temporal lobe dysfunction and electrodermal nonresponding in schizophrenia. *Biol Psychiatry, 31*, 159-170.

Katsanis, J., Ficken, J., Iacono, W.G., & Beiser, M. (1992). Season of birth and electrodermal activity in functional psychoses. *Biol Psychiatry, 31*, 841-855.

Leckman, I.F., Scholomskas, D., Thompson, W.D., Belanger, A., & Weissman, M.M. (1982). Best estimate of lifetime psychiatric diagnosis: A methodological study. *Arch Gen Psychiatry, 39*, 879-883.

Lenhart, R.E. (1985). Lowered skin conductance in a subsyndromal high-risk depressive sample: Response amplitudes versus tonic levels. *J Abnorm Psychol, 94*, 649-652.

Levinson, D. F. (1991). Skin conductance orienting response in unmedicated RDC schizophrenic, schizoaffective, depressed, and control subjects. *Biol Psychiatry, 30*, 663-683.

Mednick, S.A., Machon, R.A., Huttunen, M.O., Bonett, D. (1988). Adult schizophrenia following prenatal exposure to an influenza epidemic. *Arch Gen Psychiatry, 45*, 189-192.

Meehl, P.E. (1970). Nuisance variables and the ex post facto design. In M. Radner & S. Winokur (Eds.), *Minnesota studies in the philosophy of science, IV*, (pp. 373-402). Minneapolis: University of Minnesota Press.

Öhlund, L.S., Öhman, A., Alm, T., Öst, L-G., Lindström, L.H. (1990). Season of birth and electrodermal unresponsiveness in male schizophrenia. *Biol Psychiatry, 27*, 328-340.

Öhlund, L. S., Öhman, A., Öst, L., Lindström, L. H., & Wieselgran, I. (1991). Electrodermal orienting response, maternal age, and season of birth in schizophrenia. *Psychiatry Res, 36*, 223-232.

Öhman, A., Nordby, H., & D'Elia, G. (1986). Orienting in schizophrenia: Stimulus significance, attention, and distraction in a signaled reaction time task. *J Abnorm Psychol, 95*, 326-334.

Öhman, A., Nordby, H., & D'Elia, G. (1989). Orienting in schizophrenia: Habituation to auditory stimuli of constant and varying intensity in patients high and low in skin conductance responsivity. *Psychophysiology, 26*, 48-61.

Patterson, T. (1976). Skin conductance responding/nonresponding and pupillometrics in chronic schizophrenia: A confirmation of Gruzelier and Venables. *J Nerv Ment Dis, 163*, 200-209.

Patterson, T. & Venables, P. H. (1978). Bilateral skin conductance and skin potential in schizophrenics and normal subjects: Identification of the fast habituator groups of schizophrenics. *Psychophysiology, 15*, 556-560.

Pulver, A.E., Sawyer, J.W., & Childs, B. (1981). The association between season of birth and the risk for schizophrenia. *Am J Epidemiol, 114*, 735-749.

Roth, W.T., Goodale, J., & Pfefferbaum, A. (1991). Auditory event-related potential and electrodermal activity in medicated and unmedicated schizophrenics. *Biol Psychiatry, 29*, 585-599.

Rubens, R. L., & Lapidus, L. B. (1978). Schizophrenic patterns of arousal and stimulus barrier functioning. *J Abnorm Psychol, 87*, 199-211.

Simons, R. (1981). Electrodermal and cardiac orienting in psychometrically defined high risk subjects. *Psychiatry Res, 4*, 347-356.

Smith, G.N., & Iacono, W.G. (1986). Lateral ventricular size in schizophrenia and choice of control group. *Lancet, i*, 1450.

Smith, G.N., Iacono, W.G., Moreau, M., Tallman, K., Beiser, M., & Flak, B. (1988). Choice of comparison group and computerized tomography findings in schizophrenia. *Br J Psychiatry, 153*, 667-674.

Sommer, W. (1985). Selective attention differentially affects brainstem auditory evoked potentials of electrodermal responders and nonresponders. *Psychiatry Res, 16*, 227-232.

Storrie, M.C., Doerr, H.O., & Johnson, M.H. (1981). Skin conductance characteristics of depressed subjects before and after therapeutic intervention. *J Nerv Ment Dis, 69*, 176-179.

Straube, E. R. (1979). On the meaning of electrodermal nonresponding in schizophrenia. *J Nerv Ment Dis, 167*, 601-611.

Torrey, E.F. (1991). A viral-anatomical explanation of schizophrenia. *Schizophren Bull, 17*, 15-18.

Torrey, E.F., Rawlings, R., & Waldman, I.N. (1988). Schizophrenic births and viral diseases in two states. *Schizophren Res, 1*, 73-77.

Watson, C.G., Kucala, T., Tilleskjor, C., & Jacobs, L. (1984). Schizophrenic birth seasonality in relation to the incidence of infectious diseases and temperature extremes. *Arch Gen Psychiatry, 41*, 85-90.

Wing, J.K., Cooper, J.E., & Sartorius, N. (1974). *The measurement and classification of psychiatric symptoms*. New York: Cambridge University Press.

Yokata, T., Sato, A., & Fujimori, B. (1963). Inhibition of sympathetic activity by stimulation of limbic system. *Jpn J Physiol, 13*, 138-144.

Zahn, T. P., Carpenter, W. T., & McGlashan, T. H. (1981). Autonomic nervous system activity in acute schizophrenia. I. Method and comparison with normal controls. *Arch Gen Psychiatry, 38*, 251-258.

Zahn, T. P., Rumsey, J. M., & Van Kammen, D. P. (1987). Autonomic nervous activity in autistic, schizophrenic, and normal men: Effects of stimulus significance. *J Abnorm Psychol 96*, 135-144.

# THE LATERALITY OF ELECTRODERMAL RESPONSES:

# A NEW PERSPECTIVE ON INDIVIDUAL DIFFERENCES IN

# PERSONALITY AND PSYCHOPATHOLOGY

John Gruzelier

Laboratory of Neuro-Psychophysiology
Department of Psychiatry
Charing Cross and Westminster Medical School
St Dunstan's Road
London W6 8RF England

Currently the nature and direction of hemispheric influences on electrodermal activity are not understood. All cognitive research into the question has been based on structural models of hemispheric specialisation. Models of fixed structure assume that hemispheric specialisation, whether it be verbal/nonverbal, verbal/visuo-spatial, serial/parallel, etc, is determined by the structure of the nervous system, as seen in the morphological asymmetries of the planum temporale, larger on the left than the right in the majority of dextral subjects, and thought to underpin left hemispheric language advantages (Geschwind and Levitsky, 1968). However, while evidence in support of structural models is not uncommon in studies of the damaged brain (Beaton, 1985), attempts to demonstrate predicted cognitive advantages in normal subjects have been difficult to achieve. Plausible explanations have been offered by some theorists that factors like attentional biases, priming, practice effects, fatigue, over arousal, under arousal, and so forth, may interfere with structure-based processes. Accordingly it has been posited that dynamic processes, such as arousal and attention, may interact with structural processes to accentuate, nullify or even reverse predicted cognitive asymmetries (Cohen, 1982).

Bilateral recording of psychophysiological measures may provide an ideal opportunity to monitor dynamic processes, such as arousal and attention, and provide validation for post hoc interpretations of data which invoke dynamic processes. A study by Gruzelier and Phelan (1991) exemplifies how a dynamic process, anxiety, can reverse a putatively structure-based lexical process. Medical students were tested on two occasions, one of which was immediately before a mid-year examination and the other four weeks before or after; order of testing was counterbalanced. The ecological validity of the stressor was confirmed by increased scores of frustration-tension on the IPAT Anxiety

Scale (Krug, Scheier and Cattell, 1976), by highly significant increases in electrodermal non-specific responses, as well as by retardation of habituation to a standard series of moderate intensity tones, as had been shown earlier by Maltzman et al, (1972), also in an investigation of examination stress in students. Cerebral asymmetry for lexical processing was examined with a divided visual field tachistoscope task in which normal subjects showed a right visual field-left hemisphere advantage (Connolly et al, 1983). This asymmetry was confirmed in the non-stress condition, whereas the stressor produced the opposite hemispheric advantage, as shown in Figure 1. Twenty-two of the 33 subjects showed the reversal of hemispheric asymmetry.

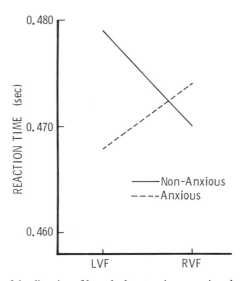

**Figure 1**. Evidence of the direction of lateral advantage in processing changing with anxiety.

The interactive model of fixed versus dynamic processes has guided our research on bilateral skin conductance, together with the consideration that electrodermal activity has historically been closely allied to processes of arousal and attention, i.e. dynamic processes, more so than with cognitive processes associated with hemispheric specialisation and fixed structure.

In this chapter we will focus on studies of individual differences in bilateral skin conductance. Investigations (Gruzelier, 1973; Gruzelier & Venables, 1974; Gruzelier et al, 1981b) showing in normals and psychiatric patients Gaussian distributions of lateral asymmetries in electrodermal orienting responses (Gruzelier, 1979), led us to consider the significance of individual differences in lateral asymmetry for both normal and abnormal psychological function.

## HABITUATION, RESPONSIVENESS AND CEREBRAL ASYMMETRY

We first discovered that individual differences in lateral asymmetry of orienting and nonspecific responses were associated with rate of habituation and the number of responses (Gruzelier, Eves and Connolly, 1981). The experiments, which were carried out in three laboratories, with different recording apparatus, experimenters and scorers, totalled 109 subjects. Orienting responses (ORs) were measured for up to 13 70 dB tones of 1000Hz and 1 sec duration with interstimulus intervals psuedorandomised between 20 and 40 secs. Nonspecific responses were all responses outside the OR interval of 0.8 and 5 secs poststimulus. The lateral asymmetry was expressed as a laterality index 2(right-left/right + left). In each experiment significant correlations were found between lateral asymmetry and both trials to habituation (mean r for all experiments = 0.41, p<0.001) and the number of nonspecific responses (mean r = 0.45, p<0.001). Similar effects were found with both variables to 90 dB, 5 sec long tones which were also examined in one of the groups (r= 0.53, p<0.01 and 0.62, p< 0.001 respectively). Importantly correlations were not significant in female subjects in all experiments (r = 0.24 for the total sample). Nor were they in sinistrals (0.42). Both are groups in whom cerebral asymmetry appears less clear cut compared with dextral males (Harris, 1979; Herron, 1980); in the case of sinistrality a result which pertains to the subgroup in which speech is located in the right hemisphere or is thought to be equally distributed in both hemispheres.

The nature of the relationship was such that fast habituation was associated with larger left hand responses and left hemispheric influences, and slow habituation with larger right hand responses and right hemispheric influences. Moderate degrees of responding were associated with symmetry. The relationship implied reciprocal hemispheric influences on habituation. This interpretation was supported by correlations obtained between trials to habituation and mean response amplitudes after removing with partial correlations the influence of habituation on response amplitude. Correlations were negative with the left hand and positive with the right hand; we reasoned that control of habituation by one hemisphere would have produced correlations with one hand only. Correlations were not significant with asymmetries in skin conductance level, ranging only between 0.06 and 0.32. Furthermore, after partialling out the influence of levels on skin conductance response amplitude, the correlations between lateral asymmetry of responses and trials to habituation were hardly altered.

Hemispheric influences on habituation rate were interpreted on the basis of two principles. First, most evidence supports a relationship between the influence of each hemisphere and the asymmetry pattern of greater responding on the ipsilateral hand compared than the contralateral hand, at least when stimuli are attended to in the passive state. Whether this is due to contralateral inhibitory influences or ipsilateral excitatory influences, or both, has not been demonstrated. Under active task conditions these relationships may reverse, and in the case of motor preparation contralateral excitatory influences may prevail in support of likely effector functions of palmar electrodermal activity. The second principle is that evidence in neurological patients with unilateral lesions which compared Wernicke's aphasics with right parietal hemi-neglect patients, indicates that the left hemisphere has an inhibitory polarity over electrodermal orienting responses while the right hemisphere has an excitatory polarity (Heilman and Watson, 1989). Thus, when left hemisphere influences predominate, inhibition will be uppermost, habituation will be fast, and right hand influences will be smaller via contralateral inhibitory effects. Under right hemisphere functional dominance the opposite effects will prevail, namely habituation will be slow and right hand responses will be greater than left hand ones. A discussion of these issues may be found in Gruzelier (1979, 1987); Gruzelier, Sergeant and Eves (1988) (see also Figure 3).

Notwithstanding the fact that the neurological evidence for these principles is limited, and their examination must be a critical direction for future research, the model is theoretically consistent (1) with evidence associating electrodermal responsivity with attention and vigilance, and (2) evidence associating attention and vigilance with hemispheric specialisation.

First, decrements in vigilance have been found to parallel reduced electrodermal responding (Ross et al, 1959; Stern, 1966), associations confirmed by careful consideration of the temporal relationships between electrodermal responses and hits and misses in detection (Surwillo and Quilter, 1965; Krupski, Ruskin and Bakan, 1971; Blakeslee, 1979). Furthermore, when habituation rates have been measured prior to vigilance tasks, an association was found between fast habituation and poor vigilance and slow habituation and superior vigilance (Coles and Gale, 1971; Siddle, 1972; Crider and Augenbraun, 1975; Kopp et al, 1987). Selective attention in the face of distractors, on the other hand, has been shown to be facilitated by prior habituation to the distractor stimulus (Waters et al, 1977).

Second, turning to hemispheric specialisation, evidence from studies with normals and attentional disabilities in patients with callosectomy have implicated the right hemisphere in sustained vigilance and the left hemisphere in selective attention. Accordingly it was proposed that "extremes in electrodermal reactivity are associated with differences in attention such that fast habituation is associated with focused, selective attention, and slow habituation with sustained, broad, vigilant attention (Gruzelier et al, 1981a). Focused selective attention is a prerequisite of analytic, sequential processing of the left hemisphere while broad vigilant attention is compatible with the parallel, holistic processing of the right hemisphere." (Gruzelier, 1987).

## HABITUATION AND THE LATERALITY OF PAIN IN MIGRAINE

Two experiments involving migraineurs with consistently lateralised pain provided additional support for the relationship between habituation and cerebral laterality (Gruzelier et al, 1987). Importantly subjects were examined in the interictal phase and therefore in the absence of head pain; with the onset of pain the dynamics of cerebral blood flow are complex (Lauritzen and Olesen, 1984). It was hypothesised that the predisposition to unilateral headache took the form of over-activation or overload of the hemisphere ipsilateral to the pain (e.g. Crisp et al, 1985).

In the first experiment bilateral electrodermal activity was recorded to a series of 20 moderate intensity flashes in 30 female subjects, 5 with left-sided migraine, 6 with right-sided migraine, 7 with bilateral tension headache, and 12 controls. In the second, 13 additional subjects, 7 with left-sided and 6 with right-sided pain, were examined with the standard moderate intensity tone habituation sequence. In both experiments those with left-sided head pain were fast habituators and those with right-sided pain were slow habituators. When the data from the two experiments were combined the clinical groups differed in their lateral asymmetry with those in the latter group being significantly more asymmetric in a right>left direction. The results for habituation are shown in Figure 2; it can be seen that laterality of pain was associated with opposite extremes of habituation in line with the model.

## FUNCTIONAL ASYMMETRY AND SUSCEPTIBILITY TO CARDIOVASCULAR DISORDERS

In a series of studies we have investigated the bilateral skin conductance of cardiac patients to shed light on the possible involvement of hemispheric imbalance in susceptibility to cardiovascular disorders. In particular we examined the role of central triggers of hyperventilation and possible distinctions between the personality of patients who hyperventilate to psychological versus physical provocation tests. We had earlier found in forty dextral cardiac patients, who presented with clinical signs and symptoms of exhaustion, that, when compared with forty controls, habituation was slower in electrodermally responsive patients, and that they were more asymmetric in the direction of larger right hand responses with longer right hand response latencies, consistent with evidence above of the relationship of habituation to lateral asymmetry. Patients also had a

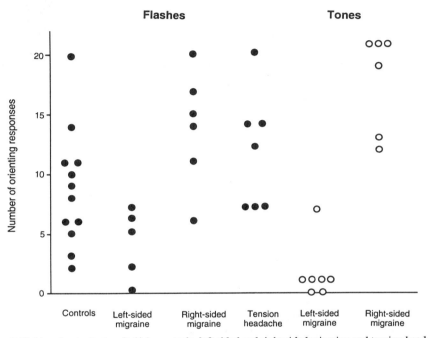

**Figure 2**. Habituation to flashes (left) in controls, left sided and right sided migraine and tension headache. Habituation to tones in another sample of right and left-sided migraine.

markedly abnormal elevation of skin conductance levels on the right hand which was representative of 75% of the sample and gave rise to a highly significant (p<0.001) asymmetry (Gruzelier, Nixon, Pugh, Liddiard and Baxter, 1986). These results suggest imbalances in functional activity, higher in the right hemisphere.

Lane and Schwartz (1987) in considering stress-induced cardiac arrhythmias proposed that individuals who produced more lateralised cortical activity during emotional arousal may generate more lateralised sympathetic input to the heart. As left-sided input is more arrythmogenic, then in view of the contralateral mediation of hemispheric influences this involves the right hemisphere. There is evidence of right hemispheric involvement in emotion, especially negative emotion, which results show is associated with right anterior activation in contrast to positive emotion which appears to involve left anterior regions (Sackheim et al, 1982; Flor-Henry, 1983; Davidson and Tomarken, 1989). Lane and Schwartz hypothesised that it is strong negative, avoidance emotion that places susceptible individuals more at risk for fatal arrhythmias. In order to elucidate their proposition of the arrhythmogenic properties of right hemispheric functional dominance, and our finding of abnormal right hemispheric activation in cardiac patients, we compared 15 cardiac patients with coronary artery disease and 15 with arrhythmias (Conway, Gruzelier, Freeman & Nixon, 1992). While in fact there was no evidence that the arrhythmia group was more asymmetric in bilateral skin conductance during a number of stress and resting conditions than the group with structural disorders, relationships were found in the total group between lateral asymmetries in the skin conductance levels and the personality measures. Correlations were obtained with Type A coronary prone behaviour (Bortner, 1969), as well as with the Managerial and Aggressive subscales of the Leary Adjective Checklist (Leary, 1957), both attributes of the Type A behaviour pattern.

In an earlier study, Conway, Freeman & Nixon (1988) showed that patients who hyperventilated to psychological stressors as distinct from physical stressors were characterised as Self Effacing and Docile on the Leary scale; a profile antipathetical to that of Type A. This result was replicated when we compared those patients who hyperventilated (a decrease of 14 mmHg $CO_2$) to the individualised psychological stressor (N=17) with those who did not hyperventilate (N=13). Here it was the electrodermal response amplitude asymmetry which correlated with the Self Effacing score in the direction of larger right hand responses. These two studies indicated that both of the personality types connected with cardiovascular dysfunction were associated with right hemispheric functional dominance (Conway et al, 1992), but levels of skin conductance activity and responses differentiated the two.

Subsequently the Self Effacing subscale of the Leary checklist administered to medical students was found to correlate with amplitude asymmetries in nonspecific responses during the tone habituation sequence in the direction of higher right hand response amplitudes (0.43, p<0.02) (Conway & Gruzelier, 1992). There were also positive correlations between this personality scale and anxiety.

Thus in clinical and normal samples support was found for a relationship between hemispheric imbalances of function, in the direction of higher right hemispheric activity, and psychological factors relevant to cardiovascular function, whether in the form of personality traits having a bearing on cardiovascular function, personally relevant stressors which produce hyperventilation, or in the characterization of cardiac patients suffering exhaustion.


## ANXIETY AND THE ALTERATION OF FUNCTIONAL ASYMMETRY

In the student study above the major effect on bilateral skin conductance responses was found to be categorisation of students according to trait anxiety on the Speilberger scale, a result which will be seen to be consistent with a series of studies in the laboratory. As shown in Figure 1 anxiety may alter structure-based cognitive asymmetries. This has also been demonstrated with asymmetries in electrodermal responses. In our first study of bilateral electrodermal activity in medical students (Gruzelier et al, 1981), slow habituators were found to have higher scores of IPAT anxiety than fast habituators, a result consistent with reports of Maltzman et al (1972) and Gruzelier and Phelan (1991), but by no means a universal relationship (O'Gorman, 1975). There were sufficient numbers of slow habituators to subdivide them according to lateral asymmetry, which disclosed that the anomalous leftward asymmetry group had the higher anxiety scores

(Gruzelier, 1987). In other words while anxiety was generally associated with right hemispheric activity, at high states of anxiety left hemispheric influences predominated. This is in keeping with Tucker's (1981) view that anxiety.places a processing load on the left hemisphere. This was inferred from evidence that anxiety was associated with a left hemisphere activational bias, as shown in superior right ear loudness judgments, which at the same time coincided with poorer left than right hemispheric processing of verbal and spatial stimuli in a divided visual-field task.

The electrodermal evidence lead to the conceptualisation of the influence of anxiety on cerebral asymmetry in terms of the inverted-U curve of arousal and performance as follows (Gruzelier, 1987). Fast habituation reflects a state of left hemispheric inhibitory control. As the excitation-inhibition balance tips towards excitation, habituation progressively slows until a state of right hemispheric activation dominance is reached along with raised anxiety. Then with higher states of anxiety the control reverts to the left hemisphere heralding the downswing of the inverted-U curve and coinciding with behavioural disorganisation. The schema is shown in Fig. 3.

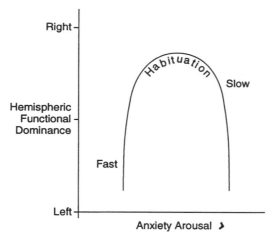

**Figure 3.** Schema relating functional hemispheric dominance and arousal/anxiety level to rate of habituation

One implication of this is that hemispheric dominance may be associated with different types of anxiety: when characterised by strong cognitive components such as obsessional thoughts and ruminations, the left hemisphere is dominant, when anxiety is generalised, free floating and nonspecific, the right hemisphere is dominant. Preliminary support for these hypotheses was found in a study of students where the IPAT subscales of frustration-tension, apprehension-worrying and suspicion were associated with left hemispheric dominance and subscales of emotional instability and lack of self control were associated with right hemispheric dominance. The inverted-U shaped relationship between anxiety and lateralisation was examined by Kopp and Gruzelier (1988) with DSM III anxiety disorders and controls who were subdivided as stable, labile or intermediate on the basis of unilateral electrodermal responsiveness during a tone habituation sequence. In controls bilateral auditory thresholds (8000 Hz) favoured the left hemisphere in stabiles and the right in labiles, consistent with the up-swing of the curve. In patients thresholds favoured the left hemisphere in stabiles and the right hemisphere in those patients with intermediate levels of responsiveness, whereas patient labiles showed a left hemisphere advantage, results which followed all three phases of the inverted-U curve and were consistent with high anxiety causing a lateral shift from right to left.

Further support was forthcoming in the studies of stressors on bilateral skin conductance in patients and students (Conway et al, 1992; Conway and Gruzelier, 1992). In the patient study those who in their medical history reported clinical anxiety (N=18) were more right asymmetric in electrodermal responses than those without anxiety (N=12). The student study involved thirty-five dextral medical students, twenty of them female, who were examined with a moderate intensity tone habituation sequence followed by voluntary hyperventilation, an individualised stressor and a recognition memory task in the presence of noise bursts, each task followed by a relaxation recovery phase and presented in a counterbalanced design. Subdivision into two groups with the Speilberger Trait anxiety scale disclosed that the low anxiety group had greater left hand response amplitudes to the orienting tones while those high in anxiety had the opposite asymmetry. Correlations between trait anxiety and lateral asymmetries in orienting and nonspecific responses were also significant (0.44, p <0.02 & 0.56, p <0.002 respectively).

Finally, in an unpublished study Holland and Gruzelier (Gruzelier, 1987) examined relationships between bilateral skin conductance activity and both IPAT anxiety and a hemisphericity scale based on hemispheric cognitive specialisation (Zenhausern, 1978). No relationships were found between electrodermal lateral asymmetries and the hemisphericity scale, whereas IPAT anxiety was related to both larger right than left orienting response amplitudes and skin conductance level asymmetries. This evidence confirms that a broader conceptualisation of hemisphere functions than the traditional cognitive dichotomies are needed.


## LATERAL IMBALANCE AND SYNDROMES OF SCHIZOPHRENIA

While many investigators have reported more rightward asymmetries in schizophrenia, (Gruzelier, 1973; Gruzelier and Venables, 1974; Gruzelier et al, 1981b; Schneider, 1983; White, Farley and Charles, 1987), this has not been universally found (Iacono, 1982). In our investigations, while the rightward shift characterised patients as a whole, there were individual patients that had larger left hand responses. We examined the significance of this in a subsequent study by classifying patients according to the direction of the lateral asymmetry to moderate intensity tones, or to louder 90dB tones in the case of non-responders to the moderate intensity sequence, and examining psychiatric ratings as the dependent variable (Gruzelier, 1981; Gruzelier and Manchanda, 1982). Forty-eight patients in all, which included a replication sample, were rated on the Brief Psychiatric Rating Scale (Overall and Gorham, 1962) and the Present State Examination (Wing et al, 1974). They were all unmedicated at the time, were short-stay hospital patients and had positive symptoms of the Schneiderian type which were integral to the PSE-assisted classification of schizophrenia. Those with larger right hand responses were distinguished by a syndrome consisting of classical negative symptoms including blunted affect, poverty of speech, motor retardation and emotional withdrawal. Those with the opposite asymmetry were distinguished by delusions, positive or labile affect, cognitive acceleration, pressure of speech and over-activity on the ward. Accordingly three syndromes were delineated in schizophrenia: two with a bearing on lateralisation. One of these consisted of a negative syndrome and characterised those with greater right than left hemispheric activation. The second, a positive syndrome excluding Schneider's symptoms, characterised those with greater left than right hemispheric activation. A third, a positive syndrome consisted of Schneiderian symptoms, particularly auditory hallucinations and was unrelalated to lateralisation. See also other three-syndrome approaches (e.g. Liddle, 1987; Friston et al, 1992). The nature of the syndromes was consistent neuropsychologically with the direction of the electrodermal lateral asymmetry. Negative affect and withdrawal have been associated with right hemispheric activation, while poverty of speech is consistent with under activation of the left hemisphere. Positive affect and cognitive acceleration including pressure of speech are consistent with left hemispheric activation, as are raised levels of behavioural activity. The two syndromes delineated by laterality as the independent variable suggest an arousal dimension depicting activity-withdrawal. Accordingly they have been labelled 'Active' and 'Withdrawn' in keeping with theoretical models distinguishing the hemispheres on the basis of motoric-sensory/passive and approach-withdrawal dimensions (Tucker and Williamson, 1984; Davidson and Tomarken, 1989).

Reviews of the literature on measures of laterality and schizophrenia disclosed evidence of psychophysiological and cognitive variables depicting asymmetries in either direction. Both direction of asymmetry and clinical correlates had affinities with the Active and Withdrawn syndromes (Gruzelier, 1983; 1984; 1985). Measures included EEG power, CNVs, ERPs, the Hoffman reflex, lateral eye movements, visual search eye movements and manual reaction time, and dichotic listening. We have also examined the Active and Withdrawn syndromes with neuropsychological tests of learning and memory validated on neurological patients with lateralised frontal, temporal and parietal lesions (Gruzelier et al, 1988; Gruzelier, 1990). Losses of function fulfilling criteria of double dissociation of function occurred in each syndrome in the hemisphere with the lower level of activation.

This investigative approach has been extended to the schizotypal personality (Gruzelier et al, 1992). In medical students a three syndrome factor structure has been found which has a strong bearing on the three syndromes in schizophrenia. Furthermore, classifying subjects on the basis of a laterality score based on the discrepancy between left and right hemisphere recognition memory scores, replicated in schizotypy the relationships obtained between the memory scores and syndromes in schizophrenia. Thus it would appear to be the individual difference in the direction of asymmetry, rather than asymmetry per se which is of importance in schizophrenia. Accordingly analyses of asymmetries of nosological categories per se are likely to be uninformative (Bernstein et al, 1981; Iacono, 1982; Öhman et al, 1989).

## ELECTRODERMAL RESPONDING AND NONRESPONDING IN SCHIZOPHRENIA

Neuropsychological investigations have also been extended to the more widely researched individual difference in electrodermal activity in schizophrenia, namely the Responder/Nonresponder distinction. This concerns whether or not electrodermal orienting responses are elicited to moderate intensity tones, research which was originally undertaken from a neuro-psychophysiological standpoint (Gruzelier and Venables, 1972; 1974). About 50% of patients, failed to elicit responses, particularly those who were institutionalised; the remainder responded, many of whom were slow habituators, a proportion that varies from study to study (Bernstein et al, 1982; Dawson, Nuechterlein and Adams, 1989). Original interest in central mechanisms concerned the involvement of limbic system pathology in schizophrenia, in particular frontohippocampal systems in the loss of habituation, and frontoamygdaloid systems in the absence of orienting. Recently there has been considerable support from neuroanatomical and neurochemical postmortem studies of limbic involvement in schizophrenia (Gruzelier & Raine, 1993).

As noninstitutionalised patients may change from one sub-group to another (Rubens and Lapidus, 1978), we selected chronic patients with persistent symptoms. Patients examined neuropsychologically were drawn from a larger group (N=42, twenty-seven male and fifteen female) with an average age in their mid 50s, age of onset twenty-five years, and total length of time in hospital twenty-two years. Neuroleptic medication expressed as the CPZ equivalent averaged 1200 mg a day, which contrasts with the considerably lower 300 mg in the early studies (e.g., Gruzelier & Venables, 1972). Of the forty-two patients 55% were nonresponders and 19% slow habituators. The first neuropsychological experiment involved sixteen patients (nine Responders and seven Nonresponders) who were tested nine months later when habituation status was remarkably similar: - $r = 0.81$, p<0.001. They were examined with tests of frontal function and tests of object recognition involving the right parietal lobe; regions which have also been shown to influence the electrodermal orienting response (Heilman and Watson, 1989; Luria and Homskaya, 1979; Bagshaw et al, 1965). Two of the object recognition tests distinguished the groups in the direction of poorer performance in Responders, namely Ghent's Over-lapping Figures and the Unusual Views test. Whereas other right parietal object recognition tests, Dot Centring, Binet's Blocks, Gollin's Graded Figures and Incomplete Letters showed no differences. Accordingly, no global object recognition or right parietal deficit was implicated. What appeared to characterise the deficiency in Responders was the inability to return figure to ground, a feature of processing that Pribram (1990) has attributed to the hippocampus.

Considering the tests of frontal function, the groups differed on the Wisconsin Card Sort (Nelson, 1986) in terms of total number of errors and perseverative errors; again Responders were the more impaired. Correlations between trials to habituation and a range of tests were found: Wisconsin perseverative errors and the number of categories sorted, verbal fluency, Trail Making, and the Stroop; the greater the habituation deficit the poorer the performance.

A second experiment was undertaken with the five object recognition tests and three tests which are compromised by damage to the hippocampus: Hebb's Digits and Corsi's Blocks, and the Cross on the Line test (Milner, 1971). The patients were similar clinically and demographically to the previous study, but were from another hospital. They consisted of 11 Responders and 16 Nonresponders and satisfied DSM-III-R diagnostic criteria. In replication of the first experiment Responders were impaired on the Overlapping Figures and Unusual Views test and, in support of predictions, were impaired in the learning of recurrent sequences in the Hebb and Corsi tests, and performed more poorly on the Cross on the Line Test.

The results are consistent with hippocampal impairment in chronic schizophrenic patients with persistent symptoms. In view of the fact that acute patients may vary in their Responder/Nonresponder status, these effects which appear to have a structural basis in the CNS may not hold for remitting patients. Not all the Nonresponders were nonhabituators, signifying that in this chronic, well-medicated sample it is the absolute difference that provides the marker, not the distinction between nonresponding and nonhabituation.


## CONCLUSION

In conclusion, electrodermal orienting and habituation processes, especially when measured bilaterally, provide valuable insights into central nervous system mechanisms which have relevance to individual differences which are of central importance to the psychology of personality and to a range of clinical conditions. The concern with individual differences cast in a neuropsychological framework has been of fundamental importance to obtaining the behavioural and replicable relationships reviewed in this chapter. Consideration of functional brain processes as distinct from processes based on fixed-structure has been shown to be critical to the elucidation of relationships between the brain and electrodermal responses. Electrodermal measurement as an adjunct to cognitive procedures can provide validation of the operation of dynamic processes, and without the awareness of this relationship will make the use of electrodermal responses as markers of group membership unreliable. As evidence of the multiple determinants of central influences on electrodermal activity grows (Gruzelier et al, 1988; Gruzelier & Raine, 1992), a greater richness in relationships can be anticipated.

## REFERENCES

Bagshaw, M.H., Kimble, D.P., and Pribram, K.H., 1965, The GSR of monkeys during orienting and habituation and after ablation of the amygdala, hippocampus and infero-temporal cortex, *Neuropsychologia* 3:111.

Beaton, A., 1985,*"Left Side, Right Side"*, Yale University Press, London.

Bernstein, A.S., Frith, C.D., Gruzelier, J.H., Patterson, T., Straube, E., Venables, P., and Zahn, T., 1982, An analysis of the skin conductance orienting response in samples of American, British, and German schizophrenics, *Biol Psychol.* 14:155.

Bernstein, A.S., Taylor, K.W., Starkey, P., Juni, S., Lubowski, J., and Paley, H. 1981, Bilateral skin conductance, finger pulse volume, and EEG orienting response to tones of differing intensities in chronic schizophrenics and controls. *J nerv Ment Dis.* 169:513.

Blakeslee, P., 1979, Attention and vigilance: performance and skin conductance response changes. *Psychophysiology* 16:413.

Bogerts, B., 1990, The neuropathology of schizophrenia, in H. Hafner and W.F. Gattaz, eds, *"Search for the Causes of Schizophrenia,"* vol 2. Springer-Verlag, London.

Bortner, R.W., 1969, A short rating scale as a potential measure of Pattern A behaviour. *J. chron. Dis.* 22:87.

Cohen, G., 1982, Theoretical interpretations of lateral asymmetries, in: *"Divided Visual Field Studies of Cerebral Organisation,"* J.G.Beaumont, ed., Academic Press, New York.

Coles, M.G., and Gale, A., 1971, Physiological reactivity as a predictor of performance in a vigilance task, *Psychophysiology* 8:594.

Connolly, J.F., Gruzelier, J.H., and Manchanda, R., 1983, Electrocortical and perceptual asymmetries in schizophrenia, in: *"Hemisphere Asymmetries of Function in Psychopathology,"* P. Flor-Henry and J. Gruzelier, eds., Elsevier/North Holland, Amsterdam.

Conway, A.V., Freeman, L.J., and Nixon, P.G.F., 1988, Hypnotic examination of trigger factors in the hyper-ventilation syndrome, *Amer. J. Clin. Hyp.* 30:296.

Conway, A.V., and Gruzelier, J.H., 1992, Lateral asymmetry in electrodermal responses in conditions of baseline, hyperventilation and laboratory stressors in relation to anxiety and cardiovascular susceptibilty factors, (in preparation).

Conway, A.V. Freeman, L.J., Gruzelier, J.H., and Nixon, P.G.F., 1992, Psychological stress, hyper-ventilation and lateralisation of electrdermal responses in the production of electrocardiogram abnormalities, (submitted for publication).

Crider, A., and Augenbraun, C.B., 1975, Auditory vigilance correlates of electrodermal response habituation speed. *Psychophysiology* 12:36.

Crisp, A.H., Karmen, J., Potamianos, G., and Bhat, A.V., 1985, Cerebral hemisphere function anf laterality of migraine. *Psychother. Psychosom.* 43:49.

Davidson, R.J., and Tomarken, A.J., 1989, Laterality and emotion: an electrophysiological approach, in: *"Handbook of Neuropsychology,"* L. Squire and G.Gainotti, eds, Elsevier, Amsterdam.

Dawson, M.E., Nuechterlein, K.H., and Adams, R.M., 1989, Schizophrenic Disorders, in: *"Handbook of Clinical Psychophysiology"*, G.Turpin, ed, Wiley, Chichester.

Douglas, R.J., 1967, The hippocampus and behaviour. *Psychol. Bull.* 67:416.

Flor-Henry, P., 1983, *"The Cerebral Basis of Psychopathology,"* John Wright, London.

Friston, K.J., Liddle, P.F., Frith, C.D., Hirsch, S.R., and Frackowiak, R.S.J., 1992, Left-parahippocampal dysfunction in schizophrenia: A PET study, *Brain*, 115:367.

Geschwind, N., and Levitsky, W., 1968, Human Brain: Left-right asymmetries in temporal speech region, *Science* 161:186.

Gruzelier, J. H., 1973, Bilateral asymmetry of skin conductance orienting activity and levels in schizophrenics. *Biol. Psychol.* 1:21.

Gruzelier, J.H., 1979, Lateral asymmetries in electrodermal activity and psychosis, in: *"Hemisphere asymmetries of Function in Psychopathology,"* J.H. Gruzelier and P. Flor-Henry, eds, Elsevier/North Holland, Amsterdam.

Gruzelier, J.H., 1981, Hemispheric imbalances masquerading as paranoid and non-paranoid syndromes. *Schiz Bull.* 7:662.

Gruzelier, J.H., 1983, A critical assessment and integration of lateral asymmetries in schizophrenia, in: *"Hemisyndromes: Psychobiology, Neurology, Psychiatry,"*, M.S. Myslobodsky, ed, Academic Press, New York.

Gruzelier, J.H., 1984, Hemispheric imbalances in schizophrenia, *Int. J. Psychophysiol.* 1:227.

Gruzelier, J.H., 1985, Central nervous system signs in schizophrenia, in: *"Handbook of Clinical Neurology, Neurobehavioural Disorders,"* vol 46, J.A.M. Frederiks, ed, P.J. Vinken, G.W. Bruyn, and H.L. Klawans, eds, Elsevier, Amsterdam.

Gruzelier, J.H., 1987, Individual differences in dynamic process asymmetries in the normal and pathological brain, in: *"Individual Differences in Hemispheric Specialisation,"* A. Glass, ed, Plenum, London.

Gruzelier, J.H., 1990, Brain localisation and neuropsychology in schizophrenia: Implications forsyndromes, sex differences and genetics, in: *"Search for the Causes of Schizophrenia,"* H. Hafner and W.F. Gattaz, eds, Springer Verlag, Bern.

Gruzelier, J.H., 1991, Hemispheric imbalance: Syndromes of schizophrenia, premorbid personality, and neurodevelopmental influences, in: *"Neuropsychology, Psychophysiology and Information Processing."* Vol 5, *"Handbook of Schizophrenia,"*, S Steinhauer, J.H. Gruzelier, and J. Zubin, eds, Elsevier, Amsterdam.

Gruzelier, J.H., and Venables, P.H., 1972, Skin conductance orienting activity in a heterogeneous sample of schizophrenics: possible evidence of limbic dysfunction, *J. Nerv. Ment. Dis.* 155:277.

Gruzelier, J.H. and Venables, P.H., 1974, Bimodality and lateral asymmetry of skin conductance orienting activity in schizophrenics: Replication and evidence of lateral asymmetry in patients with depression and disorders of personality, *Biol. Psychiat.* 8:55.

Gruzelier, J.H., Eves, F.F., and Connolly, J.F., 1981a, Habituation and phasic reactivity in the electrodermal system; Reciprocal hemispheric influences, *Physiol. Psychol.* 9:313.

Gruzelier, J.H., Eves, F.F., Connolly, J.F., and Hirsch, S.R., 1981b, Orienting, habituation, sensitisation and dishabituation in the electrodermal system of consecutive, drug-free admissions for schizophrenia, *Biol. Psychol.* 12:187.

Gruzelier, J.H., and Manchanda, R., 1982, The syndrome of schizophrenia; Relatiohs between electrodermal response lateral asymmetries and clinical ratings, *Brit. J. Psychiat.* 141:488.

Gruzelier, J.H., Nixon,P.G.F., Liddiard, D., Pugh, S. and Baxter, R., 1986, Retarded habituation and lateral asymmetries in electrodermal activity in cardiovascular disorders, *Int. J. Psychophysiol.* 3:219.

Gruzelier, J. H., Nicolaou, T., Connolly, J.F., Peatfield, R.C., Davies, P.T.G., and Clifford-Rose, F., 1987, Laterality of pain in migraine distinguished by interictal rates of habituation of electrodermal responses to visual and auditory stimuli, *J. Neurol. Neurosurg. Psychiat.* 50:410.

Gruzelier, J.H., Seymour, K., Wilson, L., Jolley, T., and Hirsch, S., 1988, Impairments on neuropsychological tests of temporo-hippocampal and fronto-hippocampal functions and word fluency in remitting schizophrenia and affective disorders, *Arch. Gen. Psychiat.* 45:623.

Gruzelier, J.H., Sergeant, J., and Eves, F., 1988, The use of bilateral skin conductance measurement in elucidating stimulus versus response processing influences on the orienting reaction, *Int. J. Psychophysiol.* 6:195.

Gruzelier, J.H., and Phelan, M., 1991, Laterality-reversal in a lexical divided visual field task under stress, *Int. J. Psychophysiol.* 11:269.

Gruzelier, J.H., Burgess, A., Stygall, J., Irving, G., and Raine, A., 1992, Hemisphere imbalance and syndromes of schizotypal personality, (submitted for publication).

Gruzelier, J.H., and Raine, A., 1992, Schizophrenia, schizotypal personality, syndromes, cerebral lateralisation and electrodermal activity, (to be published in Schiz Bull).

Harris, L. J., 1978, Sex differences in spatialability: possible environmental, genetic and neurological factors, in: *"Asymmetrical Function of the Brain,"* M. Kinsbourne, ed, Cambridge University Press, London.

Heilman, K.M., and Watson, R.T., 1989, Arousal and emotion, in: *"Handbook of Neuropsychology", vol 3.*, L.Squire and G Gainotti, eds, Elsevier, Amsterdam.

Herron, J., 1980, *"Neuropsychology of Left-Handedness,"* Academic Press, London.

Iacono. W., 1982, Bilateral electrdermal habituation-dishabituation and resting EEG in remitted schizophrenics, *J. Nerv. Ment. Dis.* 170:91.

Ketterer, M.W., and Smith, B.D., 1977, Bilateral electrodermalactivity, lateralised cerebral processing and sex, *Psychophysiology* 14:513.

Kopp, M.S., Mihaly, K., Linka, E. and Bitter,I., 1987, Electrodermally differentiated subgroups of anxiety patients. I. Autonomic and vigilance characteristics, *Int. J. Psychophysiol.* 5:43.

Kopp, M., and Gruzelier, J.H., 1988, Electrodermally differentiated subgroups of anxiety patients and controls. II. Auditory, somatosensory and pain thresholds, agoraphobic fear, depression and cerebral laterality, *Int. J. Psychophysiol.* 7:65.

Krug, S.E., Scheier, I.H.Cattell, R.B., 1976, *"Handbook for the IPAT Anxiety Scale,"* Institute of Personality and Ability Testing, Champagne.

Krupski, A., Ruskin, D.C., and Bakan, 1971, Physiological and personality correlates of commission errors in an auditory vigilance task, *Psychophysiology* 8:304.

Lacroix, J.M., and Comper, P., 1979, Lateralisation in electrodermal system as a function of cognitive/hemispheric manipulations, *Psychophysiology* 16:116.

Lane, R., and Schwartz, G.E., 1987, Induction of lateralised sympathetic input to the heart by the CNS during emotional arousal: A possible neurophysiologic trigger of sudden death, *Psychosom. Med.* 49:274.

Lauritzen, M., and Olesen, J., 1984, Regional cerebral blood flow during migraine attacks by Xenon-133 inhalation and emission tomography, *Brain* 107:447.

Leary, T., 1959, *"Interpersonal Diagnosis of Personality,"* Ronald Press, New York.

Levy, J., Heller, W., Banich, M. T., and Burton, L.A., 1983, Are variations amongst right-handed individuals in perceptual asymmetries caused by characteristics arousal differences between hemispheres, *J. Exp. Psychol.* 9:3.

Liddle, P.F., 1987, The symptoms of chronic schizophrenia: A re-examination of the positive-negative dichotomy, *Br. J. Psychiat.* 151:147.

Luria, A., and Homskaya, E.D., 1970, Frontal lobe and the regulation of arousal processes, in: *"Attention: Contemporary Theory and Research,"*, D.Mostovsky, ed, Appleton, New York.

Maltzman, I., Smith, N.J., and Cantor, W., 1971, Effects of stress on habituation of the orienting reflex, *Neuropsychologia* 19:65.

Matinez-Selva, J.M., Roman, F., Garcia-Sanchez, F.A., and Gomez-Amor, J., 1987, Sex differences and the asymmetry of specific and nonspecific electrodermal responses, *Int. J. Psychophysiol.* 5:155.

Milner, B., 1971, Interhemispheric differences in the localisation of psychological processes in man, *Br. Med. J.* 27:272.

Nelson, H.E., 1976, A modified card sorting test sensitive to frontal lobe defects, *Cortex*, 12:314.

O'Gorman, J.G., 1977, Individual differences in habituation of human physiological responses; a review of theory, method, and findings in the study of personality correlates in non-clinical populations, Biol Psychol, 5:257.

Öhman, A., Nordby, H., and D'Elia, G., 1989, Orienting in schizophrenia; Habituation to auditory stimuli of constant and varying intensity in patients high and low in skin conductance responsivity, *Psychophysiology* 26:48.

Overall, J. E., and Gorham, D.R., 1962, The Brief Psychiatric Rating Scale, *Psychol. Rep.* 10:799.

Pribram, K., 1991, Issues concerning the psychophysiology of consciousness, *Int. J. Psychophysiol.* 11:65.

Roman, F., Garcia-Sanchez, A., Martinez-Selva, J.M., Gomez-Amor, J., and Carillo, E., 1989, Sex differences and bilateral electrodermal activity. A replication, *Pavl. J. biol. Sci.* 24:150.

Roman, F., Martinez-Selva,J.M., Garcia-Sanchez,F.A., and Gomez-Amor, J., 1987, Sex differences, activation level and bilateral electrodermal activity, *Pavl. J. Biol. Sci.* 22:113.

Ross, S., Dardano, J.F., and Hackman, R.C., 1959, Conductance levels during vigilance task performance, *J. Appl. Psychol.* 43:65.

Rubens, R., and Lapidus,B., 1978, Arousal patterns and stimulus barrier functioning in schizophrenia. *J. Abn. Psychol.* 87:199.

Sackheim, H.A., Greenberg, M.S., Wynman, A.L., Gur, R.C., Hungerbuhler, J.P., and Geschwind, N., 1982, Hemispheric asymmetry in the expresion of positive and negative emotions; neurological evidence, *Arch. Neurol.* 39:210.

Schneider, S.J., 1983, Multiple measures of hemispheric dysfunction in schizophrenia and depression, *Psychol. Med.* 13:287.

Stern, R.M., 1966, Performance and physiological arousal during two vigilance tasks varying in presentation rate, *Percept. Motor Skills* 23:691.

Surwillo, W.W., and Quilter, R.E., 1966, The relation of frequency of spontaneous skin potential responses to vigilance and to age, *Psychophysiology* 1:272.

Tucker, D.M., 1981, Lateral brain function, emotion and conceptualisation, *Psychol Bull* 89:19.

Tucker, D., and Williamson, P.A., 1984, Asymmetric human control systems in human self regulation, *Psychol. Rev.* 91:185.

Waters, W.F., Macdonald, D.G., and Korenko, L., 1977, Habituation of the orienting response; a gating mechanism subserving selective attention, *Psychophysiology* 14:228.

White, C., Farley, J. and Charles, P., 1987, Chronic schizophrenic disorder I. Psychophysiological responses, laterality and social stress, *Br. J. Psychiat.* 150:365.

Wing, J.K., Cooper, J.E., and Satorius, N. *"The Measurement and Classification of Psychiatric Symptoms,"* Cambridge, University Press, London.

Zenhausern, R., 1978, Imagery, cerebral dominance and style of thinking: A unified field model, *Bull. Psychonom. Soc.* 12:381.

# BRAIN ASYMMETRY AND AUTONOMIC CONDITIONING:

## SKIN CONDUCTANCE RESPONSES

Kenneth Hugdahl and Bjørn Helge Johnsen

Department of Biological and Medical Psychology
University of Bergen
N-5009 Bergen, Norway

## INTRODUCTION

### Brain Asymmetry and Autonomic Responses

Hemispheric asymmetry, or laterality, normally implies that a mental function is lateralized within one of the cerebral hemispheres, not shared by the other hemisphere. Human hemispheric asymmetry is generally conceived of as a specialization for higher cognitive functions, like language and visuo-spatial processing (Hellige, 1990). However, recent advances in psychophysiological research have in addition revealed a number of important biological asymmetries, related to immune function (Barneoud, Neveu, Vitiello & Le Moal, 1987), neuroendocrine responses (Wittling & Pfluger, 1990), and autonomic function (e.g. Weisz, Szilagyi, Lang, & Adam, 1992; Heller, Lindsay, Metz, & Farnum, 1990). Wittling (1990) found that the cerebral hemispheres markedly differed in their capability to regulate blood pressure during emotionally laden situations. Both diastolic and systolic blood pressure was significantly increased for right hemisphere presentations of short film clips with emotional content. Similarly, Hugdahl, Wahlgren and Wass (1982) reported that habituation of the electrodermal orienting response was delayed when visual stimuli were unilaterally presented to the right as compared to the left hemisphere.

It is therefore clear that the effects of hemispheric asymmetry goes beyond the more traditional view of higher-order cognitive functions. It is further clear that vital physiological functions involving both endocrine and autonomic processes are influenced by the cortex, although the exact nature of central regulation of e.g. autonomic function is still unclear (see Cechetto & Saper, 1990 for an update on this issue). Biological asymmetry may be thought of as operating through two different mechanisms, either that the right and left hemispheres differentially regulate outflow to the periphery, or that peripheral mechanisms act asymmetric by their own action. The view taken in this chapter is that the sympathetic and parasympathetic branches of the autonomic nervous system are differently regulated from the right and left hemispheres of the brain. Predominant

*Progress in Electrodermal Research*, Edited by
J.-C. Roy *et al.* Plenum Press, New York, 1993

sympathetic activation is thought to be regulated from the right hemisphere, and parasympathetic activation regulated from the left hemisphere (cf.Werntz, Bickford, Bloom, & Shannahoff-Khalsa, 1983). Support for this comes mainly from studies showing a right hemisphere superiority for processing of emotional stimuli, and particularly for negative or aversive stimuli (e.g. Ley & Bryden, 1979), and a left hemisphere superiority for positive or pleasurable stimuli (Davidson, 1983). Furthermore, Heller, Lindsay, Metz and Farnum (1990) showed that autonomic arousal was directly related to stimulation of the right hemisphere in a visual half-field paradigm. A similar finding was reported by Hachinsky et al. (1992) where rats had either the left or right middle cerebral artery experimentally occluded. Heart rate, blood pressure, plasma epinephrine and norepinephrine were monitored, among other variables. The results clearly showed greater sympathetic consequences after right hemisphere lesions than after left hemisphere lesions.

## Brain Asymmetry and Electrodermal Activity

Electrodermal activity has since its discovery in the 19th Century by Féré (1888) and Tarchanoff (1890), been linked to autonomic arousal, and particularly to sympathetic activity because of the unique sympathetic innervation of the eccrine sweat glands (e.g. Venables & Christie, 1980). However, of equal importance is the fact that electrodermal phenomena are responsive also to cognitive processes, like attention, orienting, and learning. In a classic paper from 1929, Darrow showed that electrodermal responses were sensitive to "ideational stimuli" like the presentation of words, or questions.

Seen in this perspective it is not surprising that electrodermal responses have been frequently used in efforts to reveal the asymmetric regulation of autonomic function by the hemispheres (see Hugdahl, 1984). Basically, two approaches have been used. The first is comparison of response amplitudes between the left and right hands to various kinds of verbal and/or visuo-spatial stimuli (e.g. Lacroix & Comper, 1979). The other approach involves unilateral activation of either the right or left hemisphere by dichotic listening (Hugdahl & Brobeck, 1986), or by visual half-field presentations (Hugdahl, Broman & Franzon, 1983a). For both approaches, lateralized effects have been observed, presumably reflecting differential hemisphere regulation of electrodermal function (see also Rippon, 1985).

## Brain Asymmetry and Conditional Learning

From an information-processing perspective on lateralization in the cerebral hemispheres it should come as no surprise that research efforts initially were focused on perceptual, attentional, and emotional asymmetry (see Bryden, 1982 for a review of laterality research). However, it is surprising that so little interest has been put into the question of laterality for learning, and particularly for elementary forms of associative, or conditional learning. A main argument in this chapter is that the two hemispheres of the brain not only differ in perceptual analysis of sensory stimuli, but that they also differentially regulate the formation of an association in memory. That the hemispheres differ in their capacity to form associations may not only have a basic research interest, but may also be of critical importance for a neuropsychological understanding of learning disabilities. The behavioristic tradition is probably to blame for the neglect of research on how conditional associations are stored and retrieved in the human brain. Instead, focus has traditionally been on the stimulus-response connection, with no role for the brain in this process.

It may be of interest to recall Pavlov's (1927) original view of conditional learning as a theoretical tool to explain the functioning of the cortical hemispheres. For Pavlov, studies of conditional learning provided insights into the functional properties of the nervous system, and particularly the cerebral hemispheres.

Conditional learning involves complex interactions between perception, attention, and memory (Öhman, 1983), thus it should be possible to demonstrate an asymmetry for cortical representation of conditional associations. This was demonstrated for electrodermal responses by Hugdahl, Kvale, Nordby and Overmier (1987) who found that the left hemisphere was specialized for learning of verbal associations (words), while the right hemisphere was specialized for learning of non-verbal associations (color patches). It could be predicted that the right hemisphere should be sensitive to storage and/or retrieval of conditional learning to emotionally relevant stimuli, and particularly negative emotional stimuli. This is predicted on the basis of the huge literature on right hemisphere superiority for emotional perceptual and attentional processing (see Ley & Bryden, 1979; Strauss & Moscovitch, 1981; Suberi & McKeever, 1977).

## Conditioning to Facial Emotional Expressions

Previous research on emotional conditioning with electrodermal responses has frequently utilized faces of emotional expressions as conditioned stimuli (CSs) together with either shock or noise as the significant unconditioned stimulus (UCS) (e.g. Dimberg & Öhman, 1983; Öhman, 1986). Dimberg and Öhman have convincingly demonstrated that conditional learning to angry facial expressions are very resistant to extinction, once the connection has been made. The effect is furthermore specific for directing the gaze towards the subject, when stimulus displays where the stimulus face is looking away from the subject were used, no effect emerged.

Rapid learning of the intention of a stranger is probably one of the most powerful examples of biological preparedness (cf. Seligman & Hager, 1972). Conditioning to an emotional facial expression may thus be considered to belong to the category of prepared learning. A key feature of prepared learning is that the association occurs even with minimal, or "degraded" stimulus input. This may be exemplified with conditioning of phobic fear, where usually only one brief encounter with the fearful stimulus is enough to produce a full-blown phobia that may exist for years. Seen in a neuropsychological perspective, prepared learning must be mediated through different brain mechanisms than non-prepared learning. We would like to extend this argument and suggest that prepared learning is mediated by the right hemisphere of the brain. We thus predict that a subliminal, degraded, presentation of a facial emotional expression should more easily elicit a conditioned association from the right hemisphere. The reason is that if the right hemisphere is superior in forming a conditioned association to an emotional conditional stimulus, then this superiority should be more pronounced the more degraded the stimulus is. Using subliminal presentation times would be a way of inducing stimulus degradation. Our argument is that the right hemisphere still is able to make the association, while the left is not. We further posit that processing of emotional information may be automatic and without conscious awareness (Posner, 1978). This has been elaborated by Öhman (e.g. 1986) who argues that fear-conditioning may disengage automatic and conscious processes. Fear-conditioning engages fast automatic processes which primarily affects physiological responses. Our suggestion is that automatic emotional processes are not exclusively subcortical in origin, but that they are regulated from the right hemisphere (cf. Hugdahl, Nordby & Kvale, 1989).

Hemisphere specific presentations of the face stimuli were accomplished through the Visual Half-Field (VHF) technique (McKeever, 1986). The VHF technique allows for initial unilateral presentations because of the partial decussation of the optical fibers in optical chiasma. Specifically, when fixation is focused to the center of the visual field, stimuli presented in the left half-field will initially be projected only to the right hemisphere, and vice versa. Stimulus presentations have, however, to be brief in order to prevent saccadic eye-movements, which otherwise would destroy the unilateral stimulus input to each hemisphere.

### Bilateral Recordings of Skin Conductance

The present studies also utilized bilateral electrodermal recordings, i.e. from both hands. Differences in response amplitudes between the left and right hand recordings have been linked to differences in hemispheric activation (e.g. Lacroix & Comper, 1979). However, since other authors have not been able to replicate the first observations by Lacroix and Comper (1979), the question of whether the left and right hand recordings index hemisphere function remains open (see Hugdahl, 1984, Freixa i Baqué, Catteau, Miossec, & Roy, 1984 for critical reviews). Furthermore, using animal models, both Sequeira-Martinho, Roy, and Ba-M'Hamed (1986), and Naveteur and Sequeira-Martinho (1990) have argued that bilateral differences in EDA are mainly caused by peripheral rather than central factors.

### PILOT STUDY

In a pilot-experiment (Öhman, Esteves, Parra, Soares, & Hugdahl, 1988) subjects were conditioned to angry and happy faces with one of the faces (CS+) always followed by the shock-UCS, and the other never paired with shock (CS-). Brief (30 ms) test-trials were interspersed among the CS+ and CS- trials. After the acquisition, or learning, phase, a test, or extinction, phase occurred with brief (30 ms) presentations of the happy and angry face, immediately followed by a neutral masking face. On half of the trials, each of the previous CS+ and CS- were presented to the right hemisphere (left VHF), and on the other half of trials they were presented to the left hemisphere (right VHF). The UCS was presented for 500 ms with a 500 ms CS-UCS interval. The results from the test phase are seen in Figure 1.

Surprisingly, a significant differentiation between the CS+ and the CS- was observed only for right hemisphere presentations, that is, the left hemisphere had obviously not "learned" that it was only the CS+ that previously was associated with shock. Consequently, the left hemisphere responded as much to the CS- as to the CS+. Finally, the results showed that the right hemisphere effect was most pronounced when the angry face had been the CS+ and the happy face the CS-.

The results of this study were remarkable considering that the only difference between conditions was that on some trials the stimulus picture was moved to the right side of the screen, and on some trials it was moved to the left side. The results were furthermore remarkable in the sense that the difference between the hemispheres was obtained after learning had occurred, i.e. during the "probe" or test phase. Presenting the CS probes for only 30 ms (and followed by the mask) was obviously not enough stimulus degradation to prevent retrieval of the stored association from the right hemisphere. However, before drawing too far-reaching conclusions, Hugdahl and Johnsen decided to try to replicate the "right hemisphere" effect (see Johnsen & Hugdahl, 1991). This was part of a series of four experiments that were launched to more closely investigate the right hemisphere superiority for aversive conditional learning (see Johnsen & Hugdahl, in press; Hugdahl & Johnsen, 1991, Hugdahl, Kvale, Nordby, & Overmier, 1987).

274

## Extenction-Test phase

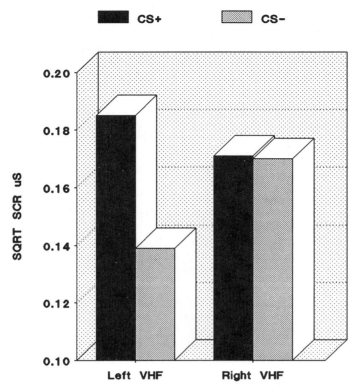

**Figure 1**. Square root transformed skin conductance responses (SCRs) during the extinction test phase. Data are averaged across trials and hands. VHF = visual half-field. Data from Öhman et al. (1988).

## ISSUES ADDRESSED

Basically, there were six issues that were addressed in these experiments. 1) Is it possible to replicate the laterality findings from the pilot study (Experiment 1). 2) Is the observed effect perceptual or associative in nature (Experiment 2). 3) Is the effect caused by priming, or sensitization, of the right hemisphere because of the shock-UCS presentations (Experiment 2). 4) If there is a genuine hemisphere difference in conditional learning, then males and females should differ in their responding, since sex differences have been found in other studies of brain asymmetry (McGlone, 1980) (Experiment 3). 5) Is it possible to observe the effect in other physiological response systems than the electrodermal system. (Experiment 4). 6) If verbal stimuli were used as conditioned stimuli, whould then a left hemisphere superiority be observed (Experiment 5)?

## COMMON METHODS

The subjects were female and male students at the University of Bergen, age varying between 19 and 35 years. All subjects were tested for right-handedness with a questionnaire containing 15 items related to manual preferences.

Bilateral phasic skin conductance responses (SCRs) were recorded on a Beckman polygraph with two Beckman SCR couplers. The couplers each supplied a constant voltage of 1.35 V. To control for possible differences in voltage between the couplers, both couplers were randomly shifted between subjects for right-hand versus left-hand recordings. Beckman 8 mm Ag/AgCl cup-electrodes were filled with a 0.05 molar NaCl Unibase concentration.

The stimuli were slides that were back-projected onto a 70x72 cm milk-glass screen inside a sound-attenuating chamber. The slides were projected from two slide-projectors, each fitted with a high-speed shutter in front of the lens. This was done in order to achieve maximum onset of slide presentation, and to control for short presentation times.

A plywood box was mounted inside the chamber, with the milk-glass screen as the posterior wall and a small rubber-mask opening for the eyes in the anterior wall. A 2 mm light-emitting diode (LED) was placed in the center of the milk-glass screen as a fixation point (when the LED was lit during a trial).

The face-stimuli were tachistoscopically projected either to the right or left side of the LED, i.e. either in the right or left VHF. Electric shocks, serving as UCSs, randomly presented to the fourth and fifth fingers of the subject, were generated from a DC shock generator. The shock generator was electrically shielded from all other equipment. Half of the subjects in each group (condition) had shock in their right hand, the other half in their left hand. The intensity of the electric shock was determined individually for each subject before the experiment started by delivering shocks of increasing intensity until the subject reported that the shock was "unpleasant but not painful". In the fifth experiment, white noise was used instead of shock as the UCS.

To control for involuntary eye-movements during a trial, electro-oculogram (EOG) was recorded from both eyes with a Beckman nystagmus coupler.

The pictures of facial emotional expressions were taken from the Ekman, Friesen, and Ellsworth (1972) standardized facial expressions set. The same model expressing either an angry (#105) or a happy (#101) expression were used. On unilateral trials, the slides were projected about 2.5 degrees of visual angle either to the right or left of the center LED.

Generally, all experiments contained three phases, a familiarization, or habituation, phase, an association, or acquisition phase when the CS was followed by the UCS, and a test, or extinction, phase.

## EXPERIMENT 1

The aim of the first experiment (Johnsen & Hugdahl, 1991) was to replicate the basic finding in the Öhman et al. (1988) study. Specifically, it was predicted that probing the right and left hemispheres separately with the CS pictures after association had occurred should result in larger responses from the right hemisphere. Second, the masking stimulus used in the Öhman et al. (1988) study was removed although CS presentations were kept to 30 ms during the probe phase. Finally, we wanted to further explore differences in SCR magnitudes between the left and right hand recordings. Since we were probing the hemispheres separately during the test phase, differences between the hands should then reflect differential autonomic outflow from the hemispheres.

A differential conditioning paradigm was used with CS+ (paired with shock) and CS- (never paired with shock) presentations. Half of the subjects had the angry face as CS+

and the happy face as CS-. The other half of the subjects had the arrangement reversed, happy face CS+ and angry face CS-.

During the association, or acquisition, phase of the experiment, both CSs were presented foveally and separately. Duration was 210 ms. Because the short time between the onset of the CS and the onset of the UCS (500 ms) did not permit the observation of conditioned responses to the CS, every third CS+ presentation was made without the UCS. These trials were used to assess the strength of the CS+/UCS association. During the probe phase, the CSs were presented for 30 ms lateralized either to the right or left of the LED. Thus, the CSs were presented **foveally** and **above** recognition threshold during the habituation and acquisition phases, but **lateralized** and **below** recognition threshold during the probe phase. There were two habituation trials, nine acquisition trials, and 32 test trials.

The results showed that reliable association occurred only to the angry face as CS+. The results for the critical test, or extinction, phase are shown in Figure 2.

The results are displayed as difference scores across trials, that is, CS- response magnitudes are subtracted from CS+ magnitudes. Since there was no significant association

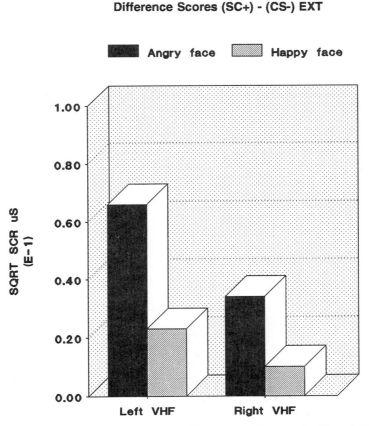

**Figure 2**. Square root transformed skin conductance difference scores between the CS+ and CS- during the extinction test phase (Ext = extinction). Data are averaged across trials and hands. Data from Johnsen & Hugdahl (1991), reprinted with permission from the publisher.

during the acquisition phase for the happy CS face, CS+/CS- differences were generally small during the test phase, which explains the rather small numbers in the Figure. The absence of a significant conditional association for the happy CS indicates that the responses to this stimulus during the test phase reflected carry-over effects of non-associative differences during acquisition.

The findings for the angry CS face were however quite interesting, with left field (=right hemisphere) presentations yielding significantly larger CS+/CS- differentiation than right field (=left hemisphere) presentations (see Figure 2). Thus, probing only the right hemisphere with the angry CS **after** association training had occurred resulted in significantly larger responses than probing the left hemisphere for the same association. It is important to keep in mind that the **only** difference between the left and right field conditions were that the CS face was presented to the left on some trials and to the right on some trials. The results basically confirmed the findings of the Öhman et al. (1988) study. The results did not generally support the view that differences in SCRs between the two hands are related to differences in hemisphere functioning. The differences that were found were small and theoretically insignificant.

## EXPERIMENT 2

An important question related to the findings in Experiment 1 is whether the CS+/UCS association was more easily encoded in the right hemisphere, or whether the angry face elicited larger responses because negative emotional expressions are more easily **perceived** by the right hemisphere. Thus, it seems important to disentangle associative from non-associative factors. We have previously argued that separating e.g. perceptual from associative factors "is not an easy question to answer" (Johnsen & Hugdahl, 1991). Perceptual CS properties are often stressed in modern cognitive theories of learning (e.g. Siddle & Remington, 1987).

However, one way to separate non-associative from associative processes would be to add a group of subjects that have everything equal to the conditioning groups, except that the shock-UCS is omitted. If the no-shock angry CS group shows the same response magnitudes as the corresponding shock group, then the effect is non-associative. However, if the groups still differ, then the effect is associative. This was tested in the second experiment. Another aspect that was added to Experiment 2 was that lateralized presentations of the CSs were moved from the test phase to the association phase, testing with foveal presentations.

The experiment consisted of four groups, two CS/shock groups and two CS/no-shock groups. The shock and no-shock conditions were identical except that no UCS-shocks were presented in the no-shock groups. For both shock/no- shock conditions, one group had the angry face presented in the right VHF with the happy face **simultaneously** presented in the left VHF. This group will be labelled the "Angry right/Happy left" group. The other group had the presentation reversed, the angry face in the left VHF and the happy face in the right VHF. This group will be labelled "Angry left/Happy right". The compound CSs were presented for 180 ms during the association phase, and the separate CSs were presented 30 ms during the test phase.

Effects of the CS/UCS pairings during the association phase were evaluated as the average of the first two presentations of the angry and happy face during the test phase. In comparison with Experiment 1, the present Experiment used **lateralized** and **above** recognition threshold presentations during the association phase, and **foveal** and **below** recognition threshold presentations during the test phase.

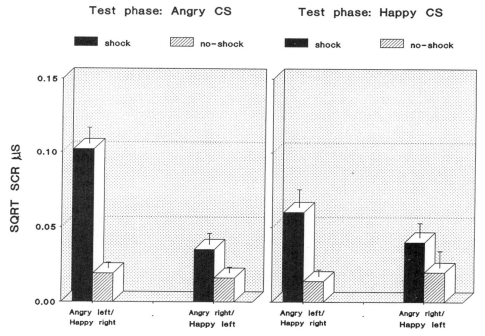

**Figure 3**. Square root transformed skin conductance responses (SCRs) during the test phase Experiment 2. Data are averaged across trials and hands, and separated for groups and conditions. Note that the "Angry right/Happy left", etc. notations refer to the visual hemi-fields. Data from Johnsen & Hugdahl (in press), reprinted with permission from the publisher.

The data showed that conditioned associations had occurred for both the angry and happy faces. The results for the test phase are shown in Figure 3. Figure 3 shows SCR magnitudes across trials, separated for groups and conditions.

The data were evaluated in a 3-way ANOVA, with a posteriori follow-up tests. The most conspicuous finding was the absence of any effects for the no- shock conditions, seen in the significant main-effect of shock vs. no-shock. There were no differences between the critical "Angry left/Happy right" and "Angry right/Happy left" no-shock groups. Furthermore, there was a huge difference between the shock and no-shock "Angry left/Happy right" groups, seen in the significant two-way interaction of Face position x Shock/no-shock during conditioning. The results thus supported an interpretation in terms of associative rather than perceptual processes.

However, although the findings in Experiment 2 supported an associative explanation, other confounding factors cannot be completely ruled out. For one thing, the shock may have uniquely primed or sensitized the right hemisphere, although half the subjects had shock in their right hand, and half in their left hand, and although there were no significant differences between these conditions. This can be tested by including a new stimulus in the test phase, that is, including a stimulus that has not been presented during the conditioning phase, and consequently never been associated with the shock-UCS. If responses to right hemisphere presentations of the new stimulus are equal to the responses to the face-stimuli then a priming confounding would exist. In a pilot study recently run in our laboratory, no clear confounding effects were found. A second argument against a priming confounding effect is that if the shock had primed the right hemisphere to respond to **any** kind of stimulus, then there should not have been a difference in response magnitudes when probing with the angry versus the happy face-CS in Experiment 2 (see Figure 3).

To summarize Experiment 2, when probing both hemispheres at the same time during the test phase for elicitation of the encoded association, largest responses were obtained for the group that **previously** during the experiment had the angry face presented to the right hemisphere, while at the same time the happy face was presented to the left hemisphere. The left hemisphere showed a much weaker associative connection between the happy face and the UCS.

## EXPERIMENT 3

Only female subjects were used in Experiments 1 and 2. For this reason sex differences were examined in Experiment 3. Hemisphere differences are often reported between males and females (McGlone, 1981). Furthermore, it has previously been shown that the prevalence of phobic fears is higher in females than in males (Geer, 1965). It was therefore predicted that females should be more right hemisphere lateralized for associative learning than males. The same experimental design was used in Experiment 3 as in Experiment 2, with the addition of two male groups.

The results showed that only the females acquired the learned association during the association phase. During the test phase there was a clear difference between the female and male groups in right hemisphere responding (see Figures 4 and 5).

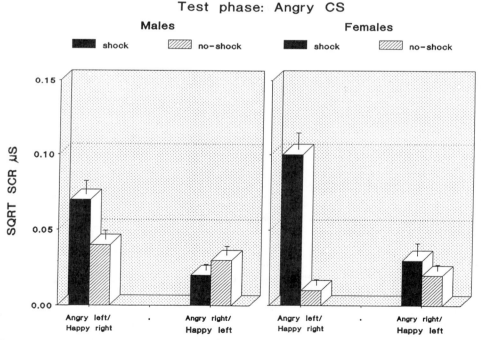

**Figure 4.** Square root transformed skin conductance responses (SCRs) to the angry face during the test phase Experiment 3. Data are averaged across trials and hands and separated for males and females. Note that all notations (left, right) refer to the visual hemi-fields.

As can be seen in Figure 4, probing the right hemisphere with the angry CS face yielded significantly larger responses in the females as compared to the males. The same occurred when probing with the happy CS face, although overall response magnitudes were smaller. This was statistically supported in the significant interaction of Sex x Face position x Emotion.

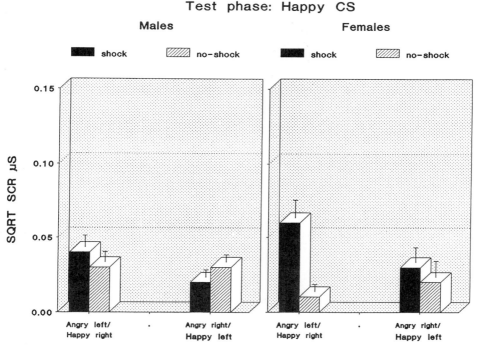

**Figure 5**: Square root transformed skin conductance responses (SCRs) to the happy face during the test face Experiment 3. Data are averaged across trials and hands and separated for males and females. Note that all notations (left, right) refer to the visual hemifields.

## EXPERIMENT 4

Heart rate changes in a typical triphasic fashion during the CS-UCS interval in autonomic conditioning studies (see Obrist, Webb & Sutterer, 1969). Typically, there is an initial deceleration 1 to 3 seconds after CS onset, followed by an acceleration for about 3-4 seconds, with a second deceleration occurring at about the time when the UCS is presented (Bohlin & Kjellberg, 1979). The acceleration in response to the CS may be considered an index of development of the conditioned response. Several authors have suggested that phasic changes in cardiac activity to sensory stimuli are regulated from the right hemisphere (e.g. Walker & Sandman, 1979; Hugdahl, Franzon, Andersson, & Walldebo,

1983b). Yokoyama et al. (1987) showed that patients with right hemisphere lesions did not reveal the typical anticipatory HR response profile in a two-stimulus paradigm. Furthermore, Rosen et al. (1982) reported that HR changes were smaller following right carotid injections of sodium amytal than those following left carotid injections. These observations fit the anatomy of the vagus nerve and the innervation of the sino-atrial (S-A) node of the heart. It is the right branch of the vagus nerve that innervates the S-A node, which is the primary pace maker for the beating of the heart (Brodal, 1981).

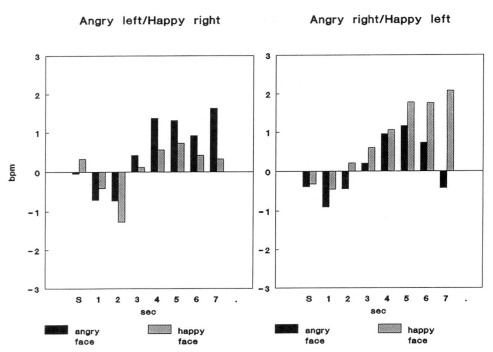

**Figure 6**. Second-by-second changes in beats-per-minute (bpm) after stimulus-presentation (S) in Experiment 4 during the test phase. Data are averaged across trials and split for the two groups in the study. Note that all notations (left, right) refer to the visual hemi-fields.

Relating these findings to the present series of experiments, it could be predicted that acceleratory changes in HR after CS presentations should differ between the groups in Experiments 2 and 3. Thus, a new study was run with the same paradigm as in Experiments 2 and 3 but where HR was also recorded. Second-by-second changes in HR was scored as deviations in beats- per-minute (bpm) from the last three seconds immediately preceding the presentation of the probe CS during the test phase.

The results are shown in Figure 6, separated for the "Angry left/Happy right" and "Angry right/Happy left" groups.

As can be seen in Figure 6, probing with the angry CS-face resulted in increased acceleration in the "Angry left/Happy right" group than did probing with the happy face. However, probing with the happy CS face resulted in increased acceleration in the "Angry right/Happy left" group. Thus, for both CS probes, projections to the right hemisphere during the conditioning phase resulted in greater acceleration to that stimulus during the extinction, test phase of the experiment. However, it is presently unclear why the results were obtained only for the HR measure. It may also be noted that the acceleratory response observed to the happy face is in conflict with other studies, usually showing HR deceleration to positive affective stimuli.

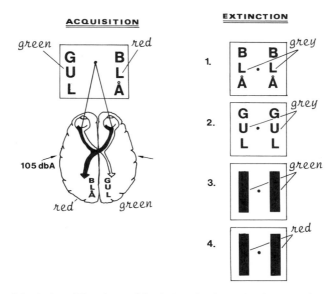

**Figure 7**. Outline of the design of Experiment 5 for the learning (acquisition) and test (extinction) phases of the experiment. From Hugdahl et al. (1987), reprinted with permission from the publisher.

## EXPERIMENT 5

Hugdahl et al. (1987) investigated whether a left hemisphere superiority for electrodermal associative conditioning could be established by using **verbal** CSs. The design of this study is seen in Figure 7.

Two color-words (yellow and blue, GUL and BLÅ in Norwegian) written in two conflicting colors (green and red) were simultaneously presented in the left and right VHF during the association phase of the experiment. The compound-CS display was paired with 105 dB white noise through earphones. During the test phase, each of the four CS cues (GUL, BLÅ , red, green) were presented foveally and separated. During the test phase, each of the four CS cues was used to probe for conditioned carry-over effects from the association phase. It was predicted that the word-element of the compound CS presented to the left hemisphere (right VHF) during association should show larger responses during the test phase than the word-element presented to the right hemisphere. Second, it was predicted that the non-verbal color-element presented to the right hemisphere during association should show greater responses during the test phase than the color-element presented to the left hemisphere.

The results for the first trial during the test phase are seen in Figure 8.

The results clearly showed that differential conditioned responding occurred depending on which hemisphere the word- and color-elements were presented to during the association phase of the experiment. There was furthermore a significant interaction with the left and right hand SCR recordings. The interaction showed a larger difference between the left and right hemi-fields for the Word CSs on the left compared to the right hand. There were no differences between the hands for the Color CSs.

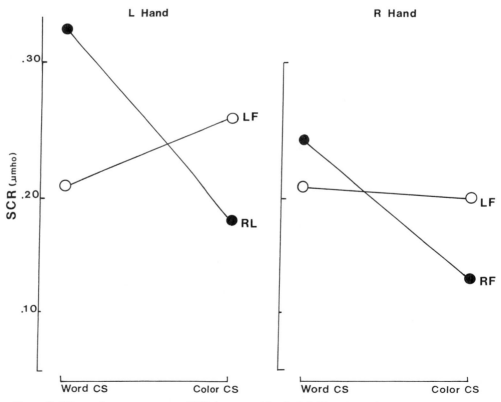

**Figure 8.** Skin conductance responses (SCRs) separated for the left (L) and right (R) hand and for the word and color cues of the CS stimulus. LF = Left visual half-field, RF = Right visual half-field. Data from Hugdahl et al. (1987), reprinted with permission from the publisher.

## SUMMARY AND CONCLUSIONS

A series of experiments are reviewed where skin conductance responses were used to index hemisphere differences in representation of learned responses to facial emotional expressions. Few studies of hemispheric specialization and lateralization have been directed to the question of laterality of simple associative learning, and that the two hemispheres of the brain may be differentially involved in the establishment of conditioned associations. Following several lines of research it is argued that associative learning to emotionally relevant conditional stimuli are represented in the right hemisphere. The connection between higher cortical structures and electrodermal reactivity is far from known. Electrodermal activity is regulated from several different cortical areas involving both the frontal and temporal lobes. The link to the frontal lobes may be important in trying to track down a right hemisphere dominance for electrodermal responses to emotional stimuli. Cechetto and Saper (1990) have argued that the medial prefrontal cortex including the infralimbic may act as an autonomic motor cortex. This is an attractive hypothesis since limbic structures clearly are involved in regulation of both electrodermal activity and emotional affect. We further suggest that it is the right infralimbic cortex that regulates electrodermal reactivity after a conditioned association has occurred, linking peripheral electrodermal activity to cortical functioning.

## REFERENCES

Bohlin, G., and Kjellberg, A., 1979, Orienting activity in two-stimulus paradigms as reflected in heart rate, in: "The Orienting Reflex," H.D. Kimmel., E.H. van Olst., and J.F. Orlebeke, eds., Erlbaum Associates, Hillsdale, N.J.

Barneoud, P., Neveu, P.J. and LeMoal, M., 1987, Functional heterogenity of the right and left neocortex in modulation of the immune system. *Physiology and Behavior*, 41:525-530.

Brodal, A., 1981, "Neurological Anatomy in Relation to Clinical Medicine. Third edition," Oxford University Press, New York.

Bryden, M.P., 1982, "Laterality. Functional Asymmetry in the Intact Brain", Academic Press, New York.

Cechetto, D.F., and Saper, C.B., 1990, Role of the cerebral cortex in autonomic functioning, in: "Central Regulation of Autonomic Functioning", A.D. Loewy and K.M. Spyer, Eds., Oxford University Press, New York.

Darrow, C.W., 1929, Electrical and circulatory responses to brief sensory and ideational stimuli, *Journal of Experimental Psychology*. 12:267- 300.

Davidson, R.J., 1983, Affect, repression, and cerebral asymmetry, in: "Emotions in Health", L. Temoshek, C. van Dyke and L.S. Zegang, eds., Grune & Stratton, New York.

Dimberg, U., and Öhman, A., 1983, The effects of directed facial cues on electrodermal conditioning to facial stimuli, *Psychophysiology*, 20:160-67.

Ekman, P., Friesen, W.V., and Ellsworth, P., 1972, "Emotion in the Human Face", Elmsford, N.Y., Pergamon Press.

Féré, C., 1888, Note sur les modifications de la résistance électrique sous l'influence des excitations sensorielles et des émotions, *Comptes Rendus de la Société de Biologie*. 5:217-19.

Freixa i Baqué, E., Catteau, M.C., Miossec, Y, and Roy, J.C., 1984, Asymmetry of electrodermal activity: A review, *Biological Psychology*, 18:219-239.

Geer, J.H., 1965, The development of a scale to measure fear, *Behaviour Research and Therapy*. 3:45-53.

Hachinsky, V.C., Oppenheimer, S.M., Wilson, J.X., Guiraudon, C., and Cechetto, D.F., 1992, Asymmetry of sympathetic consequences of experimental stroke, *Archives of Neurology*. 49:697-702.

Heller, W., Lindsey, D.L. Metz, J., and Farnum, D.M., 1990, Individual differences in right-hemisphere activation are associated with arousal and autonomic response to lateralized stimuli, *Journal of Clinical and Experimental Neuropsychology*, 13:95.

Hellige, J.B., 1990, Hemispheric asymmetry, *Annual Review of Psychology.* 41:55-80.

Hugdahl, K., Wahlgren , C., and Wass, T., 1982, Habituation of the electrodermal orienting reaction is dependent on the cerebral hemisphere initially stimulated, *Biological Psychology.* 15:49-62.

Hugdahl, K., Broman, J.-E., and Franzon, M., 1983a, Effects of stimulus content and brain lateralization on the habituation of the electrodermal orienting response (OR), *Biological Psychology.* 17:153- 68.

Hugdahl,K., Franzon, M., Anderson, B., and Walldebo, G., 1983b, Heart rate responses (HRR) to lateralized visual stimuli, *Pavlovian Journal of Biological Science.* 18:186-98.

Hugdahl, K., 1984, Hemispheric asymmetry and bilateral electrodermal recordings: A review of evidence, *Psychophysiology.* 21:371-93.

Hugdahl, K., and Brobeck, C.G., 1986, Hemispheric asymmetry and human electrodermal conditioning. The dichotic extinction paradigm, *Psychophysiology.* 23:491-99.

Hugdahl, K., Kvale, G., Nordby, H., and Overmier, J.B., 1987, Hemispheric asymmetry and human classical conditioning to verbal and nonverbal visual Css, *Psychophysiology,* 24:557-65.

Hugdahl, K., Nordby, H., & Kvale, G., 1989, Conditional learning and brain asymmetry: Empirical data and a theoretical framework. *Learning and Individual Differences,* 1:385-405.

Hugdahl, K., and Johnsen, B.H., 1991, Brain asymmetry and human electrodermal conditioning, *Integrative Physiological and Behavioral Science.* 26:39-44.

Johnsen, B.H., and Hugdahl, K., 1991, Hemispheric asymmetry in conditioning to facial emotional expressions, *Psychophysiology,* 29:154-62.

Johnsen, B.H., and Hugdahl, K., in press, Right hemisphere representation of autonomic conditioning to facial emotional expressions, *Psychophysiology.*

Lacroix, J.M., and Comper, P., 1979, Lateralization in the electrodermal system as a function of cognitive/hemispheric manipulation, *Psychophysiology.* 16:116-29.

Ley, R.G., and Bryden, M.P., 1979, Hemispheric differences in recognizing faces and emotions, *Brain and Language.* 7:127-38.

McGlone, J., 1980, Sex differences in human brain asymmetry: a critical survey, *The Behavioral and Brain Sciences.* 3:215-27.

McKeever,W.F., 1986, Tachistoscopic methods in neuropsychology, in: "Experimental Techniques in Human Neuropsychology", J.H. Hannay, Ed., Oxford University Press, New York.

Naveteur, J., and Sequeira-Martinho, H., 1990, Reliabilty of bilateral differences in electrodermal activity, *Biological Psychology,* 31:47- 56.

Obrist, P.A., Webb, R.A., and Sutterer, J.R., 1969, Heart rate and somatic changes during aversive conditioning and a simple reaction time task, *Psychophysiology.* 5:696-723.

Öhman, A., 1983, The orienting response during pavlovian conditioning, in: "Orienting and Habituation. Perspectives in Human Research", D. Siddle ed., John Wiley and Sons, Chichester, U.K

Öhman, A., 1986, Face the beast and fear the face: Animal and social fears as prototypes for evolutionary analyses of emotion, *Psychophysiology.* 23:123-45.

Öhman, A., Esteves, F., Parra, C., Soares, J., and Hugdahl, K., 1988, Brain lateralization and preattentive elicitation of conditioned skin conductance responses, *Psychophysiology.* 25:473.

Pavlov, I.P., 1927, "Conditioned Reflexes", G.V. Anrep, Translation., Dover Publications, New York.

Posner, M.I., 1978, "Chronometric Explorations of Mind", Erlbaum Associates, Engelwood Heights, N.J.

Rippon, G.M.J., 1985, Bilateral electrodermal activity: Effects of differential hemispheric activation. Paper presented at the 25th Annual Meeting of the SPR, Houston, Texas, October.

Rosen, A.D., Gur, R.C., Sussman, N.M., Gur, R.E., and Hurtig, H., 1982, Hemispheric asymmetry in the control of heart rate, *Neuroscience Abstracts,* 8:917.

Seligman, M.E.P., and Hager, J.E., 1972, "Biological Boundaries of Learning", ed., Appleton-Century-Crofts, New York.

Sequeira-Martinho, H., Roy, J.C., and Ba-M'Hamed, S., 1986, Cortical and pyramidal stimulation elicit nonlateralized skin potential responses in the cat, *Biological Psychology,* 23:85-86.

Siddle, D.A.T., and Remmington, B., 1987, Latent inhibition and human Pavlovian conditioning: Research and relevance, in: "Cognitive Processes and Pavlovian Conditioning in Humans", G.L.C. Davey ed., John Wiley and Sons, Chichester, U.K.

Strauss, E., and Moscovitch. M., 1981, Perceptual asymmetries in processing facial expressions and facial identity, *Brain and Language*. 13:308-32.

Suberi, M., and McKeever, W.F., 1977, Differential right hemispheric memory storage of emotional and non-emotional faces, *Neuropsychologia*. 15:757-68.

Tarchanoff, J., 1890, Uber die galvanischen erscheinungen an der haut des menchen bei reizung der sinnesorgane und bei verschiedenen formen der psychischen tatigkeit, *Pflugers Archiv fur die Gesamte Physiologie*. 46:46-55.

Venables, P.H., and Christie, M.J., 1980, Electrodermal activity, in: "Techniques in Psychophysiology", I. Martin, and P.H. Venables, eds., John Wiley and Sons, Chichester, U.K.

Walker, B.B., and Sandman, C.A., 1979, Human visual evoked responses are related to heart rate, *Journal of Comparative and Physiological Psychology*. 93:717-29.

Weisz, J., Szilagyi, N., Lang, E., and Adam, G., 1992, The influence of monocular viewing on heart period variability, *International Journal of Psychophysiology*. 12:11-18.

Werntz, D.A., Bickford, R.G., Bloom, F.E., and Shannahof-Khalsa, D.S., 1983, Alternating cerebral hemispheric activity and the lateralization of autonomic nervous function, *Human Neurobiology*. 2:39-43.

Wittling, W., 1990, Psychophysiological correlates of human brain asymmetry: Blood pressure changes during lateralized presentation of an emotionally laden film, *Neuropsychologia*. 28:457-70.

Wittling, W., and Pfluger, M., 1990, Neuroendocrine hemisphere asymmetries: Salivary cortisol secretion during lateralized viewing of emotion-related and neutral films, *Brain and Cognition*. 14:243-65.

Yokoyama, K., Jennings, R., Ackles, P., Hood, P., and Boller, F., 1987, Lack of heart rate changes during an attention-demanding task after right hemisphere lesions, *Neurology*. 37:624-30.

# ELECTRODERMAL AMPLITUDE ASYMMETRY AND ORIENTING RESPONSE-NON-RESPONSE IN PSYCHOPATHOLOGY

Pierre Flor-Henry

Clinical Director, Acute Psychiatry
Psychiatric Treatment Centre
Alberta Hospital Edmonton
Edmonton, Alberta. T5J 2J7
Canada

Evidence from Russian investigations in the 1960s on the verbal regulation of the orienting reflex and on the frontal lobes and the regulation of arousal, were reviewed by Venables, (1977), and Gruzelier, (1979). It showed that in neurological populations patients with temporal or parietal lesions who had no electrodermal reactivity to a neutral orienting tone stimulus became reactive to a signal stimulus - in contrast to subjects with frontal lobe lesions who remained nonresponders. Gruzelier and Venables (1973) investigated schizophrenics to tones with and without attentional significance showing that they were comparable to the temporal-parietal neurological syndromes - and not the frontal lobe disorders in this respect.

In a detailed review of studies of electrodermal psychophysiology of schizophrenia up to that time Venables (1977) considered further some of the theoretical implications of the reversed patterns of electrodermal amplitude asymmetry in nonresponders (right < left) and in responders (left < right). When one plots right and left tonic activity against increasing arousal, the nonresponding and low arousal schizophrenias fall at one end of a distribution (right < left) which shifts into the opposite pattern of asymmetry (left < right) with increasing arousal. The cross-over point corresponds to the data of Gruzelier and Venables (1974) of "transitional" schizophrenics who did not respond to neutral but responded to signal tones and in whom the electrodermal asymmetry was not significant during neutral but became significant during signal stimulus conditions. Venables proposed the model of "weak" left hemisphere which is more active than the right under low arousal while with increasing arousal transmarginal inhibition disrupts the left hemisphere and the "strong" right hemisphere then becomes predominant, thus accounting for the shifts in electrodermal amplitude asymmetry. This representation presupposes principally homolateral control of electrodermal tonic activity. Ipsilateral control of the electrodermal response had been suggested by Russian and Czechoslovakian research in the 1960s that revealed, after massive frontal lesions, the loss of electrodermal response to orienting stimuli on the side of the lesion. Repeatedly cited is the single case reported by Luria and Homskaya (1963) of a patient with a left frontal tumour whose phasic responses to a neutral stimulus were absent on the left side. Sourek (1965) also found ipsilateral reduction of EDA in all his 15 patients with resection of baso-medial frontal and medial temporal regions. He assumed an ipsilateral effect but considered the possibility of contralateral disinhibition which was the finding of Holloway and Parsons (1969) who reported an abnormal elevation of right sided amplitudes in patients with left hemisphere lesions.

At the same time American investigations with primates implied, through lesion studies, that the actual phasic components of the electrodermal response were dependent on the integrity of the amygdaloid neural systems while habituation charactertics related to the integrity of the hippocampal structures. However, as Gruzelier remarks (Gruzelier, 1979) the question of hemispheric influences on the direction of electrodermal asymmetry (EDA) is not quite resolved by the above observations because an ipsilateral decrease can be the consequence of reduced ipsilateral excitation or of increased contralateral inhibition. A report which appeared to emphasize the importance of contralateral effects was that of Myslobodsky and Rattok (1975) who in 12 male healthy subjects (10 dextrals) found that in all the dextrals verbal and numerical mentation was associated with larger EDA responses on the right whereas during visual imagery tasks the larger response was on the left hand. The directionality shift hinged mainly on the left-hand responses which increased much more in the transition from verbal to spatial (significant) cognition than the right hand's (non- significant) decrease.

Myslobodsky and Rattok (1975) favour a contralateral hypothesis to explain their results, the right hemisphere being differentially affected in the two cognitive situations. It should be noted that the visual stimulus (erotic images) was more likely to be associated with increased arousal than the emotionally neutral numerical stimuli employed and that there was a larger bilateral EDA increase in the visual than in the verbal tasks. Lacroix and Comper (1979), on the other hand, in their investigation of electrodermal amplitude characteristics during verbal and spatial mental activity in 16 normal dextral female subjects found a pattern of asymmetry exactly opposite to the one described by Myslobodsky and Rattok. Verbal thought, both before and during its expression was associated with a contralateral reduction of electrodermal response amplitude and conversely spatial thoughts (before and during their expression) with the opposite contralateral amplitude reduction. These asymmetries were independent of the state of arousal, did not habituate and were also independent of the tonic level. The same tasks administered to twelve sinistral females produced the same pattern of electrodermal responses bilaterally for both tasks. Lacroix and Comper, however, did confirm Myslobodsky and Rattok's finding of greater lability of response for the left hand of dextrals, noting in addition that in sinistrals the more labile hand was the right. Lacroix and Comper conclude that their results "provide compelling evidence for the presence of lateralized cortical influences on electrodermal responding" which they consider to be essentially contralateral and inhibitory. They acknowledge, however, that their results can equally well be explained by a model of excitatory ipsilateral mechanism.

The influence of gender on electrodermal amplitude asymmetry has been discussed by Roman et al (1986) and Martinez-Selva et al (1987). The first investigators find a pattern of right < left EDA asymmetry in males, irrespective of task condition. The same asymmetry in males is confirmed by Martinez-Selva et al who find in females the opposite asymmetry left < right in spite of the fact that they are less asymmetrical. The amplitude differences between the sexes was more pronounced for the left hand and similar asymmetries were found in skin conductance levels as well as specific and nonspecific responses. If we accept the finding of Baxter et al (1988) that in men there is relative hypermetabolic activity of the left, and in women of the right hemisphere on Positron Emission Tomography then the above patterns are consistent with the model of contralateral inhibition and ipsilateral excitation proposed by Gruzelier. A correspondence between right < left cortical EEG asymmetry and right < left EDA asymmetry was demonstrated by Rippon (1990) in 16 normal, dextral subjects studied during verbal and spatial tasks with a 28 EEG channels BEAM. Smaller amplitude of EEG (beta-2) in the right hemisphere correlated with higher EDA on the left hand. A skin conductance amplitude asymmetry (L-R/L+R) and EEG amplitude asymmetry (L-R/L+R) indices were calculated. In the verbal task, there was a significant and positive correlation between the SCR laterality index and the beta-2 laterality index. The cortical initiation of phasic electrodermal activity responses is further documented by Weitkunat et al, (1990) who report the presence of systematic high amplitude alpha bursts of 1 second duration 2 seconds before the onset of the electrodermal responses.

In their original study Gruzelier and Venables (1972) found that slightly more than half (n = 43) of 80 schizophrenics showed no electrodermal response to a 85 dB, 1000 Hz, 1 sec tone. It has been estimated that in the general population the absence of electrodermal responsivity to an orienting stimulus occurs in some 7% of adults, notably in women in the postovulatory phase of the menstrual cycle (Venables, 1977). In this way Gruzelier and Venables were able to divide schizophrenics into two groups: responders and nonresponders. Responders had higher levels of skin conductance and more spontaneous fluctuations than the nonresponders, and furthermore were slow, or failed to habituate on repeated presentation of the stimulus. Later Gruzelier and Venables (1974) showed that the responders,ie, the schizophrenics with higher arousal, scored higher on ratings for mania, paranoid hostility, attention-seeking behaviour and anxiety than did the low arousal group or non-responders. Gruzelier (1973) then examined skin conductance bilaterally in 60 schizophrenics, searching for evidence of lateral asymmetry of orienting response and bilateral differences in levels. Responders showed a significant asymmetry in electrodermal responses, with fewer responses in the left hand and a total absence of left-hand responses in three patients. In the normal group there was no instance of unilateral nonresponse, and the response incidence was similar in both hands. In addition, bilateral differences in skin conductance levels were found in the schizophrenics, with higher levels on the right hand than on the left in the responders. The nonresponders showed the opposite asymmetry, with higher electrodermal levels on the left hand than on the right hand. In addition, compared to normals, (responding) schizophrenics had higher amplitudes, shorter latencies and slower recovery times. Rippon (1979) finds that 78% of 28 nonresponding male schizophrenics show asymmetry of Skin Conductance Levels right < left as opposed to only 37% of the controls. Those non-responders who "changed" to responding with a signal stimulus are characterized by electrodermal amplitude asymmetry left < right while "non-changing" non- responders by electrodermal amplitude asymmetry right < left. 30% of unmedicated acute schizophrenics are non-responders according to Gruzelier (1981). Alm et al (1984) reports 60% non-responders in 40 schizophrenics most of whom were never treated, examined during the first illness, whose clinical characteristics were of withdrawal, conceptual disorganization and blunted affect. Neuroleptics did not effect the responding/non-responding dimension and compared to responders non-responders had; 1. lower skin conductance levels; 2. fewer spontaneous fluctuations; 3. more schizophrenic relatives; 4. more psychotic symptoms.

Gruzelier and Venables (1974) analyzed a new sample of 47 schizophrenics whom they compared to depressed patients and to individuals with personality disorders. These nonschizophrenic psychiatric controls consisted of ten unipolar psychotic depressives and a group of ten mixed personality disorders: antisocial criminal or inadequate personalities with alcohol and/or drug abuse. The psychopathic personalities showed left < right EDA asymmetry.

Raine, (1987) investigated the electrodermal correlates of psychopathy and schizotypy in criminals and found that anhedonia-psychoticism was associated with poor performance on arithmetic and digit span and reduced orienting frequency. The anhedonia-psychoticism correlated with low verbal (and consequently full scale) IQ but not with performance IQ. Raine concludes that these results suggest "a left temporal origin to the interactions existing between schizotypy, attention-distraction and electrodermal hyporesponsivity in antisocials". Of the schizophrenics, Gruzelier and Venables, (1974) 67.5% were nonresponders as opposed to 30% in the other two groups. Unilateral nonresponse was found in six of the schizophrenics, in all instances a nonresponse from the left hand. For the schizophrenic responders there was a significant laterality effect with response amplitudes higher on the right hand (compared to the left hand) while the depressive patients had the reverse asymmetry, with lower amplitudes on the right hand (compared to the left). Combining their two series of schizophrenics (Gruzelier, 1973[16]; Gruzelier and Venables, 1974) now accumulating 107 patients, unilateral nonresponding on the left side occurs in 18% of cases all of whom were dextral. Gruzelier and Hammond (1976) investigated 16 schizophrenics over a 12-week period (the first month with chlorpromazine treatment, the second month with placebo, and the third with chlorpromazine evaluating electrodermal characteristics in each phase of the trial. Exactly half (n = 8) were nonresponders and another three had spontaneous fluctuations that were unrelated to the orienting stimulus. Of the eight responders two were unilateral nonresponders for the left hand. Bilateral asymmetry of skin conductance amplitude was present, with a right-hand directionality (higher on the right) in 75% of the patients, evaluated over the three phases of the study.

Uherik (1978) in the study of 37 schizophrenics compared to controls notes the presence of a left < right EDA asymmetry as does White et al (1987) who investigated chronic schizophrenics monitored with miniaturized radio-telemetry in a variety of tasks including stressful social interactions. Bernstein et al (1985) again observed larger phasic SCR responses on the right hand in 40 schizophrenics compared to mixed affective patients and healthy controls. Further the left < right EDA asymmetry to tones was correlated with left occipital alpha power reduction in the EEG. This would suggest a pattern of ipsilateral inhibition and contralateral excitation in the cortical control systems.

Gruzelier (1979) showed that in 62 first-year medical students the distribution of electrodermal amplitudes, right and left, is Gaussian, with 75% of subjects having bilateral differences of less than 10% and the remainder equally distributed in either direction. At the same time it must be recognized that the electrodermal lateralization of skin conductance responses and skin potential responses, although quite pronounced in most normal subjects, is extremely unstable through time when tested one week apart for one month - not infrequently reversing (Naveteur and Sequeira-Martinho, 1990). In three investigations (16 surgical patients, 62 medical students, 9 sinistral subjects) totalling 87 normal subjects Gruzelier et al (1981) found that slow habituation was associated with larger right-hand responses and fast habituation with larger left-hand responses. Gruzelier (1981) next analyzed a series of 48 schizophrenic patients who satisfied the Present State Examination (PSE) criteria as well as being rated on the Brief Psychiatric Rating Scale (BPRS). The sample consisted of 30 men and 18 women whose electrodermal responses to 15, 1000 Hz tones at 90 dB for 5-second duration were measured. Twenty-nine patients had larger right- hand and 19 patients had larger left-hand responses. When the mental symptoms characteristic of the two groups were scrutinized, a clear psychopathological dichotomy was revealed: 1) Cases were the electrodermal asymmetry was right < left exhibited simple ideas of reference, hypomania, anxiety, delusions of grandeur, hypochondriasis, and depressive delusions and hallucinations on the PSE inventory. On the BPRS they showed pressure of speech and grandiosity. 2) Cases with electrodermal left < right were slow, irritable, and reticent, and exhibited motor retardation, blunted affect, and simple depression. The right < left EDA asymmetry is associated with fast habituation while the left < right EDA asymmetry is associated with slow habituation. Factor analysis showed that the most important single descriptor of the two groups was a bipolar factor of slowness, emotional withdrawal versus heightened arousal which together accounted for 56.2% of the total variance. The depressive delusions and hallucinations were found almost exclusively in the right < left group while delusions of reference and persecution were found in both groups. Simple (nondelusional) ideas of reference, however, occurred in the right < left patients.

Observations of this kind have led Gruzelier (1981) to propose the following "balance" model for the cortical control of electrodermal systems: lesions of the right hemisphere are associated with nonresponding; of the left hemisphere with hyperresponding. Consequently, in normals, the left hemisphere is inhibitory and the right hemisphere is excitatory, bilaterally. It follows further that since fast habituation implies high active inhibition, left hemisphere preponderance will be correlated with fast habituation and right hemisphere dominance with slow habituation. If superimposed on this balance control system there is simultaneously contralateral inhibition and ipsilateral excitation of electrodermal response amplitudes, then left hemisphere activation will be translated into a pattern of electrodermal asymmetry, right < left with fast habituation, and right hemisphere activation into left < right with slow habituation. These relationships between the direction of electrodermal amplitude asymmetry and habituation rates were indeed found in normal subjects (Gruzelier, 1981), with the exception of a high anxiety subgroup of normals who exhibited slow habituation with amplitude asymmetry right < left. In order to see in perspective the implications of the clinical dichotomy described above one must remember that the PSE-CATEGO diagnostic scheme is hierarchical and establishes the diagnosis of schizophrenia on the presence of first-rank symptoms. Thus mania, and to a lesser extent depression, would be classified as schizophrenia if accompanied by first-rank "schizophrenic" symptoms. Essentially the group of schizophrenia with right< left amplitude consists of the excited phase of the "unitary" concept of bipolar psychoses. These, in many investigations, are mistakenly confused with paranoid schizophrenia. In reality they are best described as thought-disordered delusional hypomanias with first-rank symptomatology. That this interpretation of the Gruzelier (1981) material is correct is further confirmed by examining the characteristic hallucinations and delusions of the patients with larger left hand electrodermal responses (right < left): delusions of grandeur and religious identification, depressive delusions, delusions of guilt, catastrophe, and nihilism. As Gruzelier concludes, the classical syndrome of schizophrenia, in the Kraepelin tradition, with blunted affect and thought disorganization electrodermally is characterized by amplitude asymmetry left < right.

Myslobodsky and Horesh (1978) had earlier demonstrated in endogenous, but not reactive, depressions an electrodermal amplitude asymmetry right < left detected both under a tone-orienting situation and during verbal-emotional tasks (where normals had the opposite asymmetry). Thus both the inhibited and excited forms of the manic-depressive syndrome of the bipolar psychoses, have the same underlying directionality of electrodermal asymmetry. Gruzelier and Venables (1974) found 30% nonresponders in both depressive patients and psychopathic personality disorders (10 of each), with right < left EDA asymmetry in depression and left < right EDA asymmetry in psychopathy. Lenhart and Katkin (1986) extracting the 10 most depressed men and the 10 most depressed women selected from 253 university students studied electrodermal amplitude and conjugate lateral eye movements in these students. The group at risk for subsyndromal bipolar disorder was characterized by EDA asymmetry right < left and an excess of lateral saccades to the left. These findings suggest a pattern of ipsilateral inhibition and contralateral excitation in the cerebral control systems. So far the evidence reviewed indicates a pattern of right < left EDA asymmetry in mood disorders, both manic or depressive, and in the case of depression both in psychotic and neurotic forms as well as subclinical forms. What is more Zahn et al (1989) showed that the children of a parent with bipolar affective illness - and who therefore are at genetic risk for affective disorder - have significantly greater electrodermal activity lateralized to the left hand during task periods.

The intensity of psychopathological symptomatology is probably a crucial aspect to the emergence of lateral asymmetry, since Iacono (1982) could find no differences from normals in a sample of 28 remitted schizophrenics, outpatients "active in the community". At the time of testing, however, none of the patients satisfied research criteria for schizophrenia, either definite or probable.

To complicate matters further de Bonis and Freixa I Baque (1980), studying the influence of stress (mild electric shock) and verbal cognitive activity on the bilaterality of electrodermal responses in normal subjects, found overwhelmingly symmetrical responses, with a common, nonsignificant trend toward right < left in both conditions. Indubitably there was, however, an increase in arousal in the stress situation, and this was associated with a bilateral increase in symmetry. This was also found by Brende (1982) who, in an unusual investigation, analyzed the electrodermal characteristics of six Vietnam veterans during the hypnotically induced recollection of psychologically traumatic war experiences. In addition, he found that unpleasant emotions were right < left: hypervigilance and aggression left < right; psychic numbing with bilateral inhibition; and voluntary efforts to control fear with right < left.

In conclusion this review suggests that there are definite and systematic asymmetries of electrodermal amplitude in various psychopathological states. The chronic, negative symptomatology forms of schizophrenia are characterized by electrodermal amplitude asymmetry left < right. On the other hand, "acute schizophrenias" with strong affective admixture, delusional manias, depressive states all show the opposite asymmetry right < left. Furthermore, first degree relatives of affective patients and normal subjects with subclinical manic depressive tendencies have the same, right < left EDA asymmetry. The precise cerebral implications, at the cortical hemispheric level of these asymmetries remain somewhat uncertain. In the view of the writer the model of contralateral inhibition and ipsilateral excitation is a reasonable hypothesis in spite of its internal redundancy. In any case, as Hugdahl (1984) concludes in his review of hemispheric asymmetry in bilateral electrodermal activity "bilateral electrodermal recordings have not been unambiguously related to hemispheric asymmetry. However, when asymmetry between the hands is clearly demonstrated, this reflects an asymmetry in the functioning of the cerebral hemispheres".

## REFERENCES

Alm, T., Lindstrom, L.H., Lars-Goran, O., and Ohman, A., 1984, Electrodermal non-responding in schizophrenia: relationships to attentional, clinical, biochemical, computed tomographical and genetic factors, *Int. J. Psychophysiol.* 1: 195-208.

Baxter, L.R., Schwartz, J.M., Mazziotta, J.C., et al., 1988, Cerebral glucose metabolic rates in nondepressed patients with obsessive-compulsive disorder, *Amer. J. Psychiat.* 145: 1560-1563.

Bernstein, A.S., Riedel, J.A., Pava, J., Schnur, D., and Lubowsky, J., 1985, A limiting factor in the "normalization" of schizophrenic orienting response dysfunction, *Schizophr. Bull.* 11#2: 230-254.

Bonis de, M. and Freixa I Baque, E., 1980, Stress, verbal cognitive activity and bilateral electrodermal responses, *Neuropsychobiology* 6: 249-259.

Brende, J.O., 1982, Electrodermal responses in post-traumatic syndromes. A pilot study of cerebral hemisphere functioning in Vietnam veterans, *J.Nerv. Ment. Dis.* 170#6: 352-361.

Gruzelier J., Eves, F., and Connolly, J., 1981, Reciprocal hemispheric influences on response habituation in the electrodermal system, *Physiol. Psychol.* 9: 313-317.

Gruzelier, J., 1981, Hemispheric imbalances masquerading as paranoid and nonparanoid syndromes? *Schizophr. Bull.* 7#4: 662-673.

Gruzelier, J., and Hammond, N., 1976, Schizophrenia: a dominant hemisphere temporal-limbic disorder? *Res. Comm. Psychol. Psychiat. Behav.* 1#1: 33- 72.

Gruzelier, J., and Venables, P., 1974, Bimodality and lateral asymmetry of skin conductance orienting activity in schizophrenics: replication and evidence of lateral asymmetry in patients with depression and disorders of personality, *Biol. Psychiat.* Vol. 8#1: 55-73.

Gruzelier, J., and Venables, P.H., 1973, Skin conductance responses to tones with and without attentional significance in schizophrenic and nonschizophrenic psychiatric patients, *Neuropsychologia* 11: 221.

Gruzelier, J.H., 1979, Lateral asymmetries in electrodermal activity and psychosis, *in: Hemisphere Asymmetries of Function in Psychopathology*, J.H. Gruzelier and P. Flor-Henry, Eds, Amsterdam, North Holland Biomedical Press, pp. 149-168.

Gruzelier, J.H. and Venables, P.H., 1972, Skin conductance responses to tones in heterogenous sample of schizophrenics: possible evidence of limbic dysfunction., *J. Nerv. Ment. Dis.* 155: 277-287.

Gruzelier, J.H., 1973, Bilateral asymmetry of skin conductance orienting activity and levels in schizophrenics? *J. Biol. Psychol.* 1: 21-41.

Holloway, F.A., and Parsons, O.A., 1969, Unilateral brain damage and bilateral skin conductance levels in humans, *Psychophysiology* 6: 138-148.

Hugdahl, K., 1984, Hemispheric asymmetry and bilateral electrodermal recordings: a review of the evidence, *Psychophysiology* 21#4: 371-393.

Iacono, W.G., 1982, Bilateral electrodermal habituation-dishabituation and resting EEG in remitted schizophrenics, *J. Nerv. Ment.Dis.* 91-101.

Lacroix, J.M., and Comper, P., 1979, Lateralization in the electrodermal system as a function of cognitive/hemispheric manipulations, *Psychophysiology* 16#2: 116-129.

Lenhart, R.E., and Katkin, E.S., 1986, Psychophysiological evidence for cerebral laterality effects in a high-risk sample of students with subsyndromal bipolar depressive disorder, *Amer.J. Psychiat.* 143: 602.

Luria, A.R., and Homskaya, E.D., 1963, Le trouble du role ré gulateur de language au cours des lé sions du lobe frontal, *Neuropsychologia*, 1: 9-26.

Martinez-Selva, J.M., Roman, F., Garcia-Sanchez, F.A., and Gomez-Amor, J., 1987, Sex differences and the asymmetry of specific and non-specific electrodermal responses, *Inter. J. Psychophysiol.*, 5: 155-160.

Myslobodsky, M.S., and Horesh, N., 1978, Bilateral electrodermal activity in depressive patients, *Biol. Psychol.* 6: 111-120.

Myslobodsky, M.S., and Rattok, J., 1977, Bilateral electrodermal activity in waking man, *Acta Psychol.* 41#4: 273-282.

Naveteur, J., and Sequeira-Martinho, H., 1990, Reliability of bilateral differences in electrodermal activity, *Biol. Psychol.* 31: 47-56.

Raine, A., 1987, Effect of early environment on electrodermal and cognitive correlates of schizotypy and psychopathy in criminals, *Inter. J. Psychophysiol.* 4: 277-287.

Rippon, G., 1979, Bilateral differences in skin conductance level in schizophrenic patients, *in: Hemisphere Asymmetries of Function in Psychopathology*, J. Gruzelier and P. Flor-Henry, Eds, Elsevier/North Holland Biomedical Press, Amsterdam; pp. 169-187.

Rippon, G., 1990, Individual differences in electrodermal and electroencephalographic asymmetries, *Inter. J. Psychophysiol.* 8: 309-320.

Roman, F., Martinez-Selva, J.M., Garcia-Sanchez, F.A., and Gomez-Amor, J., 1986, Sex differences and bilateral electrodermal asymmetry, *Psychophysiology* 23#4: 457.

Sourek, K., 1965, *The Nervous Control of Skin Potential in Man*, Prague, Nakladate istvi Ceskoslovenska Academic Ved.

Uherik, A., 1978, *Psychophysiological properties of Man*. Bratislava.

Venables, P.H., 1977, The electrodermal psychophysiology of schizophrenics and children at risk for schizophrenia: controversies and developments, *Schizophr. Bull.* 3: 28-48.

Weitkunat, R., Buhrer, M., and Sparrer, B., 1990, Cortical initiation of phasic electrodermal activity, *Inter. J. Psychophysiol.* 9: 303-314.

White, C., Farley, J. and Charles, P., 1987, Chronic schizophrenic disorder. K. Psychophysiological responses, laterality and social stress, *Brit. J. Psychiat.* 150: 365.

Zahn, T. P., Nurnberger, J.I., and Berrettini, W.H., 1989, Electrodermal activity in young adults at genetic risk for affective disorder, *Arch. Gen. Psychiat.* 46: 1120-1124.

# HEMISPHERIC DIFFERENCES AND ELECTRODERMAL

# ASYMMETRY - TASK AND SUBJECT EFFECTS.

Georgina Rippon

Department of Psychology
University of Warwick
Coventry CV4 7AL. U.K.

## ABSTRACT

As with most areas, bilateral electrodermal activity research raises both empirical and theoretical issues. With respect to the former, a basic assumption of such research is that the tasks used reliably result in differential activation of the cerebral hemispheres, and that resulting responses can be interpreted accordingly. One aspect of this paper will be a challenge to this assumption and presentation of data that illustrates particular difficulties. Further, in the selection of subjects, although some attention is paid to individual differences, by taking note of sex and handedness, it may be that researchers are doing themselves a disservice by ignoring more subtle measures of functional lateralisation. Data will be presented to illustrate this point. Finally, the interpretation of data from such studies has led to the generation of particular models concerning the cortical control of electrodermal activity; the significance of the studies reported here for the formulation of such models will be discussed.

## INTRODUCTION

Although general measures of electrodermal activity (EDA) have been widely used as an index of individual states and traits for over a century now, it is only since the 1970s that psychophysiologists have been considering the significance of bilateral measures of EDA. The research occurs in the context of interpreting such responses as measures of central nervous system activation, specifically as indices of functional hemispheric asymmetry. Much of the impetus for such research has come from the clinical field where findings of extreme or anomalous electrodermal asymmetry in psychopathological populations are interpreted in terms of abnormalities of right or left hemispheric function or abnormalities of hemispheric balance (Gruzelier and Manchanda, 1982; Gruzelier, 1984).

An underlying assumption of such research was that EDA provided a useful index of relatively inaccessible CNS activity and therefore had a useful contribution to make in

*Progress in Electrodermal Research*, Edited by
J.-C. Roy *et al.* Plenum Press, New York, 1993

elucidating issues in hemispheric specialisation research, in both normal and abnormal populations. It was an assumption that has subsequently been challenged. In the mid-1980s there were three excellent critical reviews which drew attention to the multitude of problems which had become apparent in this burgeoning field (Hugdahl, 1984, Freixa i Baqué et al, 1984, Miossec et al 1985), supplemented more recently by an updating review by Hugdahl (1988). The problems identified were both methodological and theoretical. The chief methodological problem was the selection of appropriate tasks, a common difficulty in hemispheric specialisation research. The possible problems of insufficient attention to subject characteristics was also raised. The key theoretical problem concerned the interpretation of the data and the application of models of control which had no independent validation (Miossec et al, 1985). Each of these issues will be considered in the light of data collected by the author.

## TASK SELECTION

A basic assumption in the majority of studies investigating variations in EDA asymmetry as a function of task demands is that there are "hemisphere specific" cognitive tasks. These are then employed to differentially activate the relevant hemispheres and observations made of resulting variations in EDA asymmetry (if any). Verbal tasks are used on the assumption that they will affect left hemisphere activity; tasks designed to affect right hemisphere activity are more varied, but frequently incorporate visuospatial processing. A smaller proportion of studies vary the affective valence of stimuli (e.g. Hugdahl, Wahlgren and Wass, 1982; Meyers and Smith, 1987).

The assumptions of "hemisphere specific " tasks are made on the basis of rather crude dichotomising of hemisphere specialisation. It is clearly unlikely to represent the subtlety of functional representation within and betweeen the hemispheres. It is an assumption based on earlier work of experimental and clinical neuropsychologists who themselves point out the over-simplification. Not only is it unlikely that one hemisphere will deal uniquely with anything other than the simplest of stimuli, it is also clear that both inter - and intra-hemispheric variations can occur with different processing requirements, both within and between subjects   If, then, studies are carried out with the assumption that tasks are differentially activating the hemispheres and EDA does not vary in the directions predicted by such assumptions, it may be due to the ineffectiveness of the tasks in eliciting variations in hemispheric activity rather the ineffectiveness of the EDA as an index of these variations. Rarely is any independent evidence supplied to investigate task effectiveness. The follow-ing study which has been reported in a different context elsewhere (Rippon,1990) provides an example of how the availability of such evidence could well lead to a different assess-ment of the EDA results.

The task involved the manipulation of either verbal stimuli (the selection of a synonym for a given word from a set of four alternatives) or visuospatial stimuli (the selection of an appropriate abstract shape with which to complete a given series, again from a set of four alternatives). The abstract nature of the shapes aimed to avoid naming or labelling and consequent left hemisphere activation. The tasks were matched for difficulty on the basis of ratings from 3 independent judges. There were 8 female and 8 male subjects, all right handed with no family history of sinistrality.

Stimuli were presented on slides for 5 seconds (the 'think' interval). Each stimulus slide was followed by a blank slide for 15 seconds during which the subject indicated her/his solution to the task by means of a bimanual button press (the 'respond interval). There were 10 stimuli in each type of task; the tasks were presented in counterbalanced order. EDA and EEG activity occurring during the 'think' interval were measured and mean skin conductance response amplitude and alpha and beta waveband amplitude were calculated.

Bilateral skin conductance was measured using Ag/AgCl electrodes and 0.5 KCl electrolyte; responses were recorded on a Grass Model 7 polygraph with a constant voltage system. A response was defined as a change in skin conductance of 0.02 mhos or greater, occurring in the interval 1-5 seconds after stimulus presentation. 28 channels of EEG data were collected, using a Neurosciences Series III Brain Imager. These data are subjected to Fast Fourier transform techniques and interpolation techniques used to produce topographic maps of activity in the traditional EEG wavebands. The data can also be downloaded for statistical analyses. In the studies reported here, stepwise discriminant analysis techniques identified those electrode sites which reliably discriminated between experimental variables; data from these electrodes were then subjected to analyses of variance.

Inspection of the skin conductance data could have led to the interpretation that differential hemispheric activation was having no effect on EDA asymmetries. In both conditions left hand activity was higher than right ($F=5.306$, $p=0.037$). If, however, the EEG data are also considered, it is clear that the task itself is not having the expected effect. With respect to alpha activity, there is more activity on the right hemisphere in both conditions, although the difference is not statistically significant. With respect to Beta 2, there is more activity on the left hemisphere ($F=6.925$, $p=0.019$). There is a task x hemisphere interaction ($F=9.84$, $p=0.007$), but this arises because the L>R asymmetry is greater in the picture condition (the supposedly right hemisphere task) than in the verbal condition. These data are illustrated in Fig.1.

It would appear then that the EDA measures *are* parallelling cortical activity. However, as no change in the balance of cortical activity was effected by this task it was not possible to show that EDA asymmetry varied accordingly and to draw appropriate conclusions about the nature of cortical control over the peripheral measure. Hugdahl (1984) has identified this double asymmetry as crucial in providing support for any of the relevant models of cortical-autonomic control.

It has been suggested that a more effective way of determining differential hemi-spheric activation would be to employ unilateral stimulus input (Hugdahl, 1984). Divided visual field (DVF) and dichotic listening (DL) techniques are frequently used in neuro-psychological research for the study of functional asymmetry. They have the advantage of minimising interhemispheric transfer time which may invalidate the concept of hemisphere specific processing (Miossec et al, 1985). Comper and Lacroix (1981) employed a DVF technique and reported double asymmetry findings, greater left than right hand SCRs to verbal stimuli presented to the left hemisphere and greater right than left hand SCRs to spatial stimuli presented to the right hemisphere. Hugdahl and co-workers have employed DL techniques within a Pavlovian conditioning paradigm (Hugdahl, and Brobeck, 1986; Hugdahl, Kvale, Nordby and Overmeier, 1987; Hugdahl, 1988) and report that SCRs reliably index hemisphere specific effects. However, Rippon (1989), employing indirect assessment via RT measures reported that a DVF task involving relatively simple letter stimuli was not achieving its assumed aim of differentially activating the hemispheres. While the verbal or 'left hemisphere' task was apparently successful, the 'spatial or right hemisphere task was not associated with differential hemispheric activation.

A replication of this study using BEAM techniques confirmed this . The task was to make "same/different" judgements on pairs of upper and/or lower case letters, tachisto-scopically presented in the RVF or LVF. The letters subtended an angle of $3^0$ at the eye, and were presented for 100 msec. There were two conditions for each subject. In the PHYSICAL condition, subjects had to judge whether a pair of letters was physically the same (e.g. AA) or different (e.g.Am) ; in the NOMINAL condition subjects had to judge whether a pair of letters was the same in name (e.g.Aa) or different (e.g. Ar). Conditions were counterbalanced between subjects. Psychophysiological data were collected and analysed as above.

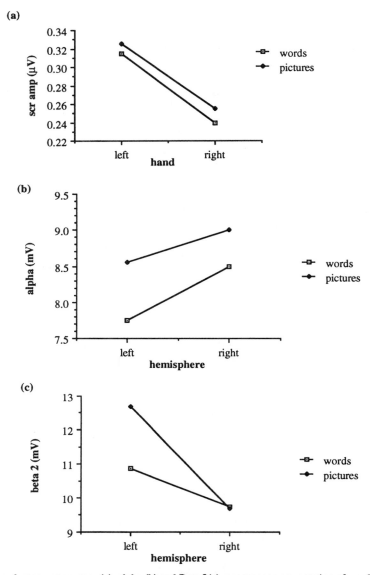

**Fig. 1.** Skin conductance responses (a), alpha (b) and Beta 2(c) responses to presentation of words and pictures.

Analysis of BEAM data demonstrated that the 2 conditions did differentially activate the hemispheres, although not quite as predicted. Significant left-right differences were found in the beta waveband for several electrode pairs. Fig. 2a shows illustrative data from TCP1/2 electrodes. Left/right comparisons showed asymmetrical activity in the verbal task, with more activity on the left hemisphere (Hemisphere F=22.049;p=0.0003; Task x Hemisphere F= 9.164, p=0.0085). Data from the spatial task showed more symmetrical responses, as had been suggested by the earlier RT findings (Rippon, 1989) which were replicated in this study. What is interesting is that the variations come from the right hemisphere, with a relative *decrement* in activity in the verbal task; i.e left hemisphere activity is comparable in both tasks, whereas right hemisphere activity is greater in the spatial task than in the verbal task. There was no effect of visual field of presentation. These EEG responses were parallelled by patterns of EDA activity, asymmetrical in the verbal task and symmetrical in the spatial task. (Hand F=9.132,p=0.009; Hand x Task, F=7.741,p=0.014)(See Fig.2b).

It is interesting to note that it was again in the beta waveband that significant task related effects were observed. Ray and Cole (1985) have suggested that beta activity can reflect cognitive processes; parallel changes in skin conductance response amplitude support the posited role of this measure as an index of task demands.

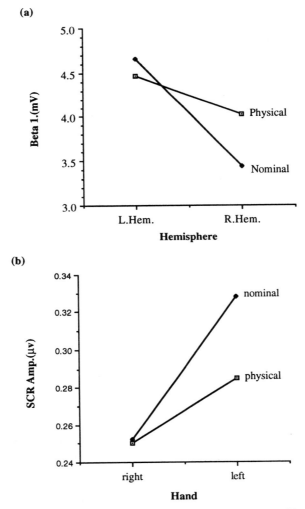

**Fig.2.** Beta 1 (a) and skin conductance responses (b) in a letter matching task.

An interpretation of these findings could be that subjects employed verbal strategies to support the supposedly spatial task, with the resultant involvement of both hemispheres. Variations in strategies employed have been an issue in cognitive approaches to hemispheric processing (Beaumont, Young and McManus, 1984) and individual variations in strategy could confound initial stimulus controls.

Another variable that requires further consideration is the processing requirements of the task. In both the above studies, active processing requirements were involved. It may well be that the success of the Hugdahl et al paradigms is that they involve fairly passive stimulus processing. Gruzelier, Sergeant and Eves (1988) have demonstrated the varying effects of stimulus and response processing influences on skin conductance.

In conclusion adequate control of task variables is clearly crucial. It is unsurprising that the fairly crude verbal/visuospatial dichotomies are inappropriate, but even in fairly tightly controlled stimulus presentation conditions, assumptions about the relative effects on hemispheric activation may be unjustified, and therefore interpretations of any accompanying EDA changes invalid.


## INDIVIDUAL DIFFERENCES

The issue of subject variables in the area of EDA asymmetry obviously requires consideration. There is strong evidence that gender and handedness are variables which affect functional hemispheric specialisation, although the relationship is clearly complex (McGlone, 1980; Annett, 1985, Bradshaw, 1990). There is further evidence of gender differences in EEG asymmetries (Beaumont et al, 1978; Trotman and Hammond, 1979; Glass et al 1984; Petsche et al, 1988); rather fewer with respect to handedness differences (Glass et al, 1984). If EDA is to be taken as an index of hemispheric activation it is to be expected that gender and possibly handedness would be shown to affect EDA asymmetry.

However, where there are any conclusive findings of the effect of handedness and/or gender on EDA they are often contradictory. With respect to sex differences, some studies report more asymmetrical responses (in the direction of L>R) in males than females (Smith and Ketterer 1982; Roman et al 1986), the reverse of that reported by other studies (Ketterer and Smith , 1977).

With respect to handedness, Robinson and Zahn (1981) report that left-handers show consistently higher levels of EDA from the left hand and right handers consistently higher levels from the right hand; Lacroix and Comper (1979) found task-related variations in EDA in dextral females not shown by sinistral females. Other studies find no difference (Gruzelier et al, 1981). Reviewers have gone so far as to say : "the only issue on which most authors agree is the absence of a relation between hand preference and EDR lateralisation" (Freixa i Baque et al, 1984, pg.228).

Some studies have considered a combination of the variables. Ketterer and Smith (1977) indicated that a family history of sinistrality was implicated in increased left hand responding, possibly interacting with the sex of the subject. Smith, Ketterer and Concannon's (1981) data indicate a complex relationship between sex and familial handedness, with males with a dextral family history and females with a partially sinistral family history showing different patterns of left and right hand responding to sinistral history males and dextral history females. It should be noted that their findings are unusual in that they partly refer to nonspecific responses and responses to blank slides following stimulus presentation.

It could be that studies investigating the effects of such variables suffered from the methodological difficulties discussed above, which would certainly have contributed to conflicting or inconclusive data. However, a study measuring EDA and electrocortical activity in parallel reported sex differences in left and right hemisphere EEG measures which were not reflected in the electrodermal measure (Rippon, 1990).

Roman's group has suggested that there is a consistent lateralisation in EDA which varies between subjects and remains constant throughout different experimental conditions. They call this the electrodermal Responsiveness Pattern (RP) and find that it is independent of gender (Roman et al, 1987,1989) and handedness (Roman et al, 1992). A similar finding was reported by Rippon (1990). When individual subjects were allocated to 'high' or 'low' asymmetry groups according to the lateralisation of their electrocortical activity a positive relationship with electrodermal asymmetry was found. That is, there was a consistent lateralisation pattern in subjects EDA which was matched by their EEG activity.

It is possible, then, that there is some kind of 'lateralisation' factor operating, affecting the asymmetry or otherwise of psychophysiological measures. An attempt to investigate the 'source' of this led the author back to handedness measures.

Annett's work (1985) has indicated that handedness is not a discrete but a continuous variable. With respect to dextrals, measures of hand preference indicate a range from mixed laterality where subjects, although nominally right handed, show very little difference between the hands with respect to a range of skills, to "strong dextrals" who show an "over-reliance" on their right hand, associated with a marked weakness of their left hand. The degree of an individuals dextrality (or lack of it) is genetically determined. Rippon (1991) reported data indicating a relationship between degrees of handedness and degrees of EEG asymmetry. So the variations in functional representation represented by variations in handedness (even within a nominally dextral population) might be associated with variations in the degree to which individuals display psychophysiological asymmetries. If this is the case, then this would provide support for the hypothesis of a link between hemispheric activity and electrodermal responses and also go some way towards explaining the frequently inconclusive findings in the literature. Even if authors only select right handed subjects for their studies, if their population varies according to the degree of their right handedness, this could affect the electrodermal activity being measured.

Handedness/electrodermal data were available on 30 subjects who had participated in the studies described above. Handedness was assessed by average time taken to complete a simple peg-moving task with each hand (the Annett pegboard, Annett 1985). Degree of dextrality is measured by subtracting right hand scores from left. Large positive scores indicate strong dextrality; small or negative scores indicate weak or mixed laterality. SCR data are mean responses from each hand during task performance. The EEG measures reported are from the TCP1/2 electrode pairs as they indicated hemispheric differences in both of the studies included here.

There were 22 males and 8 females, all right-handed with no family history of sinistrality, age range 18 - 49 years. Handedness/EDA/EEG comparisons were possible on 16 of these Ss, 11 male and 5 female. Ss were then divided into 'high' 'medium' and 'low' dextral groups on the basis of their pegboard scores, and comparisons made between the 'high' and the 'low' dextral groups. This resulted in groups of N=20 (10 x high and 10 x low) for the electrodermal comparisons and N=10 (5 x high and 5 x low) for the EEG comparisons.

Data were combined from the studies, with the synonym selection task and the Nominal task in the DVF study being categorised as 'verbal' tasks, and the pattern selection task and the Physical task in the DVF study being categorised as spatial tasks. Although one would not normally combine data from different studies in this way, it does allow one to explore the effect of a particular variable on psychophysiological measures taken under broadly similar conditions.

Figure 3a shows the pattern of electrodermal activity from the subjects as a whole. Previously reported patterns are confirmed, with L>R responses in the verbal conditions and L=R in the spatial conditions (Task x hand, F=4.368, p=0.05 ). The 'high' and 'low' groups show a clear difference in EDA activity. (Figs.3b,c ). 'High' dextrals showed a significant L>R difference in the verbal tasks, with little difference between the hands in the spatial tasks; 'low' dextrals showed little difference between the hands in either task. (Task x Hand x Dextrality interaction ; F=5.063; p=0.037).

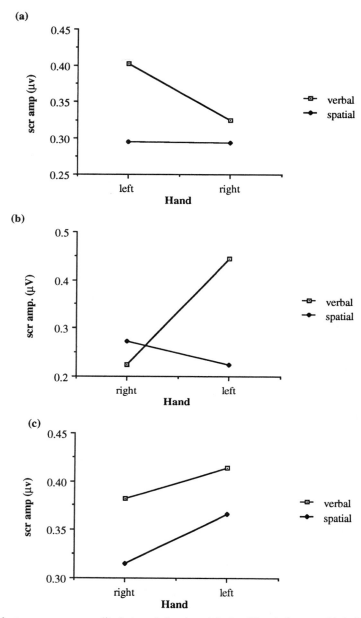

**Fig. 3.** Skin conductance response amplitude to verbal and spatial stimuli in whole group (a), in 'high' dextrals (b) and low dextrals (c).

A similar pattern emerges when considering the EEG data. Alpha activity reveals greater left than right hemisphere activity in the verbal tasks; and left/right symmetry in the spatial task.(Task x Hemisphere = 13.563; p=0.0062) 'High' dextrals show a L>R activity in the verbal tasks and R>L in the spatial tasks. 'Low' dextrals show little hemispheric difference in either task (Task x Hemisphere x Dextrality; F=10.835, p=0.0110). These data are illustrated in Fig. 4.

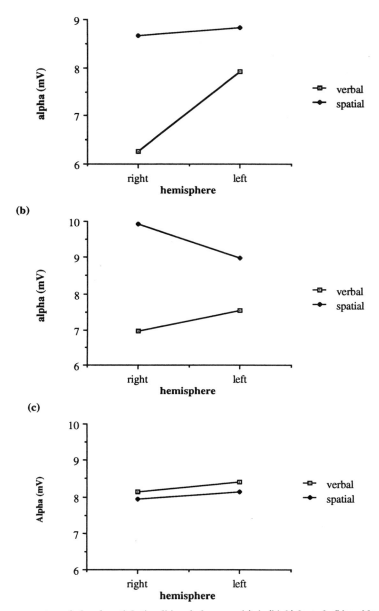

**Fig. 4.** Alpha response to verbal and spatial stimuli in whole group (a), in 'high' dextrals (b) and low dextrals (c).

The pattern is less clear in the beta waveband 1 (see Fig.5) where the Task x Hemisphere x Dextrality interaction just fails to reach significance ($F=4.794$; $p=0.06$).

In conclusion, both EDA and EEG asymmetries have been shown to vary as a function of subjects' functional lateralisation, even within a right handed population. This could counteract the rather pessimistic conclusions concerning cortical electrodermal relationships which are drawn from the lack of any apparent relationship between electrodermal measures and handedness. Any study considering handedness as a discrete rather than a continuous variable could contain sufficient variance in the different groups to swamp any EDA differences which have been consistently shown to be "small and easily distorted" (Hugdahl,1984, pg. 389). As functional lateralisation can vary independently of sex (Bradshaw,1990) this could also be a confounding factor in studies attempting to investigate sex differences in electrodermal asymmetry. Further, it is clear that attempts to control for lateralisation differences by only selecting right-handed male subject with no family history of sinistrality could well be inadequate.

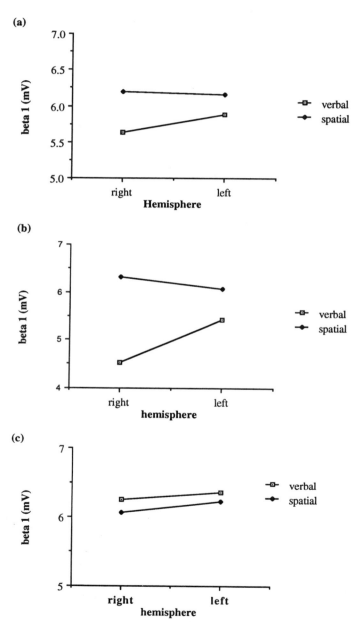

Fig. 5. Beta 1 response to verbal and spatial stimuli in whole group (a), in 'high' dextrals (b) and low dextrals (c).

## CORTICAL CONTROL OF EDA

Thus far, this chapter has avoided discussion of the nature of the cortical control over electrodermal asymmetry. The issues revolve around the question of whether the control is ipsilateral and/or contralateral, excitatory and/or inhibitory (Freixa i Baque et al ,1984). Much data is interpreted in support of a model of contralateral inhibition i.e. increase in activation in one hemisphere is associated with a decrease in electrodermal activity on the contralateral hand (Lacroix and Comper,1979; Comper and Lacroix, 1981; Boyd and Maltzman, 1982, Rippon, 1989). Reviewers have pointed out that the same data could be explained by a model of unilateral excitation  (Freixa i Baque, 1984; Miossec et al, 1984) .  Other researchers report findings indicating contralateral excitation linked with motor control (Gruzelier et al, 1988).

A key problem here, as with the methodological difficulties discussed above, is the absence of any independent measure validating the assumptions about the nature and direction of cortical activity in the relevant studies. As a conclusion to this chapter we could consider how the data presented here might contribute to this debate, given that they  provide direct measures of the cortical activity occurring during the tasks concerned.

The first study characterises nicely the problems in that the data could be interpreted either in terms of contralateral inhibition or ipsilateral excitation, as it shows L>R hemisphere activity (taking alpha increase on the right hemisphere as a measure of reduced cortical activation) parallelled by L>R hand EDA.  As the task did not effect the type of double asymmetry advocated by Hugdahl (1984), reliable interpretation is impossible.  In the second study, with respect to beta activity, left hemisphere activity remained comparable in the two task conditions; whereas right hemisphere activity varied. This was parallelled by relative stability of right hand EDA and variations in the left hand,  with *increases* in *left hand EDA* associated with *decreases* in *right hemisphere EEG* activity.  An overview of these studies as seen in the Individual differences section reveals relatively constant left hemisphere activity in the tasks; where variations do occur, they are on the right hemisphere.  Right hand responses are relatively stable independent of the degree of the subjects' dextrality or the current task; variations in left hand activity show some evidence of increases in left hand activity associated with decreases in right hemisphere activity.

These data would seem to provide support for a model of contralateral inhibition. They are, however, only tentatively offered as such support.  Even EEG measures cannot be taken as wholly accurate measures of cortical activity; more direct measures such as MRI or PET scans data are required before we can move towards a more accurate understanding of how cortical activity can be reflected in electrodermal measure (Raine et al, 1991).


## CONCLUSION

To return to the key issue, the usefulness or otherwise of EDA as an index of variations in cortical activity.  Reviews of the literature have suggested that the findings thus far are rather disappointing.  The data reported here indicate that this may partly be due to failure in the control of independent variables, with particular emphasis on task  and subject selection. Hugdahl (1984) has indicated that "bilateral differences in EDA are small and easily distorted "(pg. 389) making close attention to methodological issues even more important.

The complex role of individual differences is also clearly an issue.  Attention to these is, unfortunately likely to make the selection of appropriate subjects more difficult.  On the positive side, the links with Annett's work on degrees of handedness provide interesting overlaps with the clinical field and the possible role of genetic links to abnormalities of hemispheric balance in conditions such as schizophrenia (Gruzelier,1984).  It should be remembered that much of the impetus for electrodermal asymmetry research arose from the observation of marked asymmetries in such conditions (Gruzelier,1973).

Critics of EDA would dismiss it as a measure *too* easily distorted and lacking in reliability. Proponents of its use claim it as a subtle index providing us with a window on central activities to which we do not have easy access. It could be that the ease of acquisition of data has made researchers careless with respect to the control of conditions under which it is collected. Until more careful attention is paid to this, we cannot really rule on its utility.

## REFERENCES

Annett, M. (1985). *Left, right, hand and brain: The right shift theory.* London, Lawrence Erlbaum.

Beaumont, J.G., Mayes, A.R. and Rugg, M.D. (1978). Asymmetry in EEG alpha coherence and power: effects of task and sex. *Electroenceph. Clin. Neurophysiol.* 54:220-226.

Beaumont, J, Young, A. and McManus, I. (1984). Hemisphericity: a critical review. *Cognitive Neuropsychology* 1:191-212.

Boyd, G. and Maltzman, I. (1983). Bilateral asymmetry of skin conductance responses during auditory and visual tasks. *Psychophysiology*, 20;196-203.

Bradshaw, J. (1990). *Hemispheric specialisation and psychological function.* New York, Wiley.

Comper, P. and Lacroix, M. (1981). Lateralisation in the electrodermal system: effects of unilateral tachistoscopic presentations. *Psychophysiology* 18:149.

Freixa i Baqué, E., Catteau, M-C, Miossec, Y, and Roy, J.C. (1984). Asymmetry of electrodermal activity: a review. *Biological Psychology*,18:219-239.

Glass, A, Butler S. and Carter, J. (1984). Hemispheric asymmetry of EEG alpha activation: effects of gender and familial handedness. *Biological Pychology* 19:169-187.

Gruzelier, J. (1973). Bilateral asymmetry of skin conductance, orienting activity and levels in schizophrenia. *Journal of Biological Psychology* 1:21-41.

Gruzelier, J. (1984) Hemispheric imbalance in schizophrenia. *International Journal of Psychophysiology* 1:227-240.

Gruzelier, J. H. and Manchanda, R. (1982). The syndrome of schizophrenia: relations between electrodermal response, lateral asymmetries and clinical ratings. *British Journal of Psychiatry*, 141:488-495.

Gruzelier, J., Eves, F. and Connolly, J. (1981). Reciprocal hemispheric influences on response habituation in the electrodermal system. *Physiological Psychology*, 9:313-317.

Gruzelier, J., Sergeant, J. and Eves, F. (1988). The use of bilateral skin conductance measurement in elucidating stimulus versus response processing influences on the orienting reaction. *International Journal of Psychophysiology*, 6:195-205.

Hugdahl,K. (1984). Hemispheric asymmetry and bilateral electrodermal recordings: a review of the evidence. *Psychophysiology*, 21:371-393.

Hugdahl, K. (1988). Bilateral electrodermal asymmetry: past hopes and future prospects, *International Journal of Neuroscience*,39:33-44.

Hugdahl, K. and Brobeck, C. (1986). Hemispheric asymmetry and human electrodermal conditioning: the dichotic extinction paradigm. *Psychophysiology* 23:491-499.

Hugdahl, K., Kvale, G., Nordby, H, and Overmier, J. (1987). Hemispheric asymmetry and human classical conditioning to verbal and non-verbal visual CSs. *Psychophysiology*, 24: 557-565.

Hugdahl, K., Wahlgren, C. and Wass, T. (1982). Habituation of the electrodermal orienting reacton is dependent on the cerebral hemisphere initially stimulated. *Biological Psychology.* 15:49-62.

Ketterer, M.W. and Smith, B.D. (1977). Bilateral electrodermal activity, lateralised cerebral processing and sex. *Psychophysiology*, 14:513-516.

Ketterer, M.W. and Smith, B.D. (1982). Lateralised cortical/cognitive processing and electrodermal activity: effects of subjects and stimulus characteristics (Abstract). *Psychophysiology*, 19: 328-329.

Lacroix,M.and Comper,J. (1979). Lateralisation in the electrodermal system as a function of cognitive/ hemispheric manipulations. *Psychophysiology*, 16:116-129.

McGlone, J. (1980). Sex differences in human brain organisation:a critical survey. *The Behavioural and Brain Sciences*, 3:215-263.

Meyers M. and Smith, B. (1986). Hemispheric asymmetry and emotion: effects of nonverbal affective stimuli. *Biological Psychology,* 22:11-21.

Miossec, Y., Catteau, M.C., Freixa i Baqué, E. and Roy, J.C. (1985). Methodological problems in bilateral electrodermal research. *International Journal of Psychophysiology,* 2: 247-256.

Petsche, H., Rappelsberger, P. and Pockberger, H.(1988) Sex differences in the ongoing EEG: Probability mapping at rest and during cognitive tasks. In: G. Pfurtscheller and F.H. Lopes da Silva (Eds.) *Functional Brain Imaging.* Hans Huber

Raine, A., Reynold, G, and Sheard, C. (1991). Neuroanatomical correlates of skin conductance orienting in normal humans: a magnetic resonance imaging study. *Psychophysiology.* 28:548-558.

Ray, W.J. & Cole, H.W. (1985). EEG alpha activity reflects attentional demands and beta activity reflects emotional and cognitive processes. *Science,* 228:750-752.

Rippon,G.M.J.(1989). Bilateral electrodermal activity; effects of differential hemispheric activation. *Journal of Psychophysiology* ,3: 65-73.

Rippon, G.M.J. (1990). Individual Differences in electrodermal and electroencephalographic asymmetries. *International J. of Psychophysiology,*8 :309-321.

Rippon, G.M.J. (1991). EEG topographical mapping and laterality measures in dyslexic children." In : *Dyslexia: Integrating Theory and Practice.* Snowling. M. and Thomson, M. (Eds.) Whurr.

Robinson, T. and Zahn, T. (1981). Bilateral EDA, hand preference and hand position. *Psychophysiology,* 18:137-138.

Roman, F., Carrillo, E. and Garcia-Sanchez, F. (1992). Responsiveness patterns and handedness differences in bilateral electrodermal asymmetry. *International Journal of Psychophysiology,* 12:71-81.

Roman, F., Martinez-Selva,J., Garcia-Sanchez, F. and Gomez-Amor, J. (1987). Sex differences, activation level and bilateral electrodermal activity. *Pavlovian Journal of Biological Sciences,* 22;113-117.

Roman, F., Martinez-Selva,J., Garcia-Sanchez, F., Gomez-Amor, J.and Carrillo, E. (1989). Sex differences and bilateral electrodermal activity: a replication. *Pavlovian Journal of Biological Sciences,*24:150-155.

Roman, F.et al (1986). Sex differences and bilateral electrodermal asymmetry. *Psychophysiology,* 23

Smith, B. and Ketterer, M. (1982). Lateralised cortical/cognitive processing and bilateral electrodermal activity: effects of sensory mode and sex. *Biological Psychology,* 15:191-201.

Smith, B. Ketterer, M. and Concannon, M. (1981). Bilateral electrodermal activity as a function of hemispheric stimulation, hand preferences, sex and familial handedness. *Biological Psychology,* 12:1-11.

Trotman, S.C.A.and Hammond,G.R. (1979) Sex differences in task-dependent EEG asymmetries.*Psychophysiology,* 16:420-431.

# ELECTRODERMAL ACTIVITY IN PATIENTS WITH UNILATERAL

# BRAIN DAMAGE

Pierluigi Zoccolotti,[1,3] Carlo Caltagirone,[2,3]
Anna Pecchinenda[1] and Elio Troisi[2]

1  Department of Psychology,
University of Rome "La Sapienza"
Rome   Italy
2  Neurological Clinic, University of Rome "Tor Vergata"
Rome   Italy
3  Clinica S.Lucia
Rome   Italy

## INTRODUCTION

Electrodermal activity has been studied in patients with focal brain injury mainly to evaluate hypotheses about the relative contribution of the two cerebral hemispheres to emotional processes. Theoretical proposals on this issue originated from the clinical observations indicating different emotional reactions following damage in either hemisphere. Left brain damaged (LBD) patients display what has been defined as a "catastrophic reaction": failures in neuropsychological testing may induce crying, swearing, or declaring their impotence (Gainotti, 1969, 1972). Often this reaction has an abrupt onset and offset. Reactions of right brain damaged (RBD) patients are in sharp contrast with this pattern; often these patients appear unconcerned with their symptoms (e.g., arm paralysis) which are treated in a matter of fact fashion (indifferent reaction)[1]. At times, patients may even appear fatuous and lacking in inhibition (Gainotti, 1972). Somewhat similar reactions have been reported in the case of transient inactivation due to amytal sodium injection (e.g., Terzian and Cecotto, 1959).

Several theoretical formulations have been raised from these clinical observations. One hypothesis is that emotional processes are mediated mainly by the right hemisphere; damage to this structure would produce inappropriate and flattened affect. In contrast, the catastrophic reaction of LBD patients is viewed as the dramatic but not inappropriate

---

[1] Indifference should be clearly distinguished from anosognosia (i.e., lack of knowledge of disability), even though these two symptoms may both occur in the same patients. In the indifference reaction, patients may describe correctly their physical defect (e.g., arm paralysis) but, in spite of its widespread negative consequences on their everyday life, appear uninterested and unconcerned with it.

response of individuals suddenly facing their behavioral deficits (Gainotti, 1972). Apparently consistent with this latter idea is the observation that catastrophic reaction is most commonly seen in aphasic patients. One variety of this hypothesis is that the right hemisphere role in emotion is specific for the communication of affect; the other emotional disturbances observed in these patients would be causally related to their basic inability to comprehend and express emotions (Ross, 1984). Following this theoretical proposal, the indifference reaction shown by patients with a lesion in the right hemisphere would be an apparent emotional disturbance, the patient being unable to express an otherwise intact emotional experience. Other theoretical statements have proposed different dichotomies to explain the hemispheric contribution to emotional processes. One hypothesis claims that the right hemisphere is dominant for negative emotions and the left dominant for positive emotions (e.g., Sackeim et al., 1982). Other theorists have proposed the approach-avoidance dichotomy (Kinsbourne and Bemporad, 1985).

All these theoretical statements refer directly to processes of emotional experience. However, most of the empirical work aimed at checking these hypotheses has examined the processes involved in understanding emotionally significant stimuli. In contrast, only a comparatively small amount of research has been aimed at evaluating possible variations in emotional experience as a result of unilateral brain damage. Studies relevant to this issue include those examining autonomic responses (mostly electrodermal activity) to emotion-producing stimuli.

In general, studies dealing with autonomic parameters as indicators of emotional involvement have indicated flattened arousal in patients with a right hemisphere lesion.

Heilman et al. (1978) established individual thresholds for uncomfortable electric shocks in patients with right or left lesions and in controls. All patients in the right hemisphere group had hemi-neglect (i.e., a reduced tendency in orienting toward the space contralateral to the lesion). Indifference is relatively more frequent in those right hemisphere patients who display neglect (Gainotti, 1972). The patients in the left hemisphere group were all aphasic. Thresholds were not different among groups; however, clear differences were observed in electrodermal activity: patients with right brain damage displayed lower skin conductance levels (SCL) and skin conductance responses (SCR) than controls; patients with left parietal lesions displayed an augmented response as compared to controls, but no difference in SCL.

Heilman et al. (1978) concluded that hypoarousal to emotionally laden stimuli may be a part of the indifference syndrome shown by patients with right hemisphere lesion and neglect.

In Heilman et al. (1978) study, emotional involvement was indirectly evaluated through the use of aversive stimulation. An attempt to use a somewhat more genuinely emotional situation was made in a further study by Morrow et al. (1981). Stimuli consisted of slides depicting emotionally arousing scenes alternated with neutral scenes. Results showed that control subjects displayed greater skin conductance responses to pictures with strong emotional valence than to stimuli without emotional content; LBD patients showed the same pattern, albeit somewhat reduced. In RBD patients no difference in autonomic responses was observed between the two stimulus situations. Unlike the Heilman et al. (1978) study, no difference was observed in skin conductance levels among the three groups studied.

Following, we present a series of studies which were aimed at clarifying the nature of the contribution of the right hemisphere to emotional processes; for this purpose, autonomic measures (particularly electrodermal activity) to emotional and aversive stimulation were examined in conjunction with other aspects of emotional behavior (recognition of emotion, facial expressive behavior).

## STUDY I

In the first study (Zoccolotti et al. 1982), we decided to replicate the findings by Morrow et al. (1981). We also examined the relationship between the reduced autonomic arousal of RBD patients and their impairment in perceptual analysis of emotional stimuli. To carry this out, we tested whether the lack of autonomic arousal to emotional stimulation in RBD patients was related to an impairment in the ability to decode the emotional content of a visual stimulus, namely a facial expression.

We examined 16 RBD and 16 LBD patients. All patients were self-reported right-handed and had a vascular etiology. Patients were seen in a sub-acute phase (at least two months after the onset of symptomatology). Most were seen ca. 4-5 months after the CVA. The two groups did not differ with regard to mean age, years of schooling and time from onset of disease.

Basic electrodermal activity was taken to be the basal value of skin conductance (in mhos/cm$^2$) recorded just prior to the projection of the stimuli. The skin conductance response was taken to be the maximum phasic increase in conductance occurring during the stimulus presentation. The responses were converted into units of quadratic modification of conductance using the formula $\sqrt{\partial}$ conductance x 1000 suggested by Lubin and Johnson (1972) and used in previous research (Morrow et al., 1981). Skin conductance was recorded at 1-sec intervals. Two standard 10 mm$^2$ gold-plated electrodes were placed on the palmar surface of the index and ring finger; a ground electrode was attached to the middle finger. They were applied to the fingers of the hand ipsilateral to the brain lesion in the subjects belonging to the experimental group, and to the right hand in the case of the control subjects. Unless otherwise specified, this general recording and scoring procedure applies to all studies presented.

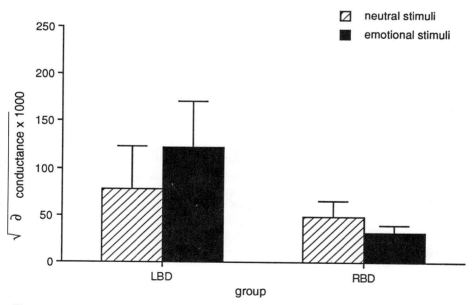

**Figure 1.** Skin conductance responses recorded for emotional and nonemotional stimuli (adapted from Zoccolotti et al., 1982). Data obtained from left brain-damaged (LBD) and right brain damaged (RBD) patients are shown separately. Vertical lines indicate standard errors.

Stimuli consisted of color slides: half of them had a highly emotional content (e.g., a cut hand, a naked woman, etc.), and half were essentially neutral (e.g., flat landscapes, buildings). See Zoccolotti et al. (1982) for further methodological details on this study.

As expected, LBD patients had higher SCRs to emotional than non-emotional stimuli, while RBD patients showed a nonsignificant opposite difference (see Figure 1). An inspection of the mean SCR per trial indicated that the patients with left hemisphere lesions exhibited skin conductance responses to emotion-arousing slides for the whole duration of the test. On the other hand, right brain-damaged patients displayed a clearcut electrodermal response only to the first (neutral) stimulus, followed by a rapid adaptation which was independent of the emotional valence of the stimulus. The existence of a response to the initial stimulus seems to exclude the likelihood that the electrodermal system is simply inactive in patients with right hemisphere lesions and instead points to the maintenance of the orientation response to new stimuli.

Skin conductance levels of both groups of patients were within the range of normal values; there was only a nonsignificant trend for RBD patients to have lower values than LBD patients.

To evaluate emotional recognition, a test of Facial Expression Recognition using pictures from the set developed by Ekman and Friesen (1975) was used. Eighteen items were used, each one consisting of a target face and a choice of two faces, one of which depicted the same expression as the target (each photo in the item portrayed a different actor). RBD patients showed fewer correct responses on this test than LBD patients. This result is consistent with findings in the literature (Cicone et al., 1980; Dekoski et al., 1980) indicating a deficit in RBD patients in the recognition of emotion. However, a covariance analysis indicated that the arousal and the recognition deficits in RBD patients were independent.

## Comments

Closely replicating the findings by Morrow et al. (1981), the results of this study indicate that damage to the right cerebral hemisphere is associated with flattened arousal: these patients fail to distinguish autonomically between emotional and neutral stimuli. It is noteworthy that differences were present only in the case of responses to emotional stimuli. SCLs of both groups were within normal limits. Furthermore, responses to the first stimulus in the trial sequence indicated a preservation of electrodermal responding to novel stimulation (orienting response) in both groups of patients. This differentiation among different indices of electrodermal activity is important in pinpointing the hemispheric contribution to emotional processes and will be further discussed below.

Similar to previous studies (e.g., Cicone et al., 1980; Dekoski et al., 1980) RBD patients showed reduced ability in recognizing emotional stimuli (facial expressions). However, this deficit was unrelated to the flattened electrodermal arousal. This finding is in keeping with the idea that processes of recognition and emotional experience are controlled by independent mechanisms. Findings consistent with this idea have also been reported by Etcoff (1989). In her study, RBD patients showed a deficit in perceiving facial expressions; this deficit was found to be specific, i.e. independent of other cognitive skills such as ability in perceiving the identity of faces or of simple geometric patterns. Confirming previous evidence (e.g., Gainotti, 1972), Etcoff (1989) also found that the RBD patients in her sample showed an indifference reaction more frequently than the LBD patients. Relevant to the present discussion is the observation that no correlation was found between different indices of degree of impairment in perceiving emotions and degree of indifference. She concludes that "production of complex emotional behaviors and the perception of facial expressions of emotions are mediated by separate circuits within the right hemisphere." Overall, these observations underscore the necessity, in testing theories of hemispheric control of emotion, that different measures of emotional involvement be used, not simply measures of emotional recognition.

## STUDY II

A second study was aimed at evaluating different indicators of response to emotional stimuli (autonomic activity, expressive behavior) within the same group of patients with unilateral hemispheric lesions (Caltagirone et al., 1989; Mammucari et al., 1988; Zoccolotti et al., 1986).

With regard to autonomic measures, we decided to record heart rate as well as electrodermal activity. The joint examination of these two parameters is important since it has been shown that, in situations of passive viewing of emotional stimuli, a directional fractionation of autonomic activity is present (Libby et al., 1973): unidirectional parameters, such as electrodermal activity or pupil dilation, show sympathetic-like activation while other bidirectional parameters, such as blood pressure or heart rate, show parasympathetic-like activity (e.g., heart deceleration).

We also decided to look at expressive measures of emotion. In the last twenty years, rediscovery of early work by Charles Darwin (1872/1965) by authors such as Izard (1971) and Ekman (1980) provided new impetus for research on the facial expression of emotion. One of the consequences of this has been the development of relatively refined systems for coding facial expressions. The Maximally Discriminative Facial Movement Coding System (MAX) by Izard (1979) and the Facial Action Coding System (FACS) by Ekman and Friesen (1978) fall into this category. They are defined as objective systems in the sense that the overall evaluation is based on a dissection of individual movements of the face muscles, which are subsequently coded according to predetermined categories. This type of coding of facial expression has a number of advantages over traditional subjective evaluations made by a group of naive judges, particularly when examining patients with hemispheric lesions. In fact, in many cases, these patients show different degrees of static and/or dynamic facial paralysis; the distortion of the face, both at rest and during movements, produced by paralysis is likely to influence subjective evaluations of naive judges in unpredictable ways (for a thorough discussion of this issue, see Zoccolotti et al., 1990). The use of subjective measures is presumably the main reason why previous research, examining facial expression in unilateral brain damaged patients, has produced mixed results (for a review see Pizzamiglio et al., 1989). Thus, one study reported reduced expressiveness in RBD patients (Borod et al., 1985) while another found a deficit in frontal patients but no laterality effect (Kolb and Milner, 1981); finally, one study has been described twice with contradictory laterality outcomes (Buck and Duffy, 1980; Duffy and Buck, 1979). No side difference in facial expressiveness has been reported after unilateral intracarotid injection of sodium amytal (Kolb and Milner, 1981)

In study II, we examined both autonomic (electrodermal activity and heart rate) and facial expression (by means of FACS) indicators in response to emotional and nonemotional film segments.

Sixty-two patients with unilateral brain damage, 23 of the right hemisphere and 39 of the left, plus 28 control subjects, took part in the study.[2] The diagnosis of damage to the hemisphere was based on clinical evidence, EEGs and neuroradiological examination (in most cases a brain CT scan had been made). Fifty-seven patients had a vascular etiology and five (3 right and 2 left brain-damaged patients) a tumoral etiology. Patients were

---

[2] Analysis of autonomic parameters was carried out on a part of the general group due to the selection of patients displaying disturbances of heart rate.

examined approximately one month after the onset of CVA (or admission to the hospital in the case of tumoral etiology). All patients were right-handed. There were no significant inter-group differences with regard to age, education and relative number of males and females.

The stimuli consisted of four short film segments: the first one showed a short sequence of a very fat man running after a very skinny one, with amusing interruptions (positive connotation); the second film segment presented the surgical cleaning of a serious burn (negative connotation); the third showed sea waves breaking monotonously on the rocks (neutral sequence); the last movie showed a puppy playing with a flower slowly moved by the hand of a person (positive connotation). The last three of these movies had been previously used in other studies (e.g., Ekman et al., 1980).

Electrodermal activity was recorded as in study I. Heart rate was recorded using a cardiotachometer which measured the length of intersystolic intervals to the closest msec.

The patients were led to a comfortable, acoustically insulated room, where they were asked to sit in an armchair in conditions of silence and dim lighting. Then, the electrodes used to record skin conductance and heart rate were applied. After an adaptation period, film segments of varying emotional intensity were rear-projected on a screen while the face of the subject was filmed using a closed-circuit television system. In order to familiarize the subject with the experimental situation, four film segments were shown which were not subsequently analyzed. Then, without any break in the continuity, the four experimental film segments were projected.

At the end of each experimental session, the subjects were interviewed in order to determine their understanding of the film sequence they had seen. Only those subjects who proved to have a good overall understanding of the sequences were included in the experiment.

Further methodological details on this study can be found elsewhere (Caltagirone et al., 1989; Mammucari et al., 1988; Zoccolotti et al., 1986; 1990).

## Autonomic Activity

In the analysis of autonomic parameters only the negative and the neutral film were considered (in general, the positive film segments produced intermediate but more variable responses).

Control subjects and LBD patients displayed greater conductance responses for the emotionally charged film segment than for the neutral one; on the contrary, the mean responses of right brain-damaged patients showed no differences linked to film type (see Figure 2). This result was substantiated by a significant patient group by film type interaction.

No difference among the three groups was found for skin conductance values preceding stimulus presentation. This result confirms those previously obtained using similar populations (Morrow et al., 1981; study I).

Heart rate (measured in terms of mean intersystolic interval in msec.) tended to decrease during film presentation as compared to the baseline period. This finding is consistent with the idea that passive viewing is associated with directional fractionation of autonomic parameters (Libby et al., 1973). Heart deceleration was considerably larger for the negative than the neutral film for both controls and LBD patients; in contrast, RBD patients showed smaller deceleration changes which did not vary significantly with the emotional nature of the film segment.

No difference among the three groups was found for mean heart rate preceding stimulus presentation.

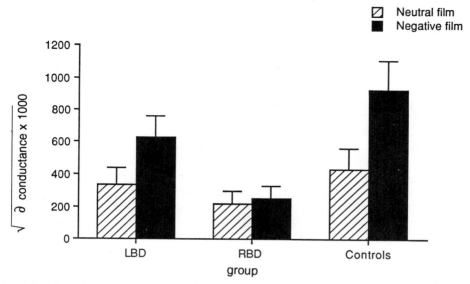

**Figure 2.** Skin conductance responses recorded during the neutral and negative film segment (adapted from Caltagirone et al., 1989). Data obtained from controls, left brain-damaged (LBD) and right brain damaged (RBD) patients are shown separately. Vertical lines indicate standard errors.

## Expressive behavior

Analysis of facial expression by means of FACS during film presentation is presented analytically in Mammucari et al. (1988); only the main results will be briefly sketched here. In general, a sizeable proportion of patients responded with facial expressions consistent with the nature of the film segments (mostly smiles in the "fat and skinny" and "puppy" film segments; a variety of negative reactions, with a predominance of disgust in the case of the "surgical toilet" film segment). In general, no difference was observed between patients with left and right hemiphheric lesions on any of the film segments. The same negative finding holds true using stricter or looser criteria for accepting facial expressions (see details in Mammucari et al., 1988).

Inspection of the videotapes revealed that a number of patients moved their gaze away from the screen during the negative film segment; this behavior was relatively frequent in LBD patients (35.9%) and controls (42.8%) and only occurred rarely in RBD patients (13.0%). This finding seems to suggest that the emotional impact of the film was less intense in these patients. It may be recalled that, in spite of continuous undisturbed looking, these patients did not display the heart rate deceleration typical of passive viewing (e.g., Sandman, 1975). Heart deceleration was less clear-cut in those LBD patients and controls displaying a gaze aversion during the negative film segment.[3]

---

[3] Interactions between gaze aversion patterns and modifications of heart rate (but not electrodermal activity) are presented in detail in Caltagirone et al. (1989).

## Comments

Autonomic measures indicated electrodermal responses associated with heart rate deceleration; this pattern has been been defined as "directional fractionation" by Lacey (1967) and is typical of passive viewing. Consistent with previous research (Libby et al., 1973) we found that both these autonomic responses were increased in the case of negative emotional stimulation as compared ot neutral stimuli.

Confirming previous investigations (Morrow et al., 1981; study I), the results of study II indicated a reduction in electrodermal reactivity to emotional stimuli in patients with lesions in the right hemisphere. The existence of a similar difference in heart rate indicates that the disturbance affecting these patients is neither specific to a single autonomic indicator nor to a single subdivision (sympathetic or parasympathetic) of the autonomic nervous system. The general nature of this conclusion suggests the hypothesis that the absence of differential autonomic arousal plays a comparatively important role in the onset of alterations to emotional behavior revealed by the clinical examination of patients with right hemispheric lesions.

It is noteworthy that all subjects were able to accurately describe the content of the film segments viewed. Therefore, the absence of variation in autonomic responses with emotional stimuli cannot be easily explained in terms of the incapacity of the RBD patients to appreciate the meaning of the stimuli.

Expressive emotional behavior showed a clear differentiation from autonomic reactivity. In fact, no difference was observed in terms of facial expression between patients with a lesion in the left or right cerebral hemisphere. Overall, these findings are inconsistent with Ross's (1984) proposal that the right hemisphere plays a specific role in the communication of affect. More generally, it suggests that different components of emotional behavior may be controlled by different neural structures, only some of which may be controlled by lateralized mechanisms.

An unexpected finding of our research is the observation that right brain-damaged patients rarely displayed a pattern of behavior commonly presented by normal controls and LBD patients when shown with a distressing visual scene. The latter often reacted by averting their gaze from the screen, whereas the former do not avert the eyes from the stressing film. Gaze aversion when the source of emotion is visual can have many meanings. Looking away may signify disinterest or boredom, or it may be part of a disgust display, or it may be a coping response to turn off the source of negative emotions. The comments of subjects who showed gaze aversion during the surgery film suggest that they could not tolerate viewing the stressful film. The absence of these movements in many of the right brain damaged patients when they viewed the surgery film could be due to an impairment in their ability to cope with negative emotion, or it might signify that their negative emotional experience was less intense.

## STUDY III

The flattening of autonomic activity in RBD patients appears relatively selective for emotional stimulation; in fact, no difference seems present in terms of SCL preceding the stimuli or SCRs to the neutral film segment. However, it may be noted that Heilman et al. (1978) observed clear electrodermal differences among left and right brain damaged patients in response to painful stimulation. Therefore, putting together their findings with those of studies I and II, one might conclude that right hemisphere involvement is implied in the case of aversive stimulation, whether noxious or emotional in nature. A clear distinction is commonly drawn between emotional and painful stimulation; however, at the same time, it is clear that, under many circumstances, painful stimuli may imply strong emotional involvement (e.g., Melzack, 1980). An examination of the procedure used by Heilman et al. (1978) suggests that this may have happened in the case of their patients. First, electric shocks (even though relatively mild producing only discomfort) may retain, at least in a number of people, a connotation of immediateness and uncontrollability; secondly, during stimulation, individuals were blindfolded, a feature that may have further enhanced the anxiety associated with the aversive stimulus.

On the basis of these considerations, we decided to reconsider this issue by modifying the experimental situation so as to reduce as much as possible the emotional "overtone" of the painful stimulation. To accomplish this, we decided to use heat stimulation. Thermal stimuli have a number of advantages over electric stimulation for our purposes: first, they have a much lower feeling of immediateness and uncontrollability than electric stimulation. Secondly, the area of stimulation can be varied in the case of heat: stimulation of a small localized area (ca. 10/20 mm$^2$) has been typically used to establish pain threshold (e.g., Benjamin, 1952); however, reliable behavioral and autonomic responses can be obtained using large surface thermodes (e.g., Jamal et al., 1985); this type of stimulation has the advantage of reducing variability of thermal thresholds (Lele, 1954). Preliminary work in our laboratory indicated that this latter method also produces a more global sensation of heat with much less feeling of aversiveness. Finally, it is well known that electric shocks produce high individual variations. On the contrary, thermal stimulation produces rather consistent responses between different individuals. This is important considering the sampling limitation due to the selection of a pathological population.

In this study, we analyzed electrodermal activity to heat stimulation in patients with a unilateral hemispheric lesion. Results from study II indicated that averting from threatening stimuli may be a factor moderating hemispheric differences. To pursue this observation, we manipulated the possibility of escaping the aversive stimulation.

Thirty-nine patients with unilateral cerebro-vascular lesions, respectively, right (RBD = 18) and left (LBD = 19); seventeen control subjects were also examined. There were no differences among the three groups on the basis of sex, age and time from onset of stroke. Patients were seen in a chronic phase approximately 4-5 months after the onset of disease. Patients were excluded who showed illness of the peripheral nervous system and upon ECG examination showed signs of cardiac arhythmia, which could influence the experimental procedure.[4] For the brain-damaged subjects, the unilaterality of the lesion was controlled using clinical and neuroradiological data (in most cases a brain CT scan had been made).

To determine thermal thresholds an apparatus was used which was comprised of a copper thermode, with a resistance linked to a rheostat which permitted changing the temperature with intervals of 0.5 degrees centigrade. Thermode area was 12 cm$^2$. A thermocouple linked to a Biolab apparatus was placed at the interface between the thermic stimulator and the stimulated skin, thus, allowing for a reading of the temperature actually applied.

Electrodermal activity was recorded as in study I.

The entire experimental procedure was sub-divided into two different sessions which both took place in a comfortable environment with little noise to insure subjects the maximum tranquility.

At the beginning of the first session, all subjects were informed of the general aims of the research. Then, each subject was administered a series of increasing thermal stimuli followed by a series of decreasing thermal stimuli. Following each application, the patient

---

[4] Heart rate was also measured. However, only findings on electrodermal activity will be presented here.

was asked to inform the examiner, the exact moment when the plate applied to the skin was felt as barely warm; thus, the value expressed in centigrade degrees resulting from the average of the two recognized values as "warm" in the two series (increasing and decreasing) was defined as the thermal threshold value. Analogously, the value expressed in centigrade degrees, derived from the average of the two recognized values as uncomfortable (not painful) by the patient was identified as the discomfort threshold value, in the course of the two series of stimulus applications. Instructions emphasized that no attempt should be made to be stoic.

During the second session, after having applied the electrodes to record cutaneous conductance and heart rate, a first sequence of six heat stimuli of different intensities were given. Three intensities were used : low (2 degrees centigrade above the thermal threshold), medium (2 degrees centigrade above the discomfort threshold) and high (5 degrees centigrade above the discomfort threshold). Each level of stimulaton was repeated twice according to a single presentation sequence. Then, a second identical series of six trials was given; this differed from the first in that it was possible for the patient to escape the stimulation (escape) thanks to a bell under his foot.

**Table 1.** Means (and SDs) of the thermal and discomfort thresholds (in degrees C°) for the three groups of subjects considered.

|                              | thermal     | discomfort   |
| ---------------------------- | ----------- | ------------ |
| Controls                     | 30.2 (1.0)  | 36.4 (1.2)   |
| Left brain damaged patients  | 30.1 (1.4)  | 36.5 (1.6)   |
| Right brain damaged patients | 30.0 (1.2)  | 36.6 (1.3)   |

The heat stimulus was applied after 25 sec for 3 sec, preceded by 5 sec of a computer acoustic signal which warned the patient of the following application of the stimulus. Each trial lasted a total of 50 sec.

Mean thresholds for thermal and uncomfortable stimuli are presented in Table 1. It is worth noting that these values are considerably lower than those classically reported in the literature for heat pain (e.g., Hardy, 1953). It is clear that no difference is present among the groups of patients for either evaluation.[5]

---

[5] To establish the reliability of these findings, we decided to replicate thermal and discomfort thresholds in a separate sample of unilateral hemispheric patients. Twenty-four RBD patients, 22 LBD patients and 19 control subjects of comparable age and education were examined. In general, thresholds were considerably similar to the values obtained in study III. Thermal thresholds were 30.7 (SD=0.7), 30.8 (1.3) and 30.3 (0.6) in RBD, LBD patients and controls, respectively; discomfort thresholds were 36.4 (1.2), 36.3 (1.4) and 36.5 (1.3) in RBD, LBD patients and controls, respectively.

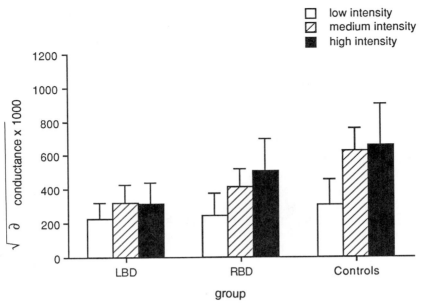

**Figure 3**. Skin conductance responses recorded during heat stimulation. Data obtained from controls, left brain-damaged (LBD) and right brain damaged (RBD) patients are separately shown. Vertical lines indicate standard errors.

Mean SCRs for the groups of patients are presented in figure 3. An ANOVA indicated that the effect of stimulus intensity was significant ($F_{(2,102)}=13.9$, p <.0001), SCRs increasing with increased temperature. However, neither the group factor (F<1) nor the group by stimulus intensity factor ($F_{(4,102)}=1.7$, n.s.) was significant. An inspection of the figure does not indicate any trend for RBD patients to show a flattened autonomic arousal to aversive stimulation; if anything, they displayed numerically greater (not smaller) electrodermal activity than LBD patients. The main effect of the escape factor ($F_{(2,102)} = 3.7$, p = .05) indicated greater SCRs in the escape condition (432) as compared to that of non-escape (375); this effect was independent of the group factor.

Reliable SCRs were observed during the warning period. An ANOVA performed on these values indicated no main effect of the group factor (F=1.4, n.s.): mean SCRs were 229 (SD=345) for the control subjects, 128 (SD=205) for the RBD patients and 89 (SD=196) for the LBD patients. Also the escape factor and the interaction between this and the group factor were insignificant (both Fs < 1).

A separate one-way analysis with the group factor as unrepeated measure was performed on skin conductance levels during the baseline period. No difference among the three groups was found for skin conductance values preceding stimulus presentation (F<1).

## Comments

For the specific purposes of our study, we determined thresholds to heat stimulation in a way that is relatively unconventional in the literature. As stated above, we wanted to obtain reliable estimates of heat thresholds in a situation with as much limited emotional connotation as possible. To achieve this, we asked our patients to tell us when the stimuli were felt as uncomfortable, not painful (Heilman et al., 1978). To the extent that the situation used is informative of perception of heat stimuli, one may conclude that unilateral hemispheric lesions do not appreciably affect thresholds for this type of stimuli: in fact, no difference was present among the three groups of patients or between the patients and the normal controls.[6] These findings of the present study are consistent with those of Heilman et al. (1978) who found no difference in terms of stimulus currents perceived as uncomfortable by RBD, LBD and controls. In another study using electric stimulation on two groups of unselected LBD and RBD patients and a matched group of controls, Cubelli et al. (1984) found that pain threshold and pain tolerance did not differentiate significantly in the three groups. Similar negative results were obtained by Neri et al. (1985)[7]. Overall, these findings indicate that, irrespective of the type of stimulation used, unilateral cortical lesions have small, if any, influence in modulating thresholds to aversive stimulation. A similar negative picture emerges from studies that looked at different pain sensitivity of the two parts of the body. In contrast to an original report by Merskey and Watson (1979) indicating a greater sensitivity of the left part of the body for pain, which they interpreted as due to right hemisphere mediation for coding pain stimuli, most subsequent studies have failed to find any significant lateral differences (for a review see Hall et al., 1981).

The main finding of the study was that the pattern of electrodermal activity associated with heat stimulation did not vary with the laterality of the lesion. Stimuli of increasing heat produced increased SCRs; however, responses were approximately the same in RBD, LBD and controls. This pattern of electrodermal activity is at variance with that observed by Heilman et al. (1978).

A number of possible reasons may account for the different outcomes of the two studies. First, one should note the differences in the selection of pathological samples. The subjects examined by Heilman et al. (1978) were acute RBD patients selected on the basis of the presence of hemi-neglect; in contrast, we examined a consecutive series of patients admitted to a rehabilitation clinic. It seems unlikely that the acute-chronic difference may account for the difference in the outcome of the two studies, since in studies I and II we used chronic and acute patients, respectively, with essentially identical results. As for the presence of hemi-neglect, only four of our patients showed signs of neglect (three in the RBD group and one in the LBD group). The small size of this subgroup prevented us from systematic analyses; however, an inspection of these records did not indicate clear-cut differences between neglect and nonneglect patients.

A second alternative is that the critical difference between the two studies lies in the type of stimuli used. We raised the possibility that electric shocks may have produced a stronger emotional overtone than heat stimuli, particularly since stimulus onset was unpredicted and the patient was blindfolded. In our procedure, we tried to limit the emotional involvement of the patients. They were instructed to report their sensations without trying to be "brave." Electrodermal activity was measured in the second session after the patient had time to become familiarized with the situation; further, stimulus onset was anticipated by an acoustical warning stimulus, thus reducing its unpredictability. If this analysis is correct, one may suggest that the presence of laterality effects is closely coupled with the emotional nature of the stimulation. Pain stimulation as such does not

---

[6] One cannot, in principle, exclude that hemispheric differences could be detected were heat stimuli in the pain range used. However, such a study may not be simple to carry out; as previously mentioned, we observed that pain threshold was difficult to define in verbal terms, the patients apparently associating the concept of pain with different emotional connotations such as distress or challenge.

[7] In both these studies, hemispheric differences were found when pain endurance (defined as difference between pain tolerance and pain threshold) was examined, with RBD patients showing higher values than those of the control subjects of those of the LBD patients. The reference to intolerance level makes it difficult to distinguish between aversive and genuinely emotional components of patients' reaction.

produce asymmetrical responding in left and right hemispheric patients; differences would only emerge if the stimuli have a clear emotional overtone.

We noted the presence of small but reliable SCRs in the warning period before the heat stimulus: no difference emerged among the three groups in these responses. This finding seems important to further pinpoint the hemispheric contribution to electrodermal activity; namely, it appears that arousal associated with stimulus expectancy is not modified to a significant extent by the presence of a focal lesion in one of the two hemispheres. Again, this finding is in keeping with the idea that right hemispheric contribution arises relatively late in the information processing sequence, when the emotional nature of the stimulus is evaluated.

In the last part of the experiment, we gave the patients the opportunity to escape the aversive stimulation if they felt it was too unpleasant by ringing a bell with their foot. As a matter of fact, this happened in 1.8% of cases over the course of the experiment, apparently confirming that the experimental manipulation was effective in reducing the emotional overtone of the aversive stimulation. At any rate, SCRs did vary slightly between the two parts of the experiment, with larger responses in the escape condition; however, this difference was present independent of the group factor. This lack of hemispheric differences may be due to different factors; effects may emerge only in emotional as compared to aversive noxious stimulation. Electrodermal activity may not be the best index of autonomic changes associated with the escape non-escape manipulation. In fact, previous research has shown that this is best measured by variations in heart rate (Sandman, 1975).

## FINAL REMARKS

Overall, the above investigations point to the idea that the right hemisphere is involved in functions of emotional arousal, intimately linked to the generation of the autonomic components of the emotional response. Findings on electrodermal activity appear particularly robust and reliable across studies (Morrow et al., 1981; study I and II).

It has been noted that hemispheric differences occur at a relatively late moment in the elaboration of stimuli. First, no difference was observed in the majority of studies for tonic measures of electrodermal activity. Second, orienting responses as well as arousal produced by warning stimuli were found to be preserved in RBD patients. Third, the results of study III showed that aversive stimulation per se does not yield hemispheric differences. Rather, RBD patients reduced arousal was found to be specific to the differentiation between emotional and nonemotional stimuli.

Furthermore, the results of the studies presented suggest that the right hemisphere's role in modulating autonomic arousal to emotional stimuli should be kept separate from other aspects of emotional functioning. In study I, recognition of emotion was found to be moderately impaired in RBD patients, a finding consistent with the vast literature on the topic. However, autonomic arousal and recognition of emotion were found to be independent. This finding militates against the idea of using data from recognition studies as a main source for evaluating theories of hemispheric functioning in emotion (for an in-depth discussion, see Gainotti et al., in press). In study II, we observed a dissociation between emotional arousal and facial expressive behavior. RBD patients failed to differentiate autonomically between emotional and nonemotional stimuli but displayed patterns of facial expressions which were consistent with the emotional connotation of the film segments and comparable to those shown by LBD patients and controls.

This general pattern of results does not seem consistent with any of the theories of hemispheric involvement in emotion. On the basis of these and related findings, Gainotti et al. (in press) proposed a division of labor between the two hemispheres in emotional processes: the right hemisphere's role would be involved in processes linked to the generation of arousal to emotionally laden stimuli; the left hemisphere would be implicated in processes of emotional control. From a clinical standpoint, the above results could help in clarifying the nature of the emotional indifference observed in right brain-damaged patients. Rather than viewing the indifference as only apparent and substantially due to a basic inability to comprehend and express emotions (e.g., Ross, 1984), they suggest that this reaction might be at least in part due to a reduced capacity to react with an appropriate autonomic response to emotionally-laden stimuli.

The majority of the patients we examined in the three studies had vascular lesions, most often ischemic strokes. In a sizeable proportion of patients these lesions affected a relatively large proportion of the hemisphere (most often in the territory of the middle cerebral artery)[8]. Consequently, it may appear surprising that no significant deficit was observed in these patients when they were compared to controls in a number of electrodermal measures such as SCL or SCRs to emotionally neutral or warning stimuli. One consideration is that different brain stem (pons) and cortical areas (pre-frontal, temporal-limbic) contribute bilaterally to the control of electrodermal activity (e.g., Raine et al., 1991); further, intact electrodermal responding has been reported in humans even in the case of bilateral amigdalectomy (Tranel and Damasio, 1989). Therefore, one may suppose that electrodermal activity can be mediated by alternative routes and relatively insensitive to unilateral focal damage.

A clear reduction in electrodermal activity has been documented in a series of patients with bilateral lesions in orbital and lower mesial frontal regions by Damasio et al. (1990). Again, the deficit was present only in the case of emotional stimulation (slides depicting social disaster, mutilation and nudity); no significant deficit was present in the case of nonemotional slides. Patients also showed normal skin potential responses to a generalized arousing stimulus (breathing) and to an orienting stimulus (proper name). The vascularization pattern of the middle cerebral artery indicates that most of our patients were not likely to have lesions overlapping those studied by Damasio et al. (1990). Therefore, one may conclude that areas within the right cerebral hemisphere and ventromedial frontal cortices independently contribute to processes of emotional arousal. Anterior-posterior and left-right dichotomies have often been discussed within the area of emotional behavior (for a discussion, see Gainotti et al., in press). Studies mapping patients with unilateral hemispheric damage intrahemispherically are needed to clarify this issue.

## REFERENCES

Benjamin, F.B., 1952, Pain reaction to locally applied heat, *J. Appl. Physiol.*, 4: 907.

Borod, J.C., Koff, E., Perlman, M. and Nicholas, M., 1985, Channels of emotional expression in patients with unilateral brain damage. *Arch. Neurol.*, 42: 345.

Buck, R. and Duffy, R., 1980, Nonverbal communication of affect in brain damaged patients. *Cortex*: 16: 351.

Caltagirone, C., Zoccolotti, P., Originale, G., Daniele, A. and Mammucari, A., 1989, Autonomic reactivity and facial expression of emotion in brain damaged patients, *in*: "Emotion and the Dual Brain," G. Gainotti and C. Caltagirone, Eds., Springer Verlag, Berlin.

Cicone, M., Wapner, W., and Gardner, H., 1980, Sensitivity to emotional expressions and situations in organic patients, *Cortex*, 16: 145.

---

[8] The characteristics of these lesions make an intrahemispheric analysis of the lesion (i.e., single lobe involvement was relatively rare) difficult. Furthermore, CT scans performed for clinical purposes typically have irregular slice spacing, a feature that limits the possibility of precise brain mapping.

Cubelli, R., Caselli, M. and Neri, M., 1984, Pain endurance in unilateral cerebral lesions, Cortex, 20: 369.

Damasio, A.R., Tranel, D. and Damasio, H., 1990, Individuals with sociopathic behavior caused by frontal damage fail to respond autonomically to social stimuli, *Behav. Brain Res.*, 41: 81.

Darwin, C. "The Expression of Emotions in Man and Animals," University of Chicago Press, Chicago, 1965 (originally published: John Murray, London, 1872).

Dekoski, S.T., Heilman, K.M., Bowers, D., and Valenstein, E., 1980, Recognition and discrimination of emotional faces and pictures, *Brain Lang.*, 9: 206.

Duffy, R.J. and Buck, R.W., 1979, A study of the relationship between propositional (pantomime) and subpropositional (facial expression) extraverbal behaviors in aphasics. *Fol. Phoniat.*, 31: 129.

Ekman, P., 1980, "The Face of Man," Garland, New York.

Ekman, P. and Friesen, W.V., 1978, "Facial Action Coding System," Consulting Psychologists Press, Palo Alto.

Ekman, P. and Friesen, W.V., 1975, "Unmasking the Face,". Prentice Hall, Englewood Cliffs.

Ekman, P., Friesen, W.V. and Ancoli, S., 1980, Facial signs of emotional experience. *J. Pers. Soc. Psychol.*, 6: 1125.

Etcoff, N.L., 1989, Recognition of emotions in patients with unilateral brain damage, *in*: "Emotion and the Dual Brain," G. Gainotti and C. Caltagirone, Eds., Springer Verlag, Berlin.

Gainotti, G., 1969, Reactions "catastrophiques" et manifestation d'indifference au cours des atteintes cerebrales. *Neuropsychologia*, 7: 195.

Gainotti, G., 1972, Emotional behavior and hemispheric side of the lesion. *Cortex* 8: 41.

Gainotti, G., Caltagirone, C., and Zoccolotti, P., in press, Left-right and cortical-subcortical dichotomies in the neuropsychological study of human emotions. *Cogn. Emot.*

Hall, W., Haiward, L. and Chapman, R., 1981, On the "lateralization of pain". *Pain*, 10: 337.

Hardy, J.D., 1953, Threshold of pain and reflex contractions to noxious stimuli. *J. Appl. Physiol.*, 5: 525.

Heilman, K.M., Schwartz, H.D., and Watson, R.T., 1978, Hypoarousal in patients with the neglect syndrome and emotional indifference, *Neurology*, 28: 229.

Izard, C.E., 1971, The Face of Emotion. Appleton-Century-Fox, New York.

Izard, C.E., 1979, The Maximally Discriminative Facial Movement Coding System (MAX). Instructional Resources Center, University of Delaware, Newark.

Jamal, G.A., Hansen, S., Weir, A.I. and Ballantyne, J.P., 1985, An improved automated method for the measurement of thermal thresholds. 1. normal subjects, *J. Neurol. Neurosurg. Psychiat.* 48: 354.

Kinsbourne, M. and Bemporad, B., 1985, Lateralization of emotion: a model and the evidence, *in*: "The Psychobiology of Affective Development," N. Fox and R.J. Davidson, Eds., Erlbaum, Hillsdale.

Kolb, B. and Milner, B., 1981, Observations of spontaneous facial expression after cerebral excisions and after intracarotid injection of sodium amytal. *Neuropsychologia*: 19: 505.

Lele, P.P., 1954, Relationship between cutaneous thermal thresholds, skin temperature and cross sectional area of the stimulus, *J. Physiol.* (London), 126: 191.

Lacey, J.I., 1967, Somatic response patterning and stress: some revision of activation theory. *in*: "Psychological Stress: Issues in Research," *in*: M.H. Appley and R. Trumbull, Eds., Appleton-Century-Crofts, New York.

Libby, W.L., Lacey, B.C. and Lacey, J.I., 1973, Pupillary and cardiac activity during visual attention, *Psychophysiology*, 10: 270.

Lubin, A. and Johnson, L.C., 1972, On planning psychological research, In: "Handbook of Psychophysiology," S. Greenfield and R.A., Sternback, Eds., Holt, Rhinehart and Winston, New York.

Mammucari, A., Caltagirone, C., Ekman, P., Friesen, W., Gainotti, G. Pizzamiglio, L. and Zoccolotti, P., 1988, Spontaneous facial expression of emotions in brain-damaged patients, *Cortex*, 24: 521.

Melzack, R., 1980, Psychological aspects of pain. *in*: Research Publications: Association for Research in Nervous Mental Disease - Pain, J.J. Bonica, ed., Raven Press, New York.

Merskey, H. and Watson, G.D., 1979, The lateralization of pain. *Pain*, 7: 271.

Morrow, L., Vrtunski, B., Kim, Y. and Boller, F., 1981, Arousal responses to emotional stimuli and laterality of lesion, *Neuropsychologia*, 19: 65.

Neri, M., Vecchi, G.P. and Caselli, M., 1985, Pain measuraments in right-left cerebral lesions. *Neuropsychologia*, 23: 123.

Pizzamiglio, L., Caltagirone, C. and Zoccolotti, P., 1989, Facial expression of emotion, *in* "Handbook of Neuropsychology," F. Boller and J. Grafman, Eds., Elsevier, Science Publisher, Amsterdam.

Raine, A., Reynolds, G.P., Sheard, C., 1991, Neuroanatomical correlates of skin conductance orienting in normal humans: a magnetic resonance imaging study. *Psychophysiology*, 28: 548.

Ross, E.D., 1984, Right hemisphere's role in language, affective behavior and emotion, *Tr. Neurosc.*, 7: 342.

Sackeim, A., Greenberg, M.S. Weiman, L., Gur, R.C., Hungerbuhler, J.P., Geschwind, N., 1982, Hemispheric asymmetry in the expression of positive and negative emotions, *Arch. Neurol.*, 39: 210.

Sandman, C., 1975, Physiological responses during escape and non escape from stress in field independent and field dependent subjects. *Biol. Psychol.*, 2: 205.

Terzian, H., and Cecotto, C., 1959, Su un nuovo metodo per la determinazione e lo studi della dominanza emisferica, *G. Psichiatr. Neuropatol.*, 87: 889.

Tranel, D. and Damasio, H., 1989, Intact electrodermal skin conductance responses after bilateral amygadala damage. *Neuropsychologia*, 27: 381.

Zoccolotti P, Scabini, D., and Violani, C., 1982, Electrodermal responses in patients with unilateral brain damage, *J. Clin. Neuropsychol.*, 4: 143.

Zoccolotti, P., Caltagirone, C., Benedetti, N. and Gainotti, G., 1986, Perturbation des reponses vegetatives aux stimuli emotionnels au cours des lesions hemispheriques unilaterales, *L'Encephale*, 12: 263.

Zoccolotti, P., Caltagirone, C., Ekman, P., Friesen, W., Gainotti, G., Mammucari, A. and Pizzamiglio, L., 1990, Methodological questions on the study of spontaneous emotional responding as compared to non verbal communication in brain damaged patients: comments on Buck's reply, *Cortex*, 26: 281.

# PARTICIPANTS

**Dr Rüdiger BALTISSEN**
Fach Psychologie
Lehrstuhl für Physiologische Psychologie
Max-Horkkeimen Str. 20
W-5600 Wuppertal
GERMANY

**Dr Vincent BLOCH**
Laboratoire de Neurobiologie de l'apprentissage
et de la mémoire (NAM). URA 1491 CNRS.
Université de Paris Sud -Bat. 446
F-91405 Orsay Cedex
FRANCE

**Dr Wolfram BOUCSEIN**
Fach Psychologie
Lehrstuhl für Physiologische Psychologie
Max-Horkkeimen Str.20
W-5600 Wuppertal
GERMANY

**Dr Michéle BROUCHON**
Département de Neuropsychologie
Centre Hospitalo-Universitaire de la Timone
F-13385 Marseille CEDEX 5
FRANCE

**Dr Andrew CRIDER**
Department of Psychology
Williams College
Williamstown, Mass 01267
USA

**Dr Bernard DELERM**
Laboratoire de Psychophysiologie SN4
Université de Lille 1-USTL
F-59655 Villeneuve d'Ascq Cedex
FRANCE

**Dr Robert EDELBERG**
U M D of New Jersey
Robert Wood Johnson Medical School
675 Hoes Lane
Pisacataway NJ 08854-5635
USA

**Dr Pierre FLOR-HENRY**
Alberta Hospital Edmonton
Psychiatric Treatement Centre
Edmonton T5J 2J7 Alberta
CANADA

**Dr Don C. FOWLES**
Department of Psychology
The University of IOWA
Iowa City IA 52242
USA

**Dr John J. FUREDY**
Department of Psychology
University of Toronto
Toronto M5S 1A1 - Ontario
CANADA

**Dr John GRUZELIER**
Charing Cross and Westminster Medical School
Department of Psychiatry - Fulham Palace Road
London W6 8RP
ENGLAND

**Dr Kenneth HUGDAHL**
Department of Somatic Psychology
Anstaveien 21
N-5000 Bergen
NORWAY

**Dr William G. IACONO**
Department of Psychology
University of Minesota
Elliot Hall
Minneapolis MN 55455
USA

**Dr Bjorn H. JOHNSEN**
Department of Somatic Psychology
Anstaveien 21
N-5000 Bergen
NORWAY

**Dr J MARQUES-TEIXEIRA**
Facultade de Psicologia e de Ciencas da Educaçao
Rua Taipas 76
4000  Porto
PORTUGAL


**Dr José MARTINEZ-SELVA**
Facultad de Psicologia
Universidad de Murcia
30071  Murcia
SPAIN


**Dr Janick NAVETEUR**
Laboratoire de Psychophysiologie SN4
Université de Lille 1-USTL
F-59655  Villeneuve d'Ascq Cedex
FRANCE


**Dr Arne ÖHMAN**
Department of Clinical Psychology
Box 1225
S-75142 Uppsala
SWEDEN


**Dr Adrian RAINE**
Department of Psychology
Seeley G.Mudd Building
University of Southern California
Los Angeles  CA 90089-1061
USA


**Dr Georgina RIPPON**
Department of Psychology
University of Warwick
Coventry  CV4 7AI
ENGLAND


**Dr Jean Claude ROY**
Laboratoire de Psychophysiologie SN4
Université de Lille 1-USTL
F-59655  Villeneuve d'Ascq Cedex
FRANCE


**Dr Florian SCHAEFER**
Fach Psychologie
Lehrstuhl für Physiologische Psychologie
Max-Horkkeimen Str.20
W-5600  Wuppertal
GERMANY


**Dr Gérard SCHMALTZ**
Laboratoire de Psychophysiologie SN4
Université de Lille 1-USTL
F-59655  Villeneuve d'Ascq Cedex
FRANCE


**Dr Anne SCHELL**
Seeley G.Mudd Building 501
University of Southern California
Los Angeles - CA 90089-1061
USA


**Dr Henrique SEQUEIRA-MARTINHO**
Département de Psychologie
Fédération Universitaire Polytechnique de Lille
60 Bd Vauban
F-59016  Lille Cedex
FRANCE


**Dr Tytus SOSNOWSKI**
University of Warsaw
Faculty of Psychology
Departement of Individual Psychology
ul. Stawki 5/7
00-183  Warszawa
POLAND


**Dr Graham TURPIN**
Department of Psychology
University of Sheffield
Western Bank
Sheffield  SL0 2TN
ENGLAND


**Dr Peter VENABLES**
Derwent Cottage
Newton on Derwent
York  Y04 5DA
ENGLAND


**Dr VERNET-MAURY**
Laboratoire de Physiologie Neurosensorielle
Bat. 404. Université Claude Bernard-Lyon 1
F-69622  Villeurbanne Cedex
FRANCE


**Dr Pierluigi ZOCCOLOTTI**
Dipartimento di Psicologia
Universita di Roma "La Sapienza"
Via degli Apuli, 8
00185  Roma
ITALY

# AUTHOR INDEX

Ackerman, P.T., 184
Ackles, P.J., 220, 287
Acocella, C.M., 212, 220
Adam, G., 271, 287
Adams, R.M., 265, 268
Adams, T., 11, 18, 19, 24, 28, 74, 88
Adelman, S., 74, 88
Aldenderfer, M.S., 125, 132
Alliger, R., 132
Alm, T., 120, 130, 132, 203, 256, 291, 294
Amaral, D.G., 99, 112
Anand, P., 85, 88
Ancoli, S., 325
Anderson, B., 281, 286
Andreasen, N.C., 125, 132
Annett, M., 302, 303, 307, 308
Anthony, B.J., 211, 212, 220
Aoyama, H., 113
Arai, H., 113
Araki, T., 110
Arena, J.G., 112, 134
Armand, J., 101, 104, 109
Asarnow, R., 133
Asberg, M., 184
Ashby, W.R., 101, 109
Attneave, F., 160, 171
Augenbraun, C.B., 175, 180, 183, 260, 267
Augustyn, G.T., 133
Ax, A., 14, 24, 137, 155, 190, 203
Ba-M'Hamed-Bennis, S., 74, 88, 113, 274, 287
Bach, L.M.N., 81, 82, 91
Bacon, S.J., 84, 88

Bagshaw, M., 96, 100, 109, 111, 116, 118, 124, 132, 133, 134, 188, 203, 204, 252, 254, 266, 267
Bailes, K., 53, 57, 197, 205
Bakan, 260, 269
Ballantyne, J.P., 325
Baltissen, R., 34, 40, 159, 160, 171
Bamford, J.L., 14, 24, 190, 203
Banich, M. T., 269
Barchas, J.D., 142, 155
Bard, P., 100, 109
Barlow, D.H., 232, 233, 234
Barneoud, P., 271, 285
Baron, M., 189, 203
Barr, M.L., 122, 133
Bartfai, A., 26, 94, 109, 120, 121, 130, 133, 229, 236, 254
Basbaum, A.I., 84, 85, 88
Basset, M., 101, 109
Bauer, R.M., 140, 155
Bauer, R.S., 52, 58
Baugher, D.M., 175, 183
Baxter, L.R., 290, 294
Baxter, R., 261, 268
Beaton, A., 257, 267
Beattie, J., 95, 109
Beaumont, J., 302, 308
Bechterew, W.V., 93, 109
Beers, J.R., 150, 155, 208, 220
Beiser, M., 134, 217, 239, 246, 247, 253, 254, 255, 256
Belanger, A., 256
Bell, B., 189, 199, 203, 204, 205
Bell, C., 76, 88
Bemporad, B., 312, 325

Damasio, A.R., 80, 92, 96, 101, 109, 116, 133, 140, 157, 324, 325
Damasio, H., 109, 113, 124, 133, 134, 325, 326
Daniele, A., 324
Danilewsky, B., 93, 110
Dardano, J.F., 270
Darrow, C.W., 5, 7, 8, 10, 14, 23, 25, 52, 57, 73, 74, 84, 89, 100, 101, 108, 110, 116, 133, 190, 204, 272, 285
Darwin, C., 315, 325
Davey, G.C.L., 150, 153, 155
Davidson, R.J., 262, 265, 267, 272, 285
Davies, P.T.G., 268
Davis, C., 62, 69
Davison, M.A., 77, 84, 89, 90, 95, 110
Dawson, M.E., 51, 57, 110, 118, 132, 133, 134, 150, 155, 173, 174, 179, 183, 185, 186, 207, 208, 209, 212, 215, 216, 217, 218, 220, 221, 232, 235, 237, 245, 251, 252, 253, 254, 255, 265, 268
DeArmond, S.J., 128, 133
Degreef, G., 112, 134, 197, 205
Dekoski, S.T., 314, 325
Delamater, A.M., 224, 226, 235
Delerm, B., 73, 77, 81, 89, 91, 112
Delgado, J.M.R., 93, 100, 110
Delorme, F., 87, 89
Delpezzo, E.M., 212, 220
Delsaut, M., 89
DeMyer, M.K., 125, 133
DeMyer, W.E., 133
Dengerink, H.A., 224, 235
Dengerink, J.A., 64, 69
Dennig, H., 99, 110
Denti, A., 83, 91
Depue, R.A., 244, 253, 255
Deuschl, G., 74, 89
Devito, J.L., 101, 109
Dewey, M.M., 133
Digman, J.M., 177, 183
Dimberg, U., 14, 25, 138, 145, 147, 149, 152, 155, 156, 157, 273, 285
Dishman, J., 227, 236
Doctor, R.F., 181, 183
Dodd, D.F., 55, 57
Doerr, H.O., 256
Donchin E., 89
Doob, A.N., 64, 70

Douglas, R.J., 268
Duffy, R.J., 315, 324, 325
Dupont, R.M., 133
Dykman, R.A., 53, 58, 175, 184
Early, C.E., 54, 57
Edelberg, R., 7, 8, 9, 10, 11, 12, 13, 14, 15, 16, 18, 20, 21, 22, 23, 24, 25, 31, 32, 33, 35, 36, 40, 52, 63, 64, 69, 74, 84, 89, 101, 108, 110, 116, 118, 122, 123, 128, 131, 133, 190, 192, 204, 222, 223, 235, 255
Edinger, H.M., 95, 110
Edman, G., 174, 184, 254
Edwards, D.L., 112
Ekman, P., 68, 71, 276, 285, 314, 315, 316, 325, 326
Elder, H.Y., 26
Elithorn, A., 101, 110
Ellsworth, P., 276, 285
Emese, L., 184
Endicott, J., 216, 221
Endo, K., 103, 110
Erlenmeyer-Kimling, L., 193, 194, 204
Esteves, F., 71, 91, 137, 144, 145, 147, 149, 155, 157, 274, 286
Etcoff, N.L., 314, 325
Euler, M., 34, 40
Eves, F.F., 255, 259, 268, 269, 295, 302, 308
Eysenck, H.J., 176, 177, 184, 186, 227, 233, 234
Eysenck, S.B.G., 177, 184
Fagius, J., 75, 76, 89, 92
Fairchild, S.B., 91
Farley, J., 264, 270, 296
Farnum, D.M., 271, 272, 286
Farr, D., 255
Feltz, D.L., 52, 58
Féré, C., 3, 4, 5, 49, 73, 89, 272, 285
Fernee, K.M., 12, 27
Ferreira, A.J., 53, 57
Ficken, J.W., 125, 128, 133, 189, 217, 239, 251, 255
Fields, H.L., 85, 88
Filion, D.L., 150, 155, 186, 207, 208, 209, 212, 215, 216, 218, 220, 232, 235, 237
Fitzgerald, H.E., 15, 24
Flak, B., 255, 256
Flanigan, H.F., 112, 134

Hustmyer, F.E., 181, 184
Huttunen, M.O., 256
Hygge, S., 23, 26
Hyman, B.T., 113, 124, 134
Iacono, W.G., 120, 121, 125, 128, 130,
    131, 133, 134, 164, 165, 171, 184,
    187, 189, 204, 217, 239, 243, 244,
    245, 246, 247, 248, 252, 253, 254,
    255, 256, 264, 265, 269, 294, 295
Ikenoue, K., 92
Illert, M., 74, 89
Inglis, G.B., 58
Irving, G., 269
Isamat, F., 96, 111, 113, 116, 134
Ishii, T., 114
Ison, J.R., 211, 221
Ito, T., 84, 90
Izard, C.E., 142, 156, 315, 325
Jackson, J.H., 93, 111
Jackson, R.K., 133
Jacobs, L., 256
Jacobsen, R., 194, 204
Jaeger, J., 205
Jamal, G.A., 319, 325
James, W., 137, 141, 156
Janes, C.L., 15, 26
Jänig, W., 74, 75, 76, 90, 108, 111
Jeje, A., 17, 26
Jenkinson, D.M., 11, 26
Jennings, J.R., 220, 287
Johnsen, B.H., 271, 274, 276, 277, 279,
    286
Johnson, G., 11, 21, 26
Johnson, J.E., 52, 53, 54, 57
Johnson, L.C., 35, 36, 40, 79, 90, 140,
    156, 184, 185, 313, 325
Johnson, M.H., 256
Johnstone, E.C., 184
Jolley, T., 268
Jones, H.E., 177, 178, 184, 229, 232, 236
Jouvet, M., 89
Juni, S., 254, 267
Juniper, K., 53, 58
Jurgensen, E., 52, 58
Kaada, B.R., 93, 100, 111
Kahneman, D., 138, 141, 142, 156, 208,
    221
Kaiser, C., 181, 184
Kanner, A.D., 141, 156
Karmen, J., 267

Karnes, E., 181, 184
Karplus, J.P., 93, 94, 111
Karst, H., 112
Kaswan, J.W., 183
Katalin, M., 184
Katic, M., 64, 70
Katkin, E.S., 10, 26, 176, 185, 293, 295
Katsanis, J., 119, 120, 121, 130, 131,
    134, 250, 252, 255
Katsumi, M., 94, 95, 111
Katzoff, E.T., 14, 26
Keizer, K., 101, 102, 103, 111
Kell, J.F., 111
Kelly, A., 150, 155, 208, 220
Kerr, B., 208, 221
Kerslake, D., 12, 24
Ketterer, M.W., 269, 302, 308, 309
Kety, S.S., 193, 204, 205
Kilpatrick, D.G., 176, 184
Kimble, D.P., 96, 101, 109, 110, 111,
    116, 124, 133, 134, 188, 203, 204,
    254, 267
Kimmel, H.D., 160, 171, 176, 184, 221
Kinsbourne, M., 312, 325
Kircher, J.C., 67, 71
Kita, R., 89
Kiyosumi, H., 114
Kjellberg, A., 281, 285
Klajner, F., 64, 70
Klein, D., 255
Klein, R.F., 195, 205
Kleinknecht, R.A., 52, 53, 54, 57, 58
Kley, I.B., 188, 205
Kligman, A.M., 13, 27
Knight, R.T., 124, 134
Koe, B.K., 87, 90
Koehler, T., 52, 53, 54, 58, 59
Koehler, W., 168, 171
Koff, E., 324
Kohno, K., 111
Kolb, B., 315, 325
Kondo, M., 29
Koon, D., 17, 26
Kopp, M.S., 181, 184, 260, 263, 269
Korenko, L., 270
Koresko, R.L., 142, 157
Korr, I.M., 34, 41
Koss, M.C., 74, 75, 77, 84, 85, 88, 89,
    90, 94, 95, 110, 111

Lundberg, A., 82, 90
Lunn, R., 174, 175, 177, 178, 183
Luria, A.R., 100, 112, 116, 134, 266, 269, 290, 295
Lykken, D.T., 13, 26, 31, 33, 38, 40, 43, 63, 67, 69, 71, 133, 164, 165, 171, 184, 225, 230, 233, 236, 248, 255
Lynn, R., 142, 156, 159, 171
Mac Dowell, K.A., 91
Macdonald, D.G., 270
Machon, R.A., 109, 133, 197, 203, 256
MacIndoe, I., 230, 236
MacKinnon, P.C.B., 53, 54, 57, 58
Magni, F., 103, 112
Magoun, H.W., 76, 81, 90, 91, 95, 112
Malmo, R.B., 53, 58, 138, 156
Maltzman, I., 224, 225, 227, 237, 258, 262, 269, 307, 308
Mammucari, A., 68, 71, 315, 316, 317, 324, 325
Manchanda, R., 264, 267, 268, 297, 308
Mandel, A.J., 81, 82, 91
Mandler, G., 137, 141, 142, 156
Mann, L.S., 135
Marcel, A., 144, 156
Marcus, J., 196, 204
Marcuse, Y., 193, 204
Marcy, R., 181, 184
Maricq, H.R., 14, 17, 27, 190, 204
Marks, I.M., 148, 156
Martens, R., 52, 54, 58
Martin, I., 9, 27, 36, 40, 41, 53, 58, 59, 175, 177, 184
Martinez-Selva, J.M., 269, 270, 290, 295, 296, 309
Maser, J., 237
Massaro, D.W., 144, 156
Masterton, R.B., 101, 104, 112
Mathis, H.I., 226, 236
Matsushima, R., 112
Matsuyama, K., 84, 91
Mayer-Gross, W., 233, 236
Mayes, A.R., 308
Mazziotta, J.C., 294
McAllen, R.M., 77, 91
McCleary, R.A., 27, 80, 90
McCrae, R.R., 177, 178, 185
McDonald, D.G., 142, 157, 181, 185
McGlashan, T.H., 29, 190, 205, 256
McGlone, J., 275, 280, 286, 302, 308

McGuiness, D., 95, 112
McKeever, W.F., 273, 286, 287
McKiever, B.L., 173, 174, 185
McMachlan, E.M., 95, 108, 112
McManus, I., 302, 308
McNally, R.J., 147, 156
Meador, K.J., 112, 134
Medley, I., 134
Mednick, S.A., 14, 27, 28, 109, 133, 185, 188, 189, 190, 192, 193, 195, 196, 198, 199, 203, 204, 205, 223, 236, 237, 252, 256
Meehl, P.E., 189, 204, 253, 255, 256
Megargee, E.I., 223, 236
Melamed, B.G., 52, 54, 58
Melzack, R., 319, 325
Meriaux, H., 89
Merskey, H., 322, 325
Mesmer, F., 1
Metz, J., 271, 272, 286
Meyers, M., 298, 309
Michaelewski, H.A., 57
Mihaly, K., 269
Miller E.N., 183
Miller, G.A., 246, 255
Miller, R.D., 26
Milner, B., 266, 269, 315, 325
Mineka, S., 150, 157
Minniti, R., 183
Mintz, J., 221
Miossec, Y., 110, 286, 298, 299, 307, 308, 309
Mirsky, A.F., 195, 204
Mitchell, D.A., 197, 199, 205
Mizuno, N., 99, 112
Moffitt, .T.E, 205
Mok, K.H., 100, 101, 113
Monk-Jones, M.E., 57
Montagu, J.D., 13, 27, 34, 37, 41
Montgomery, I., 26
Moore, M., 133
Mordkoff, A.M., 10, 27
Moreau, M., 255, 256
Mori, S., 91
Moroji, T., 114
Morrissette, J.R., 116, 134
Morrow, L., 312, 313, 314, 316, 318, 323, 325
Moruzzi, G., 76, 91
Moscovitch, M., 273, 287

Romer, M., 56, 57
Ronday, H.K., 111
Rosen, A.D., 282, 287
Rosenberry, R., 11, 26
Rosenthal, D., 193, 204, 205
Ross, E.D., 312, 318, 324, 326
Ross, S., 260, 270
Rossi, A., 128, 134
Rossmann, R., 180, 186
Roth, M., 233, 236
Roth, W.T., 256
Rowe, R., 186
Roy, J.C., 7, 73, 77, 79, 80, 81, 82, 83,
        86, 87, 88, 89, 91, 93, 103, 105,
        109, 110, 112, 113, 116, 128, 132,
        133, 134, 135, 188, 274, 286, 287,
        308, 309
Rubens, R.L., 174, 185, 256, 266, 270
Rubin, E., 74, 91
Rudy, T.A., 86, 92
Rugg, M.D., 308
Rumsey, J.M., 256
Rushmer, R.F., 12, 13, 27
Ruskin, D.C., 260, 269
Russell, J.A., 139, 157
Rust, J., 36, 41, 175, 177, 184
Rutschmann, J., 193, 204
Sackeim, A., 312, 326
Sackheim, H.A., 262, 270
Sagberg, F., 34, 41
Sakai, L.M,., 185
Salzman, L.F., 195, 205
Sandman, C.A., 281, 287, 317, 323, 326
Sandrew, B.B., 99, 112
Saper, C.B., 95, 109, 112, 271, 285
Sarkany, I., 12, 27
Sartorius, N., 256
Sartory, G., 145, 157
Sato, A., 92, 114, 134, 256
Sato, K., 10, 17, 28, 84, 91
Satoda, T., 112
Satorius, N., 270
Satz, P., 203, 204
Sawyer, J.W., 256
Scabini, D., 326
Scerbo, A., 131, 134
Schachat, R., 59
Schachter, S., 137, 157, 236
Schacter, J., 186
Schaefer, F., 40, 43, 46, 160, 171

Schaeffer, C., 142, 155
Schalling, D., 26, 109, 133, 178, 179,
        184, 186, 223, 224, 229, 230, 232,
        233, 234, 235, 236, 254
Scheier, I.H., 258, 269
Scheier, M.F., 54, 57
Schell, A.M., 150, 155, 161, 171, 174,
        177, 183, 185, 186, 207, 208, 209,
        212, 215, 217, 218, 220, 232, 235,
        237, 255
Scher, H., 62, 70
Schiffmann, K., 65, 67, 70, 71, 150, 157
Schmauk, F.J., 224, 226, 237
Schmidt, K., 224, 226, 237
Schmueli, J., 196, 204
Schneider, R.E., 11, 20, 22, 23, 26
Schneider, S.J., 254, 264, 265, 270
Schneirla, T.C., 139, 157
Schnur, D.B., 94, 112, 120, 121, 130,
        134, 197, 205, 254, 295
Scholomskas, D., 256
Schooler, C., 135
Schrell, U., 95, 113
Schulsinger, F., 14, 27, 109, 133, 185,
        193, 195, 196, 197, 198, 199, 203,
        204, 205
Schulsinger, H., 185, 188, 189, 190, 192,
        193, 205
Schultz, R.H., Jr., 55, 57
Schulz, I.J., 12, 17, 28
Schwartz, G.E., 261, 262, 269
Schwartz, H.D., 110, 325
Schwartz, H.G., 100, 106, 113
Schwartz, I.L., 17, 23, 28
Schwartz, J.M., 294
Schwartzbaum, J., 116, 134
Scull, J., 66, 70, 161, 171
Sedvall, G., 254
Seidman, D., 198, 203, 254
Seidman, L.J., 188, 205
Seligman, M.E.P., 142, 147, 157, 273,
        287
Senter, R.J., 178, 184, 224, 227, 236
Sequeira-Martinho, H., 7, 91, 93, 103,
        108, 112, 113, 116, 132, 134, 188,
        274, 286, 287, 292, 295
Sergeant, J., 189, 203, 259, 269, 302, 308
Seymour, K., 268
Shagass, C., 237
Shannahof-Khalsa, D.S., 272, 287

SUBJECT INDEX

Active coping hypothesis (of Obrist), 231
Adaptiveness of signal-elicited SCR, 66
Adoption study, 193
Adrenalin, 84, 225
Affective disorders, 119, 125-128, 132
Amygdala, 95-98, 116, 123-125, 132
Anhedonia, 179, 198, 202, 228, 244
Animal fear, 148
Anticipation, 162, 167, 225-228, 230-232
Antisocial behavior, 178, 226-228
Anxiety, 140, 142, 225-230, 257, 262-264
    alarm reaction, 232-233
    anxious apprehension, 230, 232
    conditioned, 226, 227, 230
    fight/flight response, 233
    generalized anxiety disorder, 232
    panic, 233
    psychic, 233
    somatic, 233
    versus fear, 232-233
Arousal, 76-83, 137-143, 146, 190
Associative learning, 171, 280, 285
Asymmetry
    cortical, 303
    electrodermal, 106, 108, 258-265, 271-
        273, 275, 289-294, 297-299,
        302, 306, 307
Attachments and socialization,
        development of conscience, 234
Attention, 77, 137, 140-143, 149, 154,
        164, 166, 207, 208, 211-213,
        216, 219, 243, 258, 260
Auditory thresholds, 264
Automatic processing, 141,207, 215, 216,
    219
Autonomic activity, 137, 138, 315, 316,
    318

nervous control, 84, 85, 93
Autonomic conditioning, 281
Autonomic nervous system, 73, 93, 271,
    318
Avoidance
    active, 230
    passive, 230
    two-factor theory, 230
Awareness, 145, 150, 154, 273

Backward masking, 143-146, 149, 154
Balance model, 293
Behavioral activation system (of Gray),
    231-232
Behavioral inhibition system (of Gray),
    231-234
Between-versus within-subjects designs,
    63
Bilateral electrodermal activity, 257-270,
    294, 297
Bilateral measures, 106, 297
Borderline state, 189
Brain damage, *see* Unilateral brain
        damage, lateralization models
Brain imaging, 115, 117-119

Capacitance, 11, 13, 34, 35, 44, 45, 48
Cardiovascular disorders, 261-262
Cat footpad, 9, 11
Catecholamines, 75, 84, 96, 99
Cerebral laterality, 257-270
Cingulate cortex, 96, 98, 101, 116
Classical conditioning, 147, 150, 151,
        207, 208, 211, 223, 226, 227,
        230, 273, (*see also* Pavlovian
        conditioning)
Clinical psychophysiology, 49

and attention, 232

Palmar sweat index, 49, 51, 52
    clinical utility, 50, 52
    image analysis, 56
    relationship to EDA, 50
    reliability and stability, 52, 53
    subject variables, 53
    validity, 53, 54
Palmar-dorsal differences, 8, 10, 14, 15
Parasympathetic versus sympathetic
    influences, 62
Patterning of SCRs, 162, 163, 167-169
Pavlovian conditioning, 147, 150, 151
    (*see also* Classical conditioning)
Pericruciate cortex, 101, 104
Personality, 189, 228, 262
Personality traits, 176-179
    agreeableness, 177-178
    anhedonia, 179
    extraversion, 176
    introversion, 176
    schizoid, 178-179
Phase angle, 43, 45, 47, 48
Phobic stimuli, 142, 145
Pons, 116, 123, 124, 132
Poral closure, 12
Poral valve model, 16
    reabsorption, 22, 23
    sequence, 20
Positive emotion, 264, 265
Positive skin potential response, 14, 19,
    20, 23
Positron emission tomography (PET),
    117, 129, 291
Preattentive processes, 140-142, 154
Preattentive processing, 211, 212, 215,
    218
Predictability, 166, 167
Prefrontal cortex, 100, 101, 116, 118,
    123-128
Preparedness, 142
Prepulse inhibition, 211, 218, 219
Probe reaction time (RT), 150, 151, 217
Psyche of psychophysiology, 61
Psychological and physiological
    processes, 62
Psychopath (also sociopath), 223-234
    noninstitutionalized, 226
    primary, 224, 226

neurotic, 226
    schizoid, 228, 232, 233, 234
Psychopathy
    and EDR lability, 178-179
Punishment *see* Stressor, anticipation of
Pyramidal tract, 103-107

Reabsorption, 9, 14, 20, 22
Reaction time, 223, 227
    and EDR lability, 181
Recording method, 34
Recording site (for EDA), 129
Recovery rate, 14, 19, 20, 23
    antecedent activity, 15, 24
    response patterns, 15
Reduced ipsilateral excitation, 290
Refractoriness, 160
Reinstatement, 66
Relational perception, 167
Repetitive stimulation, 225
Resistance, 32-39, 43-47
Resistance (units), 38
Response generalization, 226
Response specificity, 10
    cations, 8
    components, 8
    elevated temperature, 8
    exsanguination, 8
    high currents, 8, 23
    skin potential response, 8
Responsiveness pattern, 303
Reticular formation
    mesencephalic, 76, 95, 104
    bulbar, 80-82
Reticulospinal fibers, 83, 103

S-S versus S-R learning positions, 65
Schizophrenia, 96, 119-121, 127, 187,
    203, 216, 217, 242, 247, 254,
    264, 265
    and EDR lability, 179
    and the prediction of relapse, 51
    and the Palmar Sweat Index, 51
    negative symptom, 198, 201
    positive symptom, 198, 201
    responder/non-responder, 245-266,
    289-292
Schizophrenics, 289, 291-294
Schizophreniform disorder, 247, 249,
    250, 254

THIRD EDITION

# ANTHROPOLOGISTS AT WORK

### An Introductory Reader

**NICHOLAS F. BELLANTONI**

Museum of Natural History
University of Connecticut

**LUCI L. FERNANDES**

Department of Anthropology
University of Connecticut

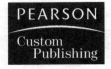

PEARSON

Custom
Publishing

Cover photographs by John Spaulding.

Coffin lids recovered from the Bulkeley Family Tomb, Colchester, Connecticut. Brass tacks on the lids provide information on the initials, age of death, and year of death of each individual. In this case, the coffins represent Peter Bulkeley (1712-1798) and Rhoda (Jones) Kellogg Bulkeley (1750-1807).

Printed in the United States of America

6 7 8 9 10 VOZN 15 14 13

ISBN 0-536-98005-5

2005540031

AP/NR

Please visit our web site at www.pearsoncustom.com

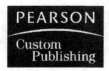

PEARSON CUSTOM PUBLISHING
75 Arlington Street, Suite 300, Boston, MA 02116
A Pearson Education Company